Congenital and Perinatal Infections

Infectious Disease

SERIES EDITOR: *Vassil St. Georgiev*
National Institute of Allergy and Infectious Diseases
National Institutes of Health

Congenital and Perinatal Infections

A Concise Guide to Diagnosis

Edited by

Cecelia Hutto, MD

Division of Infectious Diseases, Department of Pediatrics
University of Alabama School of Medicine, Birmingham, AL

HUMANA PRESS ✳ TOTOWA, NEW JERSEY

ANSI Z39.48-1984 (American Standards Institute) Permanence of Paper for Printed Library Materials.

Production Editor: Robin B. Weisberg

Cover design by Patricia F. Cleary

Cover illustration from Fig. 3B, Chapter 4, "Placental Histopathology," by Edwina J. Popek.

For additional copies, pricing for bulk purchases, and/or information about other Humana titles, contact Humana at the above address or at any of the following numbers: Tel.: 973-256-1699; Fax: 973-256-8341; E-mail: orders@humanapr.com; or visit our Website: www.humanapress.com

Printed in the United States of America. 10 9 8 7 6 5 4 3 2 1
eISBN 1-59259-965-6

Library of Congress Cataloging-in-Publication Data

Congenital and perinatal infections : a concise guide to diagnosis / edited by Cecelia Hutto.
    p. cm. -- (Infectious disease)
 Includes bibliographical references and index.
 ISBN 1-58829-297-5 (alk. paper)
 1. Communicable diseases in the fetus--Diagnosis. 2. Neonatal infections--Diagnosis. I. Hutto, Cecelia. II.Series: Infectious disease (Totowa, N.J.)
 RG629.I53D53 2005
 618.3'2075--dc22

                                                                2005006205

Dedication

To the memory of my parents, Thelma and Haywood Hutto

Acknowledgment

I wish to acknowledge the dedication, patience, and hard work of Terri Hicks without whom this book would not have been possible.

—CH

Preface

A concise clinical reference that facilitates the diagnosis of intrauterine and perinatally acquired infections was the goal in creating the *Congenital and Perinatal Infections: A Concise Guide to Diagnosis*. Information about the natural history, management, and outcome of these infections is well detailed in many other sources and so has not been included. Rather, the focus of the book is diagnosis. The initial chapters provide general information about serological and nonserological assays that are used for the diagnosis of infections, and a chapter about the placenta includes details about histopathological findings that can be helpful with the diagnosis of congenital infections. The remainder of the book is devoted to the diagnosis of specific congenital and/or perinatal infections. As illustrated in the chapters about specific infections, the approach to diagnosis of a congenital or perinatally acquired infection in the neonate begins, when possible, with consideration and diagnosis of infection in the pregnant woman, knowledge of how the infection is transmitted, and the risk of that infection for the woman and her fetus or neonate. The possibility of congenital or perinatal infection in neonates is usually considered because of the diagnosis of, or concern about a specific infection in, a mother during pregnancy that can be transmitted to the neonate or because of clinical findings in the neonate at birth that suggest an infectious cause. Diagnosis is then made using both knowledge about the most appropriate assays for detection of that infection and the timing of these assays.

This book includes chapters about microorganisms that are both common and uncommon causes of congenital and perinatal infections. Some are considered infrequent causes of infection in the United States, but may be common in other areas of the world. With increasing global travel, even these less common infections must be considered at times, particularly in large urban areas. The book is not comprehensive in its coverage of microorganisms that have been reported to cause congenital and perinatal infections. It may, however, serve as a reminder to the clinician caring for pregnant women and their neonates of the increasing diversity of microorganisms that may be transmitted from a pregnant woman to her infant and result in congenital and perinatal infections.

It is hoped that the information provided in *Congenital and Perinatal Infections: A Concise Guide to Diagnosis* will be useful to all clinicians providing care to pregnant women and/or their infants for determining when women and their neonates are at risk for these infections and which assays are most appropriate to use for their diagnosis.

Cecelia Hutto, MD

Contents

Contributors

MARK J. ABZUG, MD • *Division of Pediatric Infectious Diseases, Department of Pediatrics, University of Colorado School of Medicine and The Children's Hospital, Denver, CO*

DAVID BERMAN, DO • *Division of Pediatric Infectious Diseases, All Children's Hospital, St. Petersburg, FL*

SURESH B. BOPPANA, MD • *Division of Infectious Diseases, Department of Pediatrics, University of Alabama at Birmingham, Birmingham, AL*

WILLIAM BORKOWSKY, MD • *Department of Pediatrics, New York University School of Medicine, New York, NY*

YVONNE BRYSON, MD • *Department of Pediatrics, Children's Hospital, UCLA School of Medicine, Los Angeles, CA*

KEVIN A. CASSADY, MD • *Division of Infectious Diseases, Department of Pediatrics, University of Alabama at Birmingham, Birmingham, AL*

AIDA CHAPARRO, MD • *Division of Infectious Diseases and Immunology, Department of Pediatrics, University of Miami School of Medicine, Miami, FL*

TIMOTHY J. CLEARY, PhD • *Departments of Pathology and Microbiology & Immunology, Jackson Memorial Medical Center, University of Miami School of Medicine, Miami, FL*

ENID J. GARCÍA-RIVERA, MD • *Dengue Branch, Centers for Disease Control and Prevention, San Juan, Puerto Rico*

ANNE A. GERSHON, MD • *Division of Infectious Diseases, Department of Pediatrics, Columbia University Medical Center, New York, NY*

MARGARET R. HAMMERSCHLAG, MD • *Division of Pediatric Infectious Diseases, State University of New York Health Science Center at Brooklyn, Brooklyn, NY*

CECELIA HUTTO, MD • *Division of Infectious Diseases, Department of Pediatrics, University of Alabama School of Medicine, Birmingham, AL*

RAVI JHAVERI, MD • *Division of Pediatric Infectious Diseases, Duke University Medical Center, Durham, NC*

DAVID W. KIMBERLIN, MD • *Division of Infectious Diseases, Department of Pediatrics, University of Alabama at Birmingham, Birmingham, AL*

KATHERINE M. KNAPP, MD • *Department of Infectious Diseases, St. Jude Children's Research Hospital, Memphis, TN*

CHARLES T. LEACH, MD • *Division of Infectious Diseases, Department of Pediatrics, University of Texas Health Science Center at San Antonio, San Antonio, TX*

CHARLES D. MITCHELL, MD • *Division of Infectious Diseases and Immunology, Department of Pediatrics, University of Miami School of Medicine, Miami, FL*

EDWINA J. POPEK, DO • *Department of Pathology, Baylor College of Medicine, Texas Children's Hospital, Houston, TX*

MOBEEN H. RATHORE, MD • *Division of Pediatric Infectious Diseases and Immunology, Wolfson Children's Hospital, University of Florida College of Medicine, Jacksonville, FL*

JOSÉ G. RIGAU-PÉREZ, MD, MPH • *Epidemiology, Entomology and Prevention Activity, Dengue Branch, Centers for Disease Control and Prevention, San Juan, Puerto Rico*

PABLO J. SANCHEZ, MD • *Department of Pediatrics, University of Texas Southwestern Medical Center at Dallas, Dallas, TX*

DAVID SCHNURR, PhD • *Viral and Rickettsial Disease Laboratory, Division of Communicable Disease Control, California Department of Health Services, Richmond, CA*

GWENDOLYN B. SCOTT, MD • *Division of Infectious Diseases and Immunology, Department of Pediatrics, Miller School of Medicine, University of Miami, Miami, FL*

MASAKO SHIMAMURA, MD • *Division of Infectious Diseases, Department of Pediatrics, University of Alabama at Birmingham, Birmingham, AL*

KIM CONNELLY SMITH, MD, MPH • *Department of Pediatrics, The University of Texas-Houston Medical School, Houston, TX*

JEFFREY R. STARKE, MD • *Department of Clinical Pediatrics, Texas Children's Hospital, Baylor College of Medicine, Houston, TX*

SITHEMBISO VELAPHI, MD • *Department of Pediatrics, Chris Hani Baragwanath Hospital, University of the Witwatersrand, Johannesburg, South Africa*

KEN B. WAITES, MD • *Division of Laboratory Medicine, Department of Pathology, University of Alabama at Birmingham, Birmingham, AL*

PATRICIA WHITLEY-WILLIAMS, MD • *Department of Pediatrics, UMDNJ-Robert Wood Johnson School of Medicine, New Brunswick, NJ*

CHARLES WOOD, PhD • *Nebraska Center for Virology and School of Biological Science, University of Nebraska, Lincoln, NE*

The Tools of Diagnosis

I

1
Diagnostic Assays
Serology

William Borkowsky

INTRODUCTION

Prior to the advent of highly sensitive antigen and nucleic acid detection methods, the diagnosis of acute infection was based on the measurement of the appearance of pathogen-specific antibodies, which most commonly were immunoglobulin G (IgG). A variety of assays were initially used, including complement fixation, hemagglutination, hemagglutination inhibition, immunofluorescence assays, radioimmunoassay (RIA), and eventually enzyme-linked immunosorbent assay (ELISA). Complement fixation, hemagglutination, hemagglutination inhibition, and immunofluorescence assays are usually titrated by assessing the highest dilution of serum that results in a positive response. In the case of RIA and ELISA, a quantitative value is determined at a single dilution of serum.

RIA quantitation is done by assessing counts per minute of an isotope (often ^{125}I), which is used to label a pathogen-specific antibody. The scale of this quantitation can be on the order of several logs.

In the case of ELISA, a colorimetric change resulting from the action of an enzyme on a clear substrate is measured in a spectrophotometer as an optical density (OD), measured at a wavelength appropriate for the specific substrate. The OD reading is generally at a range of 0–2 or 3. These OD values are not linear but semiquantitative. Thus, changes in "positive" ELISA values are not accurate. Positive responses are generally those that exceed some cutoff value. This cutoff is often determined by performing the test in a noninfected population and by adding several (e.g., 3) OD standard deviation values to the mean OD value. For example, if the uninfected population has a mean OD of 0.2 and a standard deviation of 0.04, a cutoff of 0.2 and 3($\times$)0.04 would result in a value (0.32) that statistically represents the 99th percentile. Only 1% of uninfected individuals would have OD values that exceeded the cutoff.

This false-positivity rate, perhaps because of nonspecific antigen–antibody reactions, is acceptable in certain situations but not others, such as screening for human immunodeficiency virus (HIV) infection. In such cases, a more specific test (e.g., a Western blot assay) that assesses true interaction of antibody with microbe-specific

From: *Infectious Disease: Congenital and Perinatal Infections: A Concise Guide to Diagnosis*
Edited by: C. Hutto © Humana Press Inc., Totowa, NJ

antigens is necessary to confirm infection. These shortcomings limit the usefulness of ELISAs to screening tests and not to changes in antibody present in the biologic fluid tested.

DIAGNOSING INFECTION BY SEROLOGIC MEANS

When there is no preinfection serologic IgG titer, the presence of significant changes (i.e., greater than fourfold increases or decreases of antibody for all tests except RIA and ELISA) within a 2- to 6-week period of time would constitute significant antibody production. Although this technology is reasonably specific and sensitive when dealing with adult infection, the ability to utilize this strategy in the diagnosis of congenital infections is compromised by the fact that the transplacental passage of IgG is highly efficient in the last months of gestation *(1)*. Thus, a full-term newborn was likely to "inherit" titers of specific IgG comparable to what was present in the maternal circulation. Transport of the other immunoglobulin classes does not occur because the passage of antibody from the maternal side of the placenta to the infant side results from the expression of only IgG Fc receptors (FcγRIII or CD16) on the syncytiotrophoblast. Expression of these receptors begins at 3 months of gestation and increases during gestation. Bound IgG can then be internalized in the placental cell and eventually released into the fetal/infant circulation. Consequently, the measurement of pathogen-specific IgG antibody in the newborn can only be interpreted as a surrogate for evidence of maternal infection. Pediatricians and other health care providers are then left to turn to a tincture of time to utilize this information as a diagnostic tool. Three of the four IgG subclasses have half-lives of about 23 days (IgG3, which represents only 7% of the total IgG, has a half-life of 9 days). By waiting for several half-lives, maternal antibody would be expected to decline significantly. A stable titer of antibody for 6 or more months, which does not drop as expected, is presumably caused by intrinsic antibody production by the fetus or newborn.

When maternal titers of antibody are high (e.g., HIV-infected mothers may have anti-HIV titers that exceed 1 million), the time required for sufficient half-lives to pass to render an ELISA assay negative may take as long as 15–18 months. For example, an HIV ELISA test often is performed at a 1/100 dilution of serum. If the maternal titer is 4 million at birth, a 33,000 reduction in titer (which represents 15 half-lives or $15 \times 23 = 345$ days) would still yield a positive assay. In fact, the average time to deplete maternal HIV and hepatitis C antibody in the infant is about 9 months.

Even in an earlier era, when the only treatable congenital infections were syphilis and toxoplasmosis, waiting for several months to make a diagnosis of congenital infection was not tolerable for physicians and parents of affected or at-risk children. In the case of treponemal infection, the empiric treatment of all children born to mothers with serologic evidence of syphilis (positive serum rapid plasma reagin and fluorescent treponemal antibody-absorption tests) is sufficiently simple that actual diagnosis of infection in the child was not usually necessary for initiating therapy. Moreover, the utility of the strategy of testing cord blood and neonatal sera also appears to be inferior to maternal sera for detecting prenatal exposure to syphilis *(2)*.

In contrast to the situation with congenital syphilis, therapy for congenital toxoplasmosis is very long and should not be offered to those without definitive infection. With the advent of potentially effective therapies for infections with rapidly replicating agents such as cytomegalovirus (CMV) or HIV, the need to make a rapid diagnosis increased in importance. In the following sections, various strategies used to diagnose congenital infections, particularly those comprised by the TORCH (*t*oxoplasmosis, *o*ther infections, *r*ubella, *C*MV, and *h*erpes simplex virus [HSV]) agents, are explored. It should become obvious that they all have shortcomings. As a consequence, and with the development of more rapid and specific nucleic acid detection methods, assays utilizing polymerase chain reaction amplification of specific pathogen-related nucleic acid has largely supplanted serologic methods.

Nonspecific Assays

Initial efforts were directed at the measurement of immunoglobulin classes IgM and IgA, which are produced by the fetus and do not cross the placenta. The simple measurement of total IgM in newborn serum has been applied to the diagnosis of congenital infection *(3)*. Alford and colleagues were able to attribute a 40-fold increased risk of congenital syphilis, CMV, and toxoplasma infection in infants with elevated cord blood IgM *(4)*. Unfortunately, the usefulness of this approach is limited by the fact that as many as 10% of "normal" newborns have levels this high. In addition, in a study of congenital rubella, cord blood IgM was not increased unless the infected child had three or more abnormalities *(5)*.

Elevated cord blood IgA has also been used to test nonspecifically for possible congenital infection. In a study of congenital CMV infection, nine of nine infected infants had increased IgA in their cord sera *(6)*. Unfortunately, 7% of normal newborn sera also had elevated IgA. As for the measurement of IgM in cord blood specimens, contamination with maternal blood is always a worry.

Specific Assays

The measurement of specific antibody might improve the specificity of diagnostic serology. Ideally, an assay that is both very sensitive and very specific could even be adopted as a neonatal screening tool to detect clinically inapparent infections that would escape detection. The measurement of pathogen-specific IgM would be a reasonable choice to fulfill these criteria. When this strategy was applied in a Massachusetts neonatal screening program for congenital toxoplasmosis, 100 of 635,000 infants tested had positive screening tests. Congenital toxoplasma infection was confirmed in 52 infants, 50 of whom were identified only through neonatal screening and not through initial clinical examination. However, after the serologic results became available, more detailed examinations revealed abnormalities of either the central nervous system or the retina in 19 of 48 infants evaluated *(7)*. The ability to perform a variety of serologic assays on dried filter paper makes neonatal screening feasible *(8–10)*.

Maternal Screening

In contrast to routine neonatal screening, more typically physicians first try to identify women who underwent primary infection with a pathogen such as toxoplasma, CMV, HSV, rubella virus, or parvovirus during pregnancy. This can be accomplished by screening early and late in pregnancy and comparing titers of IgG to specific pathogens or by measuring pathogen-specific IgM. In the case of CMV infection, specific IgM is produced in more than 75% of pregnant women within 8 weeks of seroconversion *(11)*. Unfortunately, one may not have the luxury of having an early natal or prenatal serum titer. IgM, although produced in acute infection, may also persist for long periods of time, as evidenced by detection of toxoplasma-specific IgM in 7% of pregnant women who were infected prenatally *(12)*. IgM may persist for more than 1 year after acute infection *(13)*. In addition, for viruses that cause chronic infection (i.e., the herpesviruses), exacerbations of latent infection or reinfection with another strain of virus may also result in IgM production. It is important to differentiate primary infection from secondary infection for some pathogens in that the former is associated with a higher likelihood of congenital infection *(14)*.

To complicate matters even further, not all IgM measurements are alike. For example, detection of specific antitoxoplasma IgM by immunofluorescence is seen less often (e.g., in 25% of congenitally infected) than with a double sandwich ELISA or by a similar agglutination assay *(15,16)*. The interpretation of test results requires knowledge about the sensitivity and specificity of each assay, including its performance within a given laboratory. This has provided an impetus to explore other avenues to differentiate new from old infection.

Some investigators have utilized IgG avidity as a tool to better specify primary from recurrent infection. Primary infection typically results in low-avidity antibody (i.e., antibody that does not bind strongly to antigen under extreme conditions); recurrent infection produces high-avidity antibody. In these assays, binding is often assessed in the presence of chaotropic (denaturing) agents, such as urea. When serum samples from 5 patients with recent primary toxoplasma infection were compared with those from 21 subjects with preexisting toxoplasma immunity, patients with primary infection exhibited a low avidity of toxoplasma-specific IgG, which persisted for several months after the onset of symptoms of toxoplasmosis. In contrast, all subjects with past immunity had a high avidity of toxoplasma-specific IgG *(17)*. This assay has been evaluated in controversial serology results in a reference lab and has been found to be the best discriminator for the evaluation of acute toxoplasma infection *(18)*. Another approach to differentiating remote from recent toxoplasmosis infection in a pregnant woman utilizes the fact that acute infection results in greater agglutination of acetone-fixed tachyzoites than with formalin-fixed tachyzoites *(19)*. This differential agglutination assay is only available in the laboratory of Jack Remington (Toxolab@PAMF.org).

In one study of CMV infection during pregnancy, even in the presence of an IgM-positive result, a CMV IgG avidity index above 65% on serum obtained during the first trimester of pregnancy could reasonably be considered a good indicator of past CMV infection *(20)*. In acute infections, avidity indices below 50% were seen. Often, combining IgM detection with IgG avidity results in better predictor of acute maternal infection *(21,22)*. The predictive value of IgG avidity in one study was quite significant in that the determination of anti-CMV IgG avidity at 6- to 18-week gestation could identify all women who would have an infected fetus/newborn (100% sensitivity) *(23)*. Antibody avidity is also useful when trying to diagnose congenital rubella late in the first year of life, when maternal IgG of possible high avidity has waned, leaving low-avidity IgG in the infant.

The ability to make neutralizing antibody to a pathogen is well correlated with antibody avidity. In the case of acute CMV infection in pregnancy, neutralizing antibody is not seen until 15 weeks after infection, but it persists thereafter *(24)*. Consequently,

Table 1
Characteristics of Immunoglobins That Affect Serologic Diagnosis

Immunoglobin class	Crosses placenta	Half-life	Requires quantitation	Sensitivity	Specificity
IgG	Yes	23 days	Yes	>90%	Good but complicated by maternal transplacental IgG
IgA	No	7 days	No	60–75%	Good
IgM	No	5 days	No	60–75%	Fair; decreased by rheumatoid factor
IgE	No	2.3 days	No	25%	Good

when there is lab expertise to perform this assay, the neutralization assay can be used as a reliable method for discriminating acute primary from previous or recurrent infection in a single serum sample.

Infant Testing

In theory, the measurement of IgM and IgA can be achieved by immunofluorescence when a specific pathogen-infected cell is available or by ELISA techniques when a relatively purified antigen is available. In practice, as indicated in the discussion of maternal screening, there are problems. A comparison of the characteristics of the various antibody classes in diagnostics is shown in Table 1.

In addition, because the immune system of the fetus is relatively immature, particularly early in gestation, the ability to make specific antibody in utero may be impaired. In congenital rubella infection prior to 10 weeks of gestation, no antibody production may occur (25). Fewer than 50% of fetuses with congenital parvovirus infection have measurable IgM (26), and less than 50% of fetal blood from toxoplasma-infected fetuses was IgM positive (27). Even if antibody production occurs, competition from the presence of high titers of maternal IgG antibodies in the serum or plasma may obscure the antigen and prevent binding of the child's IgG or IgM (28). In addition, if there is rheumatoid factor (e.g., IgM anti-IgG) present in the pediatric serum, the detection of non-IgG antibodies binding to the pathogen antigen in the infant serum may represent antimaternal IgG (perhaps specific for the pathogen of interest) rather than actual antibody directed at the micro-organism itself. The rheumatoid factor may result from fetal immunization with maternal IgG allotypes.

To improve the specificity of IgM measurement in the child, a number of strategies have been employed. These include (1) chromatographic separation of IgG and IgM from serum (29); (2) the treatment of the serum with goat or rabbit anti-IgG antibodies (30); (3) mercaptoethanol treatment of sera to disrupt IgM (31); (4) pretreatment of the sera with staphylococcal protein A (32) (a protein to which all IgGs and some IgMs bind); (5) pretreatment of the sera with streptococcal protein G (33) (an even more selective IgG-binding protein); and (6) the use of antigen capture techniques (34). In this last assay, nonhuman anti-IgM antibody is used to capture human IgM. The specificity of this IgM is determined by adding a labeled microbial antigen, which can be detected by ELISA.

A different but related approach to the serologic diagnosis of congenital infection attempts to measure pathogen-specific IgA or IgE. Although IgM production may occur prior to the development of IgA, this should not be a factor when infection has occurred in utero. When pathogen-specific IgM and IgA were compared for sensitivity and specificity in the diagnosis of congenital toxoplasmosis, they were comparable, with a sensitivity of about 60% in neonatal blood specimens and excellent specificity (IgM 98%; IgA 100%) *(35)*. In other studies, the sensitivity of IgA may either exceed that of IgM *(36–38)* or be less than what is seen with IgM *(39,40)*. Even when used together, the measurement of IgM and IgA will still miss about 25% of children with congenital toxoplasmosis *(41)*. Toxoplasma-specific IgE was detected in 86.6% of patients with toxoplasmic seroconversion, and it was produced as early as IgA and IgM *(42)*. The relatively short kinetics of IgE (it is rarely detectable beyond 4 months) can be a useful tool to date the infection more precisely. For the diagnosis of congenital toxoplasmosis, specific IgE was detected less frequently than IgM or IgA (25 vs 67.3%). An immune capture IgE assay for toxoplasmosis has also been evaluated in congenitally infected infants *(43)*.

The ability to measure IgM and IgA is still problematic as a diagnostic tool when trying to diagnose a congenitally infected child after 6 months of age. In this situation, these immunoglobulins that were present at birth may no longer be so. In this scenario, the ability to assess IgG avidity may yield useful information. In a study of congenital rubella infection, low-avidity specific IgG persisted in two children until age 23–31 months *(44)*.

For many congenital infections, the ability to detect IgM or IgA in infected infants is considerably less sensitive than detection of pathogen-specific nucleic acid *(45)*. However, for parvovirus, the sensitivity of serologic diagnosis may approach that of polymerase chain reaction positivity when newborn sera are tested *(46)*. In some situations, such as diagnosing enterovirus infections, the number of different serologically unique strains capable of producing disease makes serologic testing impractical. In most studies, the application of serologic techniques to cord blood rather than to neonatal sera results in a decrease in specificity, perhaps because of contamination with maternal blood.

When perinatal infection occurs, such as HIV infection, production of either IgM or IgA is delayed for several months after infection *(47–50)*. This virtually precludes the use of serology for the very early diagnosis of perinatal HIV infection.

In Vitro Antibody Production

A different approach to serologic diagnosis of newborn infection is to measure in vitro antibody production by lymphocytes isolated from the child and washed free of maternal antibody prior to culture. Specific antibody can be measured by Enzyme-linked ImmunoSPOT (ELISPOT), ELISA, or Western blot. In ELISPOT, lymphocytes are added to antigen-coated plastic or nitrocellulose and incubated for some period of time; after the cells are washed away, local antibody production is measured by detecting "spots," resulting from adherent antibody, by enzymatic-colorimetric techniques *(51)*. For the other two assays, the supernatants of cultured lymphocytes are added to wells or nitrocellose strips containing antigens, much the way diluted sera are tested by conventional serology. The presence of color changes in the ELISA plates or the presence of bands consistent with known antigen determinants on strips from electrophoresed crude antigens is diagnostic of pediatric infection.

Such techniques have been utilized to diagnose HIV infection in young infants *(52–55)*. Unfortunately, the production of antibody to HIV in infants is not usually seen until 3–6 months of age. Because viral replication or nucleic acid can be measured before 2 months of age, these techniques, as well as the simpler, more conventional measurement of serum IgM and IgA to HIV, have largely been abandoned as diagnostic tools.

Antibodies to Neonate-Specific Antigens

One largely unexplored serologic avenue for the diagnosis of congenital infections involves the demonstration of antibodies in congenitally infected fetuses or neonates to microbial antigens that are not present in maternal serum. This strategy was employed in a study of Chagas' disease. In most cases, IgG specificities in the newborns mirrored those of their mothers, but congenitally infected newborns in addition had IgG antibodies to *Trypanosoma cruzii* antigens that were undetectable in their mothers. The new IgG specificities observed most frequently were against a shed acute phase antigen and less frequently against nine different parasite antigens *(56)*.

Finally, serologic testing is also useful for screening children with evidence of potential congenital infection (e.g., children with mental retardation and chorioretinitis or chorioretinal scars) who test seronegative for traditional TORCH agents. In one study, lymphocytic choriomeningitis virus (LCMV) was responsible for visual loss in two of four children, secondary to chorioretinitis in a population of severely retarded children *(57)*. The diagnosis was realized by detecting elevated levels of IgG to LCMV in these children, a finding also noted by a French study of two children with chorioretinal scars for whom LCMV was detected by ELISA and confirmed by Western immunoblotting *(58)*.

REFERENCES

1. Gitlin D. Development and metabolism of the immune globulins. In Kagan BM, Stiehm ER, eds. Immunologic Incompetence. Chicago: Year Book, 1971:3–13.
2. Chhabra RS, Brion LP, Castro M, Freundlich L, Glaser JH. Comparison of maternal sera, cord blood, and neonatal sera for detecting presumptive congenital syphilis: relationship with maternal treatment. Pediatrics 1993;91:88–91.
3. Alford CA, Stagno S, Reynolds DW. Diagnosis of chronic perinatal infections. Am J Dis Child 1975;129:455–463.
4. Alford CA, Schaefer J, Blankenship WJ, et al. A correlative immunologic, microbiologic and clinical approach for the diagnosis of acute and chronic infections in newborn infants. N Eng J Med 1967;227:437–449.
5. McCracken GH, Hardy JB, Chen T, et al. Serum immunoglobulin levels in newborn infants. II. Survey of cord and follow-up sera from 123 infants with congenital rubella. J Pediatr 1969;74:383–392.
6. Mason EO, South MA, Montgomery JR. Cord serum IgA in congenital CMV infection. J Pediatr 1976;89:945–946.
7. Maguire, J, Lynfield H, Stechenberg R, et al. Neonatal serologic screening and early treatment for congenital *Toxoplasma gondii* infection. The New England Regional Toxoplasma Working Group. N Engl J Med 1994;330:1858–1863.
8. Eaton RB, Petersen E, Seppanen H, Tuuminen T. Multicenter evaluation of a fluorometric enzyme immunocapture assay to detect toxoplasma-specific immunoglobulin M in dried blood filter paper specimens from newborns. J Clin Microbiol 1996;34:3147–3150.

 9. Paul M, Petersen E, Pawlowski ZS, Szczapa J. Neonatal screening for congenital toxoplas-
    mosis in the Poznan region of Poland by analysis of *Toxoplasma gondii*-specific IgM anti-
    bodies eluted from filter paper blood spots. Pediatr Infect Dis J 2000;19:30–36.
10. Petersen E, Eaton RB. Control of congenital infection with *Toxoplasma gondii* by neonatal
    screening based on detection of specific immunoglobulin M antibodies eluted from phe-
    nylketonuria filter-paper blood-spot samples. Acta Paediatr Suppl 1999;88:36–39.
11. Stagno S, Tinker MK, Elrod C, Fuccillo DA, Cloud G, O'Beirne AJ. Immunoglobulin M
    antibodies detected by enzyme-linked immunosorbent assay and radioimmunoassay in the
    diagnosis of cytomegalovirus infections in pregnant women and newborn infants. J Clin
    Microbiol 1985;21:930–935.
12. Jenum PA, Stray-Pedersen B, Melby KK, et al. Incidence of *Toxoplasma gondii* infection
    in 35,940 pregnant women in Norway and pregnancy outcome for infected women. J Clin
    Microbiol 1998;36:2900–2906.
13. Liesenfeld O, Montoya JG, Tathieneni NJ, et al. Confirmatory serologic testing for acute
    toxoplasmosis reduces rates of induced abortions among women reported to have positive
    toxoplasma immunoglobulin M antibody tests. Am J Obstet Gynecol 2001;184:140–145.
14. Stagno S Pass RF, Cloud G, Britt W, Henderson J, et al. Primary cytomegalovirus infec-
    tion in pregnancy. Incidence, transmission to fetus, and clinical outcome. JAMA
    1986;256:1904–1908.
15. Naot Y, Remington JS. An enzyme-linked immunosorbent assay for detection of IgM an-
    tibodies to *Toxoplasma gondii*: use for the diagnosis of acute acquired toxoplasmosis. J
    Infect Dis 1980;142:757–766.
16. Naot Y, Desmonts G, Remington JS. IgM enzyme-linked immunosorbent assay test for the
    diagnosis of congenital toxoplasma infection. J Pediatr 1981;98:32–36.
17. Hedman K, Lappalainen M, Seppaia I, Makela O. Recent primary toxoplasma infection
    indicated by a low avidity of specific IgG. J Infect Dis 1989;159:736–740.
18. Liesenfeld O, Montoya JG, Kinney S, Press C, Remington JS. Effect of testing for IgG
    avidity in the diagnosis of *Toxoplasma gondii* infection in pregnant women: experience in
    a US reference laboratory. J Infect Dis 2001;183:1248–1253.
19. Dannemann BR, Vuaghan WC, Thulliez P, et al. The differential agglutination test for
    diagnosis of recently acquired infection with *Toxoplasma gondii*. J Clin Microbiol
    1990;28:1928–1933.
20. Bodeus M, Goubau P. Predictive value of maternal-IgG avidity for congenital human cy-
    tomegalovirus infection. J Clin Virol 1999;12:3–8.
21. Lazzarotto T, Varani S, Guerra B, Nicolosi A, Lanari M, Landini MP. Prenatal indicators
    of congenital cytomegalovirus infection. J Pediatr 2000;137:90–95.
22. Lazzarotto T, Varani S, Gabrielli L, Spezzacatena P, Landini MP. New advances in the
    diagnosis of congenital cytomegalovirus infection. Intervirology 1999;42:390–397.
23. Lazzarotto T, Varani S, Spezzacatena P, et al. Maternal IgG avidity and IgM detected by
    blot as diagnostic tools to identify pregnant women at risk of transmitting cytomegalovi-
    rus. Viral Immunol 2000;13:137–141.
24. Eggers M, Metzger C, Enders G. Differentiation between acute primary and recurrent hu-
    man cytomegalovirus infection in pregnancy, using a microneutralization assay. J Med
    Virol 1998;56:351–358.
25. Meitsch K, Enders G, Wolinsky JS, Faber R, Pustowoit B. The role of rubella-immunoblot
    and rubella-peptide-EIA for the diagnosis of the congenital rubella syndrome during the
    prenatal and newborn periods. J Med Virol 1997;51:280–283.
26. Dieck D, Schild RL, Hansmann M, Eis-Hubinger AM. Prenatal diagnosis of congenital
    parvovirus B19 infection: value of serological and PCR techniques in maternal and fetal
    serum. Prenat Diagn 1999;19:1119–1123.
27. Foulon W, Pinon JM, Stray-Pedersen B, et al. Prenatal diagnosis of congenital toxoplas-
    mosis: a multicenter evaluation of different diagnostic parameters. Am J Obstet Gynecol
    1999;181:843–847.

28. Cohen IR, Norins LC, Julian AJ. Competition between, and effectiveness of, IgG and IgM antibodies in indirect fluorescent antibody and other tests. J Immunol 1967;98:143–149.
29. Gupta JD, Peterson V, Stout M, Murphy AM. Single sample diagnosis of recent rubella by fractionation of antibody on Sephadex G-200 column. J Clin Pathol 1971;24:547–550.
30. Thomas HIJ, Morgan-Capner P, Connor NS. Adaptation of a commercial rubella-specific IgG kit to assess specific IgG avidity. Serodiagn Immunother Infect Disease 1993;1:13–16.
31. Millian SJ, Wegman D. Rubella serology: applications, limitations, and interpretations. Am J Public Health 1972;62:171–176.
32. Tuomanen EI, Powell KR. Staphylococcal protein A adsorption of neonatal serum to facilitate early diagnosis of congenital infection. J Pediatr 1980;97:238–243.
33. Akerstrom B, Brodin T, Reis K, Bjorck L. Protein G: a powerful tool for binding and detection of monoclonal and polyclonal antibodies. J Immunol 1985;135:2589–2592.
34. Yolken RH, Leister FJ. Enzyme immunoassays for measurement of cytomegalovirus immunoglobulin M antibody. J Clin Microbiol 1981;14:427–443.
35. Wallon M, Dunn D, Slimani D, Girault V, Gay-Andrieu F, Peyron F. Diagnosis of congenital toxoplasmosis at birth: what is the value of testing for IgM and IgA? Eur J Pediatr 1999;158:645–649.
36. Bessieres MH, Berrebi A, Rolland M, et al. Neonatal screening for congenital toxoplasmosis in a cohort of 165 women infected during pregnancy and influence of in utero treatment on the results of neonatal tests. Eur J Obstet Gynecol Reprod Biol 2001;94:37–45.
37. Foudrinier F, Marx-Chemla C, Aubert D, Bonhomme A, Pinon JM. Value of specific immunoglobulin A detection by two immunocapture assays in the diagnosis of toxoplasmosis. Eur J Clin Microbiol Infect Dis 1995;14:585–590.
38. Naessens A, Jenum PA, Pollak A, et al. Diagnosis of congenital toxoplasmosis in the neonatal period: a multicenter evaluation. J Pediatr 1999;135:714–719.
39. Foulon W, Pinon JM, Stray-Pedersen B, et al. Prenatal diagnosis of congenital toxoplasmosis: a multicenter evaluation of different diagnostic parameters. Am J Obstet Gynecol 1999;181:843–847.
40. Gorgievski-Hrisoho M, Germann D, Matter L. Diagnostic implications of kinetics of immunoglobulin M and A antibody responses to *Toxoplasma gondii*. J Clin Microbiol 1996;34:1506–1511.
41. Wallon M, Dunn D, Slimani D, Girault V, Gay-Andrieu F, Peyron F. Diagnosis of congenital toxoplasmosis at birth: what is the value of testing for IgM and IgA? Eur J Pediatr 1999;158:645–649.
43. Pinon JM, Toubas D, Marx C, et al. Detection of specific immunoglobulin E in patients with toxoplasmosis. J Clin Microbiol 1990;28:1739–1743.
44. Herne V, Hedman K, Reedik P. Immunoglobulin G avidity in the serodiagnosis of congenital rubella syndrome. Eur J Clin Microbiol Infect Dis 1997;16:763–766.
45. Revello MG, Zavattoni M, Baldanti F, Sarasini A, Paolucci S, Gerna G. Diagnostic and prognostic value of human cytomegalovirus load and IgM antibody in blood of congenitally infected newborns. J Clin Virol 1999;14:57–66.
46. Koch WC, Harger JH, Barnstein B, Adler SP. Serologic and virologic evidence for frequent intrauterine transmission of human parvovirus B19 with a primary maternal infection during pregnancy. Pediatr Infect Dis J 1998;17:489–494.
47. Gaetano C, Scano G, Carbonari M, et al. Delayed and defective anti-HIV IgM response in infants. Lancet. 1987;1:631.
48. McIntosh K, Comeau AM, Wara D, et al. The utility of IgA antibody to human immunodeficiency virus type 1 in early diagnosis of vertically transmitted infection. National Institute of Allergy and Infectious Diseases and National Institute of Child Health and Human Development Women and Infants Transmission Study Group. Arch Pediatr Adolesc Med 1996;150:598–602.
49. Weiblen BJ, Lee FK, Cooper ER, et al. Early diagnosis of HIV infection in infants by detection of IgA HIV antibodies. Lancet 1990;335:988–990.

50. Schupbach J, Tomasik Z, Jendis J, Boni J, Seger R, Kind C. IgG, IgM, and IgA response to HIV in infants born to HIV-1 infected mothers. Swiss Neonatal HIV Study Group. J Acquir Immune Defic Syndr 1994;7:421–427.

51. Nesheim S, Lee F, Sawyer M, et al. Diagnosis of human immunodeficiency virus infection by enzyme-linked immunospot assays in a prospectively followed cohort of infants of human immunodeficiency virus-seropositive women. Pediatr Infect Dis J 1992;11:635–639.

52. Pollack H, Zhan MX, Moore T, Krasinski K, Borkowsky W. Ontogeny of anti-HIV antibody production in HIV-infected infants. Proc Natl Acad Sci U S A 1993;90:2340–2344.

53. Amadori A, De Rossi A, Chieco-Bianchi L, Giaquinto C, De Maria A, Ades AE. Diagnosis of human immunodeficiency virus 1 infection in infants: in vitro production of virus-specific antibody in lymphocytes. Pediatr Infect Dis J 1990;9:26–30.

54. Wang XP, Paul M, Tetali S, et al. Improved specificity of in vitro anti-HIV antibody production: implications for diagnosis and timing of transmission in infants born to HIV-seropositive mothers. AIDS Res Hum Retroviruses 1994;10:691–699.

55. Pahwa S, Chirmule N, Leombruno C, et al. In vitro synthesis of human immunodeficiency virus-specific antibodies in peripheral blood lymphocytes of infants. Proc Natl Acad Sci U S A 1989;86:7532–7536.

56. Reyes MB, Lorca M, Munoz P, Frasch AC. Fetal IgG specificities against *Trypanosoma cruzii* antigens in infected newborns. Proc Natl Acad Sci U S A 1990;87:2846–2850.

57. Mets MB, Barton LL, Khan AS, Ksiazek TG. Lymphocytic choriomeningitis virus: an underdiagnosed cause of congenital chorioretinitis. Am J Opthalmol 2000;130:209–215.

58. Brezin AP, Thulliez P, Cisneros B, Mets MB, Saron MF. Lymphocytic choriomeningitis virus chorioretinitis mimicking ocular toxoplasmosis in two otherwise normal children. Am J Opthalmol 2000;130:245–247.

2

Nonserologic Assays for Detection of Bacteria and Other Nonviral Infections

Timothy J. Cleary

INTRODUCTION

Many of the old microbiology techniques continue to play an integral part in the laboratory diagnosis of infectious diseases. However, in the past several years advances in technology enabled the clinical microbiology laboratory to respond rapidly to the needs of patients and clinicians for the identification of possible infections. Three topic areas are discussed in this chapter. The first outlines specimen collection guidelines, various culture protocols for the isolation of organisms, identification protocols, and the value of antimicrobial susceptibility testing. The second broad category covers methods for the immunological detection of nonviral infectious processes. The final section introduces the expanding area of molecular microbiology.

The organisms that are considered neonatal pathogens include a vast array of bacteria, a few fungi, and parasites. This chapter does not focus on any specific organism or give guidelines for their identification in the laboratory, but rather paints a broad picture of what the practitioner should expect of the clinical microbiology laboratory.

CULTURE AND IDENTIFICATION PROCEDURES

Specimen Collection

The importance of proper specimen collection for the diagnosis of infectious diseases cannot be overstated. There are several excellent references that provide guidelines for specimen collection (1). Adherence should be to the following principles:

1. All specimens must be properly labeled with the patient's name and hospital number. Attached to each specimen must be a key-plated voucher bearing the same patient name, hospital number, and the name of the requesting physician. The requisition must also indicate the required test or tests, the source of the material, time of collection, plus the name of any particular organism suspected.
2. When possible, specimens should be obtained before antibiotics or other antimicrobial agents have been administered.
3. The specimen must be adequate in volume for desired tests. All specimens that are collected by swab must include two swabs if a Gram stain or other microscopy is requested.
4. Specimens must be received in a clean, sterile container and be sent to the laboratory

From: *Infectious Disease: Congenital and Perinatal Infections: A Concise Guide to Diagnosis*
Edited by: C. Hutto © Humana Press Inc., Totowa, NJ

expeditiously or should be stored at a temperature that will not affect the growth of the pathogenic micro-organism. Use appropriate transport medium when required.

5. Avoid contamination from the indigenous bacterial flora.

Most of the reference guidelines available refer to specimen collection from older patients rather than the very young. For blood cultures, for example, most recommendations indicate that 10 mL blood must be collected for each bottle submitted to the laboratory for culture. Definitive criteria are not available for the very young. There are no clinical studies that address the collection of specimens in the neonate. It is important to get the best specimen as often as possible to submit for diagnostic procedures. All microbiologists bend the rules for this patient population, out of either empathy or the realization that "it's all that you are going to get under certain conditions." We also know from the literature that septic neonates often have very high bacterial loads. Therefore, the volume provided is not as important as proper collection techniques to avoid contamination in the blood culture bottle. The last point, the importance of proper collection techniques, is critical, particularly when the infected child is evaluated for suspected sepsis because of the frequent occurrence of blood cultures growing organisms that represent contamination associated with the collection procedure.

There is a saying that I heard for years (I do not know the original source): "Garbage in, garbage out." Often abbreviated as GIGO, this is a famous computer axiom meaning that if invalid data are entered into a system, the resulting output will also be invalid. Although originally applied to computer software, the axiom holds true for all systems, including specimen collection of patient samples for microbiology culture.

Microscopy

The most important basic microbiology information for a patient often depends on a well-performed microscopic procedure. There are two parts to any microscopic procedure: The first and most critical is the preparation of the smear, and the second is the actual staining procedure. The cytocentrifuge is an excellent procedure for the preparation of smears from sterile fluids. It has been found that the sensitivity of the cytospin Gram stain from cerebrospinal fluid specimens equals or exceeds that for the traditional bacterial antigen detection. In addition, the cytocentrifuge may be used to prepare bronchoalveolar lavage and nasopharyngeal wash slides for subsequent staining with specific reagents for the detection of pathogenic organisms (e.g., respiratory viruses, *Bordetella pertussis*).

In addition to the Gram stain, the acridine orange stain is particularly useful in the rapid screening of normally sterile specimens in which few organisms may be present. It is also useful in the rapid examination of blood/buffy coat smears or preparations containing proteinaceous material in which differentiation of organisms from background material may be more difficult. Acridine orange is a fluorochromatic dye that binds to nucleic acids of bacteria and other cells. Bacteria and fungi uniformly stain bright orange, whereas human epithelial and inflammatory cells and background debris stain pale green to yellow. The only drawback to this procedure is that a fluorescent microscope is needed to visualize the organisms.

Culture Procedures

The majority of organisms that are involved in infections in the neonate will grow on the common isolation media used in the laboratory. These media include a general purpose broth medium and agar-based medium (usually supplemented with 5% sheep blood or horse blood), an enriched medium (chocolate agar), and a selective medium (MacConkey agar). Special media have been developed for the cultivation of many fastidious organisms; the laboratory needs to be advised of special requests to ensure optimal recovery of these organisms.

By far the most important patient specimens sent to the laboratory in neonates are for evaluation for sepsis *(2)*. Group B streptococcus (*Streptococcus agalactiae*) and *Escherichia coli* continue to be the most common pathogens isolated from septic infants. Increased automation in the laboratory has facilitated the recovery of pathogenic microorganisms. Current blood culture instruments continuously monitor individual blood culture bottles for the growth of micro-organisms every 10–15 minutes. The method for detecting growth varies with the automated system in use, but they generally rely on the production of a gas or pressure changes within the bottle. Growth is indicated by a change in the slope of the growth curve for the product that is monitored. Because each bottle is monitored around the clock, these systems will detect a positive sample 1–1.5 days faster than manual systems. Most significant cultures are detected within 24 hours of incubation. In addition, the culture bottles have been refined to optimize the growth of organisms. Most experts agree that a blood-to-broth-medium ratio of 1:5–1:10 should be maintained for the optimal recovery of the micro-organism. Pediatric blood culture bottles have a smaller volume of broth medium and enriched medium to meet these criteria. Antibiotic-binding resins, activated charcoal, and other formulations are often added to the blood culture bottle to neutralize compounds that may inhibit or retard the growth of organisms.

Special Culture Procedures

For the isolation of fastidious organisms, selective media and methods are needed. The isolation of *Mycobacteria tuberculosis* requires an enriched medium that contains a number of antibiotics to inhibit rapidly growing commensal bacteria that may contaminate the specimen. An automated detection system, similar to the instrument used for blood cultures, is used for detection of these organisms. Likewise, *Mycoplasma hominis* and *Ureaplasma* spp require special media and cultivation methods for isolation. Because these organisms are sensitive to environmental conditions, appropriate transport media should be used to enhance their recovery from clinical material. In vitro growth of the organisms requires that the medium be supplemented with serum and other nutrients. These media are commercially available. The chlamydia species (*Chlamydia trachomatis* and *Chlamydia pneumoniae*) are rarely isolated in the laboratory because cell culture procedures are needed for cultivation. The majority of these infections are detected using molecular techniques *(3,4)*.

Identification of Organisms

As with the monitoring systems for the detection of organisms, automated systems are rapidly displacing conventional methods for the identification and antibiotic susceptibility testing of bacteria and yeasts *(5)*. These systems usually consist of miniature wells that contain biochemical substrates and varying dilutions of antibiotics. Most bacteria and yeasts that are involved in infections are reliably identified by these systems. The antimicrobial susceptibility testing profiles that are generated can be reported as the minimal inhibitory concentration of the drug or by the category of susceptible, intermediate, or resistant. These data can be available within 8–10 hours for most of the rapidly growing micro-organisms. For those organisms that are not reliably identified in the systems, specialized identifications systems are available. In the future, newer molecular methods will make their way into the laboratory to achieve this goal *(3–5)*; these methods in some instances will be faster than the conventional procedures for the identification of the organisms.

IMMUNOLOGICAL PROCEDURES

Immunoassays play a critical role in diagnostic microbiology *(6)*. These assays belong to two major categories based on whether examining for the presence of antibodies (immunoglobulins) or a specific analyte associated with a micro-organism (antigens). Serologic methods for the diagnosis of infectious diseases are addressed in Chapter 1. In this section, I examine immunological assays used for the direct detection or identification of micro-organisms from clinical specimens or organisms isolated on a culture plate. Advances in antigen detection are parallel to the advances made in the development of monoclonal antibodies (characterized with respect to their specificities and binding affinities). The immunological methods used include agglutination tests for bacterial antigens, enzyme immunoassay (EIA) antigen tests, and direct immunofluorescence assays (DFAs) and indirect immunofluorescence assays.

Bacterial Agglutination Test

A bacterial agglutination test is available for the detection of *Streptococcus pneumoniae*, *S. agalactiae*, *Haemophilus influenzae* type B, and *Neisseria meningitidis*. The assay uses latex particles coated with specific antibodies to structural antigens and can detect soluble antigens in urine, cerebrospinal fluid (CSF), and serum. The sensitivity and specificity of these tests in urine samples is extremely unreliable, and the tests should not be used on this specimen. For sterile body fluids, the tests are highly sensitive and specific for *H. influenzae*, but their sensitivity for other bacteria is much lower, particularly for *N. meningitidis*. It is important to note that the sensitivity of this assay was essentially identical to Gram stain smears prepared using a cytospin preparation of the fluid. Most laboratories have discontinued the use of this test. Those laboratories that still offer the latex particle agglutination tests will usually perform the procedure only on patients with sufficient white blood cells in the CSF.

There are a number of agglutination tests for the identification of organisms that are isolated on culture plates. Most laboratories use this procedure for the identification of β-hemolytic streptococci (groups A, B, C, D, F, G), *Salmonella* and *Shigella* typing, and the identification of *E. coli* O157.

Immunoassay Detection of Antigen

EIA systems are performed in microwells, in test tubes, or on solid membranes and incorporate an enzyme-substrate indicator system. These tests play a prominent role in viral diagnostics for the detection of influenza virus, rotavirus, and respiratory syncytial virus. The most commonly used bacterial test is for the detection of group A streptococci in pharyngeal specimens. A number of waived tests and moderately complex tests are on the market; the best tests have a sensitivity and specificity around 90–95%. Newer antigen assays for the detection of *Legionella pneumophila* and *S. pneumoniae* in urine have been introduced.

Until now, the accepted laboratory practice for the diagnosis of malaria was the microscopic examination of Giemsa or- Wright-stained blood films. An EIA has been developed to detect a plasmodium antigen. For the detection of malaria in blood samples, the assay is designed to detect an antigen (histidine-rich protein-2) associated with malaria parasites (especially *Plasmodium falciparum* and *Plasmodium vivax*) or to detect plasmodium-associated lactate dehydrogenase or aldolase. The monoclonal antibodies against these markers are immobilized in the nitrocellulose matrix; blood lysates are allowed to migrate over the membrane and are captured. The complex is visualized by the addition of the second antibody. The test lines are located at specific points on the strip to aid in the interpretation of positive results. Each test strip also contains two internal process control dotted lines that appears as positive confirmation of procedure and reagent viabilities. When compared to microscopy and clinical history, the assay has a sensitivity and specificity of 96 and 99%, respectively, for histidine-rich protein-2 detection for *P. falciparum*, with discrepant results having less than 100 parasites/µL (0.002% parasitemia).

DFAs and Indirect Immunofluorescence Assays

DFAs are commonly used in immunology, microbiology, and virology laboratories to directly detect the presence of micro-organisms. They are fast, easy to perform, and very specific but require well-trained personnel and a fluorescent microscope. An important advantage of this type of assay is that it provides results quickly. After fixation of the specimen on the slide, results are available within 1 hour. In the DFA procedure, clinical specimens such as nasal washes, sputum, CSF, or culture material are centrifuged using a cytocentrifuge and are fixed on glass slides (usually by heat or cold acetone fixation). The slides are then reacted directly with a specific antibody probe that is labeled with a fluorochrome (fluorescein isothiocyanate). After washing excess fluid from the slide, mounting oil and a coverslip are added, and the slides are examined using a fluorescence microscope.

The *C. trachomatis* DFA is an alternative method for detection of *C. trachomatis* in urogenital and rectal specimens, in conjunctival specimens for the differential diagnosis of acute conjunctivitis, and in nasopharyngeal specimens for the differential diagnosis of afebrile pneumonia or lower respiratory tract infections in infants. Because most laboratories are unable to culture this organism, this test is often the only option available for the rapid identification of this infection. Newer probe and amplification assays are more sensitive than DFA testing.

To increase sensitivity, indirect fluorescent antibody methods can be used to offer a more versatile application. In this method, a primary immunoglobulin G antibody (unlabeled) is reacted with the fixed clinical sample, which may contain the specific antigen on a microscope slide. After a wash to remove the primary antibody, a second fluorescent-labeled antibody with specificity to the primary immunoglobulin molecule is added to the slide.

MOLECULAR MICROBIOLOGY

Conventional culture and immunoassay are gradually giving way to molecular methods for detecting bacterial and viral pathogens in the clinical microbiology laboratory *(3,4)*. These assays are becoming commercially available, and the technical staff of the laboratory are easily adapting to these procedures. The molecular expertise was initially gained by working with specimens from patients infected with human immuno-deficiency virus (HIV). That experience has now evolved to include a broader range of infectious pathogens. In addition, the evolution of newer technical procedures has played an important role in the acceptance of the molecular techniques *(3,4,7)*.

Four major improvements have occurred in recent years: (a) commercially available automated nucleic acid extraction devices; (b) improvements in nucleic acid hybridization assays, which will allow clinical microbiology laboratories to use hybridization assays for the detection of potential pathogens directly from clinical specimens or from isolated colonies grown in culture; (c) adoption of real-time polymerase chain reaction (PCR) cyclers by clinical laboratories, which allows huge time and labor savings; (d) new technology to provide clinical laboratories with the ability to sequence nucleic acids on a timely basis *(8)*. With new gel electrophoresis equipment, the identity of most micro-organisms can be made available within 24–48 hours of isolation.

Nucleic Acid Probes

With the exception of viruses, ribosomes are an integral part of the cell of all prokary-otic and eukaryotic micro-organisms. The 70S ribosome of prokaryotic cells is com-posed of two subunits, which contain 16S and 23S ribosomal ribonucleic acid (rRNA). Likewise, the 80S ribosome of eukaryotic cells contains 18S and 28S rRNA. Research into the comparative ribosomal deoxyribonucleic acid (rDNA) gene sequences of mi-croorganisms has been ongoing for the past 30 years and has become an accepted method for establishing phylogenetic relationships among species. Currently, *Bergey's Manual of Systematic Bacteriology* is undergoing revision based on 16S rRNA se-quence comparisons *(9)*. Likewise, the taxonomy of yeasts is undergoing a revision based on a comparative 26S rDNA sequence analysis.

The sequence information of these ribosomal genes has been used in the clinical laboratories for diagnostic purposes. They are well suited for this purpose for several reasons. There are both highly conserved and variable regions along the length of these molecules. The conserved area allows the identification of a specific organism (species specific) or class of organisms (genus specific); the variable regions allow for discrimi-nation among members of the group. Reports have demonstrated the detection of sub-species of organisms based on subtle differences in the rRNA. In addition, rRNA is usually present in large quantities, allowing for greater sensitivity in the assay. The amount of rRNA relates to an organism's growth rate. Slow-growing bacteria, such as *M. tuberculosis*, have 10^2–10^3 copies of rRNA per cell, whereas fast-growing faculta-tive anaerobic bacteria may have as many as 10^4–10^5 molecules.

There are many different assays on the market. The Gen-Probe System (Gen-Probe Inc., San Diego, CA) uses chemiluminescence-labeled, single-stranded DNA probes that are complementary to the rRNA of the target organisms. After the rRNA is re-leased from the organisms, the labeled DNA probes combine with the rRNA of the target organisms to form stable DNA:RNA hybrids. The labeled DNA:RNA hybrids are separated from the nonhybridized probes and are measured in the luminometer. The test results are calculated as the difference between the response of the specimen and the mean response of the negative reference. This method has been in place for over a decade for the detection of pathogenic organisms directly from clinical samples (including *C trachomatis* and *Neisseria gonorrhoeae*) or the culture confirmation of organisms grown in the laboratory.

Another method used for detection and identification of micro-organisms is fluorescent *in situ* hybridization *(4)*. These probes are short sequences of single-stranded DNA that are complementary to the DNA target sequences. These probes hybridize, or bind, to the complementary DNA and, because they are labeled with fluorescent tags, allow the direct visualization of the cell that contains the specific sequence. The technique has been employed in the histopathology laboratory to aid in the diagnosis and management of a variety of solid tumors and hematologic malignancies in the clinical setting. It has been used in the clinical microbiology laboratory for the detection of micro-organisms directly from clinical material or as a procedure for culture confirmation.

Peptide nucleic acid (PNA) probes mimic DNA in many aspects but differ in the basic backbone that is used to tie the nucleotide bases together. The backbone of the PNA probes is made up of repeating *N*-2-aminoethyl glycine units linked by amine bonds instead of the sugar phosphate backbone characteristic of DNA. The resulting structure of PNA molecules allows normal base pair formation; however, there is no electric charge in the backbone of the probe, which results in very fast and strong hybridization. In addition, these probes are more resistant to protease and nuclease degradation in a cell environment, which assists in minimizing any enzymatic attack during the hybridization process. All of these factors make hybridization assays that use PNA probes more robust than other probe hybridization protocols.

Amplification Methods

The year 2003 saw the celebration of the 50th anniversary of the discovery of the molecular structure of DNA by the collaborative work of Watson, Crick, Franklin, and Wilkins. Since that time, we have witnessed an astounding growth in the area of molecular biology. No less of an achievement was the invention of the PCR method by Mullis in 1983. Since the initial description of his method, PCR methods have become the standard against which newer procedures are compared.

Traditional PCR

The PCR method is used for the specific amplification of a targeted DNA or RNA sequence. For DNA targets, the double-stranded DNA is rendered single stranded by denaturing with heating to 95°C for 2–10 minutes. The reaction vessel is rapidly cooled to between 55 and 65°C in the presence of short (15–20 bases) complementary oligonucleotides (primers), which bracket the targeted DNA to be amplified. During this step, the primer oligonucleotides hybridize to the DNA target molecule. Once the primers are bound, the temperature is raised, and the Taq DNA polymerase enzyme adds nucleotides to the $3'$ end of the primer. This occurs on both strands of DNA, resulting in the production of a new copy of double-stranded DNA. The sequence of temperature changes is repeated for up to 45 cycles, resulting in the production of (at the theoretical maximum efficiency) up to 10^{13} copies from a single copy of template DNA.

For RNA molecules, the sequence of events is initiated by the reverse transcription of the target RNA (messenger RNA for certain viruses) to generate complementary DNA. Following this step, the reaction proceeds as for DNA molecules.

Traditional PCR requires that the amplified product be further manipulated in the laboratory for detection. This detection can be performed by electrophoretic separation of the amplican on agarose gel followed by visualization with a labeled probe or by hybridization of the product to a specific probe using an enzyme-labeled immunoassay protocol.

Table 1
Micro-Organisms Identified by Real-Time Amplification Protocols

Bacteria
    Staphylococcus aureus
    Streptococcus pyogenes
    Streptococcus agalactiae
    Enterococcus species
    Listeria monocytogenes
    Cornynebacteriun diphtheriae toxin
    Mycobacterium tuberculosis
    Haemophilus influenzae
    Neisseria gonorrhoeae
    Neisseria meningitides
    Moraxella catarrhalis
    Bordetella pertussis
    Bordetella parapertussis
    Mycoplasma pneumoniae
    Mycoplasma genitalium
    Chlamydia pneumoniae
    Chlamydia trachomatis
Fungi
    Candida species
    Aspergillus fumigatus
    Pneumocystis jiroveci
Parasites
    Plasmodium vivax
    Plasmodium falciparum
    Plasmodium malariae
    Plasmodium ovale
    Toxoplasma gondii
    Trichomonas vaginalis
Viruses
    Herpes simplex virus
    Varicella-zoster virus
    Cytomegalovirus
    Epstein-Barr virus
    Parvovirus B19
    Influenza A virus
    Influenza B virus
    Respiratory syncytial virus
    Adenovirus
    Human metapneumovirus
    Severe acute respiratory syndrome virus
    HIV-1 virus
    HIV-2 virus
    Enteroviruses
    Hepatitis B virus
    Hepatitis C virus

Real-Time Amplification

In traditional PCR, the amplicans or products of the PCR reaction are detected after the completion of the PCR cycle. For real-time amplification, the products are detected as they are made. There are several methods available for the amplification of the microorganism, and the basic protocols differ in the method used for amplification *(10–15)*. The amplification methods are PCR, nucleic acid sequence-based amplification, and transcription-mediated amplification. The real-time amplification systems are based on the detection and quantitation of a fluorescent reporter molecule in the system. By recording the amount of fluorescence emission at each cycle, it is possible to monitor the amplification reaction during the exponential phase, in which the first significant increase in the amount of product correlates with the initial amount of target template. A list of organisms that have been detected by real-time methods is found in Table 1.

REFERENCES

1. Miller JM. A Guide to Specimen Management in Clinical Microbiology. Washington, DC: ASM Press, 1996.
2. Buttery JP. Blood cultures in newborns and children: optimising an everyday test. Arch Dis Child Fetal Neonatal Ed 2002;87:F25–F28.
3. Bankowski MJ. Real-time nucleic acid amplification in clinical microbiology. Clin Microbiol Newslett 2004;26:9–15.
4. Persing DH, Tenover FC, Versalovic J, et al., eds. Molecular Microbiology: Diagnostic Principles and Practice. Washington, DC: ASM Press, 2004.
5. Tang TW, Von Graevenitz A, Waddington MG, et al. Identification of coryneform bacterial isolates by ribosomal DNA sequence analysis. J Clin Microbiol 2000;38:1676–1678.
6. Murray PR, Baron EJ, Pfaller MA, Tenover FC, Yolken RH, eds. Manual of Clinical Microbiology, 7th ed. Washington, DC: ASM Press, 2003.
7. Farkas DH, Kaul KL, Wiedbrauk DL, Kiechle FL. Specimen collection and storage for diagnostic molecular pathology investigation. Arch Pathol Lab Med 1996;120:591–596.
8. Randhawa JS, Easton AJ. Demystified ... DNA nucleotide sequencing. Mol Pathol 1999;52:117–124.
9. Garrity GM, Boone DR, Castenholz RW (eds.). Bergey's Manual of Systemic Bacteriology, 2nd ed. New York, Springer-Verlag, 2001.
10. Leone G, van Schijndel H, van Gemen B, Kramer FR, Schoen CD. Molecular beacon probes combined with amplification by NASBA enable homogeneous, real-time detection of RNA. Nucleic Acids Res 1998;1:26:2150–2155.
11. Bergeron MG, Danbing M, Menard C, et al. Rapid detection of group B streptococci in pregnant women at delivery. N Eng J Med 2000;243:175–179.
12. Tang YW, Ellis NM, Hopkins MK, Smith DH, Dodge DE, Persing DH. Comparison of phenotypic and genotypic techniques for identification of unusual aerobic pathogenic Gram-negative bacilli. J Clin Microbiol 1998;3674–3679.
13. Kraus G, Cleary T, Miller N, et al. Rapid and specific detection of *Mycobacterium tuberculosis* using fluorogenic probes and real-time PCR. Mol Cell Probes 2001;15:375–383.
14. Moody A. Rapid diagnostic tests for malaria parasites. Clin Microbiol Rev 2002;5:66–78.
15. Cleary T, Roudel G, Casillas O, Miller N. Rapid and specific detection of *Mycobacterium tuberculosis* using the Smart-Cycler instrument and a fluorogenic probe. J Clin Microbiol 2003;41:4783–4786.

3

Diagnosis of Viral Infections by Viral Isolation and Identification or by Direct Detection

David Schnurr

INTRODUCTION

Laboratory diagnostic tests for viral infections play an important role in the management of infections during pregnancy and in the newborn infant. There are three basic laboratory approaches to diagnosis of viral infection: (1) isolation and identification, (2) serology, and (3) direct detection. The choice of approach depends on the agent suspected, the specimen submitted, and the resources of the laboratory. Isolation is considered the "gold standard," but not all viruses grow well or at all in currently available culture systems. Serology is the method of choice when the virus is no longer likely to be present or cannot be cultured. Direct detection provides clinically relevant information in a minimum amount of time. The approach can be both highly sensitive and specific.

Isolation is the process of growing a virus from a clinical specimen in an appropriate host system. The inoculated host system is observed for evidence of viral growth. If growth occurs, specific identification of the agent is achieved by immunological or molecular methods. Alternatively, the culture may be probed with antibodies for specific agents prior to the development of cytopathology. The process is somewhat analogous to bacterial isolation except that with bacterial culture the problem frequently involves separating potential pathogens from normal flora. In the case of viruses, there is no normal flora to contend with, and thus the culture of any agent is potentially significant.

Serologic assays are dependent on the host response to the viral infection. Recent infection is recognized by a fourfold or greater rise in titer when acute and convalescent sera are run in the same assay at the same time. The presence of specific immunoglobulin (Ig) M is evidence of recent infection. Because IgG but not IgM can cross the placenta, assays for specific IgM are especially important in diagnosis of infections of the fetus and newborn. Serology is discussed in Chapter 1.

Direct detection is the identification of an agent in a clinical specimen without amplification by culture. Agents that cannot be cultured or are no longer viable are amenable to direct detection. Methods vary wildly in their sensitivity and specificity, but all provide the advantage of rapid results that can be used in patient management.

From: *Infectious Disease: Congenital and Perinatal Infections: A Concise Guide to Diagnosis*
Edited by: C. Hutto © Humana Press Inc., Totowa, NJ

ISOLATION AND IDENTIFICATION

Isolation and identification is the gold standard technique for detection of many viral agents. The power of isolation is that a particular agent is not targeted and that, as the result of viral multiplication, even one infectious particle may be amplified millions of times, greatly facilitating the identification.

Specimens

The selection, transport, storage, and processing of the specimen are crucial for isolation attempts to be meaningful. The ideal specimen is taken from the site of the lesion or symptoms as early in the course of the illness as possible. The risk of fetal exposure or infection is determined by the status of the mother. Herpes I or II, enterovirus, rubella, and varicella-zoster virus (VZV) are some of the viruses that may be isolated and that are clinically relevant to the fetus or newborn. Other important agents such as hepatitis B virus, HIV, and parvovirus B-19 are either extremely difficult to culture or cannot be cultured.

In some cases, specimens taken from sites other than the site of the symptoms are useful. For example, enterovirus infections are frequently diagnosed from stool or respiratory specimens, which may then provide useful information on the etiology of systemic symptoms such as myocarditis or encephalitis.

It is advisable to inoculate culture systems immediately after obtaining the specimen or as soon as possible for isolation attempts to be successful. If the specimen will be inoculated within 48 hours of collection, it should be held at 4°C. However, when inoculation will be delayed for longer periods, stools and rectal swabs should be stored frozen at –20°C and respiratory and other specimens at –70°C. To select the optimal host system for culture, it is crucial that information on the symptoms of the patient, the date of onset, the date the specimen was taken, the disease suspected, and other relevant information accompany the specimen.

Specimens such as stools and cerebrospinal fluid (CSF) should be placed in a sterile container for holding and shipment. Swabs should be placed in a container with sterile viral transport media. The transport media may be purchased from a commercial supplier or may be prepared in-house. A transport media satisfactory for most purposes consists of a sterile buffered broth or balanced salt solution with approx 0.5% gelatin.

Specimen processing depends on the type of specimen. Specimens that are sterile, such as CSF, are inoculated directly into a suitable host system. Stools and rectal swabs are put into solution, and antibiotics are added. Penicillin and streptomycin in combination or gentamicin are satisfactory. Gentamicin is used by many laboratories because it has a broad spectrum of action and can be stored at 4°C. Fungizone (amphotericin B) is added to control fungal growth. Antibiotics are added directly to respiratory wash specimens. Tissue obtained at autopsy or biopsy tissue is ground and resuspended to 10 or 20% in an appropriate diluent and then inoculated.

Viral Culture Systems

Viruses are obligate intracellular parasites; therefore, cultivation requires an appropriate living host system. There is no one host system suitable for cultivation of all viral agents. In the historical development of diagnostic virology laboratory tests, the discovery and utilization of new host systems were critical events in advancing the discipline. The first host systems were laboratory or experimental animals. In the 1930s, embryonated eggs were first used to cultivate viruses. They supported the growth of nearly all viruses known at the time. However, the real breakthrough was the use of cells in culture. The report of growth of poliovirus in cultured, nonneural cells with the production of cytopathic effects (CPEs) in 1949 *(1)* marked the start of the age of cell culture for in vitro cultivation of viruses, which resulted in the discovery of a number of new viruses.

Suckling mice may still be used and are the only or best host for certain of the group A coxsackieviruses *(2)*. Otherwise, they are not used for isolation. Embryonated eggs may have some limited use, but for the most part are of historical interest only. Cell cultures have replaced the other host systems and are the host of choice for growing most viruses. Because no single cell type is permissive for all of the viral agents that could be cultured, relevant clinical information is necessary to choose the appropriate cell types.

Cells grown in culture are the in vitro progeny of cells obtained from living tissue. Cultures are started from dissociated pieces of tissue placed in nutrient media in a sterile culture vessel. Cells may grow in suspension or adhere to the surface of the vessel. Adherent cultures form sheets of cells attached to a clear glass or plastic surface. Primary culture is the first passage of the cells outside the parent organism. When cells are removed from the surface of the growth vessel and transferred into two or more vessels, they are said to be *passaged* or *subcultured*. Once subcultured, cells are called *cell lines*. Cell lines may be *finite*, capable of a limited number of doublings, or *infinite*, capable of an unlimited number of doublings. Finite cell lines are diploid and exhibit contact inhibition. Examples are the human fetal diploid cells MR5 and WI38. Continuous cell lines, theoretically capable of infinite growth in culture (e.g., HeLa, Hep2, RK13, and A549), are less expensive and easier to maintain. Among the cells types most frequently used for viral isolation are primary monkey kidney cells, human fetal diploid cells, and a variety of continuous cell lines. Despite the ongoing effort to identify better host systems, permissive hosts for many important viral agents, such as those causing hepatitis and gastroenteritis, have not been found.

Viral Culture

Viral isolation attempts are initiated by inoculating specimen aliquots into tubes or bottles of cell cultures. Companion control and inoculated cells are incubated at 33°C for growth of respiratory viruses and at 36°C for optimal growth of other viruses. For some viruses, growth is enhanced by continuous slow rotation of the tubes. The cultures are examined microscopically at periodic intervals for CPE or hemadsorption (HAd). CPE is the degeneration of cells caused by the growth of virus. The type of CPE is characteristic for a given group of viruses, as for example herpes causes a ballooning of cells, enterovirus causes rounding up and lysis, and respiratory syncytial virus (RSV) causes syncytia formation. From the appearance of the CPE, the cells in which the virus grew, the time from inoculation until the CPE appeared, and the rate of progression it is possible to make an informed guess about which virus has been isolated. Although CPE is characteristic for particular virus groups, the CPE alone is not sufficient evidence to establish the identity of the virus. It is important to be aware that cell degeneration may occur for reasons other than the growth of a virus. Toxicity caused by the inoculum, culture medium, or aging of cells may be confused with CPE. Contaminants such as mycoplasma or parasites that can cause effects not easily differentiated from those caused by viruses are occasionally introduced with the specimen. Primary monkey cells frequently carry indigenous viruses that grow in the culture and can cause CPE or hemadsorb *(3)*.

HAd is the attachment of red blood cells from various species to the cells in culture. It is useful as a marker for the growth of viruses that modify the cellular membrane by inserting viral-coded proteins, which attach to red blood cells. HAd does not identify which virus is present, but it is a good indicator for growth of members of the Myxo (influenza virus) or Parmyxovirus families. It is important to be aware that HAd in primary monkey kidney cells can be caused by an indigenous monkey virus.

Interference of viral CPE is used to monitor for the growth of rubella, a virus that does not cause CPE or HAd. At the California Department of Health, Viral and Rickettsial Disease Laboratory, when rubella is suspected, RK13 and BSC-1 cells are inoculated. Other cells that are susceptible include Vero and African green monkey kidney. Following several days of incubation, echovirus 11, a cytopathic enterovirus, is added to inoculated and control cultures. The failure of the enterovirus to cause CPEs in inoculated cultures is evidence that rubella has grown. Interference is not proof that rubella is present, but if interference does not occur, it proves that rubella has not grown. Rubella can then be identified using a specific labeled antibody.

Shell Vials

Another approach to make culture more rapid and to identify if a particular agent is present prior to the appearance of CPE or detectable HAd is the shell vial technique. The specimen is centrifuged onto the cell sheet, incubated for 24 or 48 hours, and then stained with specific antibodies. The technique is especially useful for detection of cytomegalovirus (CMV), which requires days or weeks to grow and may require subculture before viral growth can be recognized. Monoclonal antibody (MAb) to CMV early antigens, which are synthesized before CPE develops, allow for detection of viral infection before CPE is apparent *(4)*. Shell vials are also used for herpes I and II, VZV, enteroviruses, and respiratory viruses. This method makes the identification of virus more rapid, but because it requires staining for specific agents, it cannot detect all the agents that might be present.

Virus Identification

Some laboratories identify the virus group based on CPE, the cells the virus grew in, and the fact that the CPE can be passed. However, as mentioned in the Viral Culture section, there are problems with the identification of viruses when relying on the presence and type of CPE. The identification is subjective, and even the most experienced virologist may make errors in the reading and interpretation of the cause and type of CPE. Confirmation of the identification for all isolates is highly recommended.

The identification is accomplished by a specific test for viral antigen or nucleic acid or by the morphology seen by electron microscopy (EM). Identification by nucleic acid and by EM is discussed in the section on direct detection. The most common method for viral identification is by specific antibodies from either polyclonal serum or MAbs. The discovery and utilization of MAbs have had a major impact on diagnostic virology. They can be selected to have a high sensitivity and specificity, and the identical

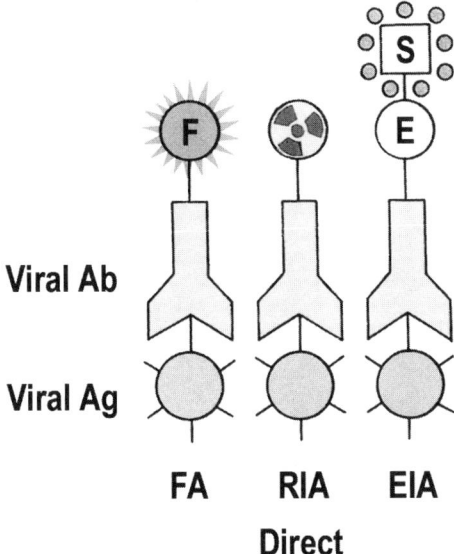

Fig. 1. Direct assay using labeled antibody. F, fluorescence; S, substrate; E, enzyme; Ag, antigen; FA, fluorescent assay; EIA, enzyme immunoassay; RIA, radioimmunoassay.

antibody is potentially available in unlimited supply. The reproducibility and unlimited supply have made it possible to develop highly standardized reagents and tests. The high specificity of MAbs can result in false-negatives because of antigenic variation, but this can be overcome using mixtures of MAbs.

Unlabeled Antibody Assays

Depending on the assay, the antibody may be unlabeled or labeled with a fluorescent molecule, a radioisotope, an enzyme, or biotin. In assays using unlabeled antibody, a specific antibody–antigen reaction is detected by a resultant biological effect. Examples of assays that use unlabeled antibodies are hemagglutination inhibition (HI), complement fixation, and neutralization. HI is the standard test for strain typing of influenza isolates but otherwise now has little use in virus identification. Complement fixation has been used for typing enteroviruses, adenoviruses, and others, but like the HI test is only infrequently used for virus identification. In the neutralization test, viral infectivity is interfered with or blocked by the reaction of specific antibody with the virus. The failure of the virus to infect cells results in the cells remaining healthy without exhibiting CPE or cell death. Neutralization is highly specific and is the standard test for typing of entero- and adenoviruses. Tests identifying viruses by specific neutralization are still important but possibly are being replaced by more rapid tests.

Labeled Antibody Assays

Labeled antibodies are versatile and may be used in a variety of formats. An important distinction in the use of labeled antibodies is the difference between the direct and indirect formats. In the direct format (Fig. 1), the labeled antibody is specific for the target antigen. For instance, to identify a suspected herpes, virus cells suspected to be infected with the virus are fixed onto a glass slide and stained with labeled antibodies to herpes I and herpes II. At the same time, uninfected cells and herpes I and herpes II

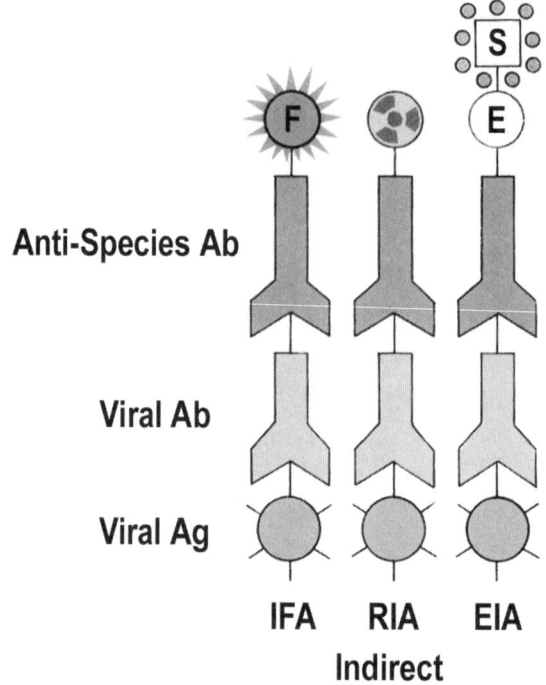

Fig. 2. Indirect assay using labeled antibody. EIA, enzyme immunoassay; IFA, indirect fluorescence assay; RIA, radioimmunoassay.

infected control cells are also stained. If the controls react properly (i.e., no staining of uninfected cells and specific staining of herpes I and herpes II controls with the proper conjugates), then the test can be read.

In the indirect format, the labeled antibody is specific for immunoglobulin of the species in which the primary antibody was made (Fig. 2). This is sometimes known as the sandwich technique because the specific antibody is sandwiched between the fixed target antigen and the labeled antispecies antibody. Because the detecting antibody is antispecies immunoglobulin, a single conjugate can be used to detect a variety of primary antibodies specific for different viruses. The direct method is relatively more specific and less sensitive than the indirect method.

In the fluorescent antibody method, fluorescein isothiocyannate (FITC) or another fluorescent molecule is conjugated to antibody molecules specific for a given antigen without destroying the binding activity of the antibody. With FITC-labeled antibodies, specific staining for herpes will be seen as crisp, green fluorescence in the nucleus and cytoplasm of infected cells. In addition to high specificity and sensitivity, another important advantage of the fluorescent-labeled antibody technique is that the morphology of staining is read; that is, one is able to determine if the staining occurs only in the nucleus or cytoplasm or both. Particular staining patterns are typical of a given virus. Disadvantages are that reading requires a fluorescent microscope, and that when using the standard glycerol-based mountants, the slide preparations are not permanent. At the Viral and Rickettsial Disease Laboratory a polyvinyl alcohol, glycerol mountant that preserves full fluorescence for up to a year or more is used.

Enzyme-labeled antibodies are also versatile reagents used in a variety of assays. Similar to assays using fluorescent-labeled antibodies, enzyme immunoassays are highly sensitive and specific. They are used in one of two formats for antigen detection: *in situ* detection and solid-phase, quantitative assays. For the *in situ* detection of antigen, horseradish peroxidase is used in the immunoperoxidase assay. This assay is analogous to the immunofluorescent assay. Following the reaction of the peroxidase-labeled antibody with the test specimen and controls, the enzyme substrate is added so that the action of the enzyme on the substrate results in the production of a colored product. The product is insoluble, so it precipitates at the site of the of the enzyme substrate reaction. The colored precipitate can be viewed by light microscopy. Advantages of this assay over FA assay is that it does not require a fluorescent microscope and it provides a permanent record. Quantitative solid-phase assays are described in the section on direct detection.

Antibodies may also be conjugated with the low molecular weight molecule biotin. Because of its relatively small size, biotin is less likely to interfere with the antibody-to-antigen binding reaction than the larger enzyme molecules. Avidin or strepavidin both bind with a high affinity to biotin and can be labeled with enzyme. The direct reaction has two steps: (1) addition of biotin-labeled primary antibody, and (2) addition of avidin enzyme complex. The substrate is then added, and color development is monitored. In theory, these assays are extremely sensitive because one biotin molecule binds four avidin enzyme complexes.

Assays using radioisotope label are not in general use because of safety and disposal problems. The use of these and other assays such as latex agglutination and time-resolved fluoroimmunoassay for detection of viral antigen are discussed in an excellent chapter on the subject *(5)*.

Interpretation

When a virus is isolated and identified, the significance of the isolate is based on the known association of the agent with the patient's syndrome and the site from which the virus was isolated. For instance, enteroviruses are known to be possible etiological agents of encephalitis. However, an isolate from stool is much less significant than one from a central nervous system specimen. Failure to isolate an agent in no way rules out the possible role of the agent in the syndrome

For many viruses, isolation and identification are the "gold standard" methods for detecting virus in a specimen. They offer the important advantages that the agent is greatly amplified, that a particular agent does not need to be targeted, and that successful culture provides a live replicating virus for further characterization. However, not all viruses grow in culture. Cell culture is time consuming and expensive and requires special expertise and training.

DIRECT DETECTION

Because of the rapid nature of the tests, direct detection of viral agents is the method of choice for producing results that have clinical relevance. Direct detection is accomplished by a variety of methods, including histopathology, EM, immunohistopathology, enzyme-linked immunosorbent assay, fluorescent antibody assays, and molecular methods, particularly polymerase chain reaction (PCR). Each method has certain advantages and disadvantages.

Histopathology

Examination of tissue or cells by light microscopy allows the pathologist to obtain information on the disease process and in some cases to determine if a viral infection has occurred and even which virus might be involved *(6)*. *Histopathology*, the analysis of sections prepared from fixed solid tissue, or *exfoliative cytology*, preparations of cells or groups of cells, are the two methods for specimen preparation. The tissue or cells are fixed to a glass slide, stained with various dyes to emphasize morphological detail, and observed with the light microscope. The viewer searches for a variety of effects, from inflammation in tissue sections or inclusion bodies in individual cells to more subtle changes in cell morphology. Inclusion bodies are sites of viral-assembled protein and nucleic acid seen within infected cells. In the absence of suspicion of a specific agent, the types of inclusion body or altered cellular morphology are indicators of viral infection. For example, the characteristic greatly swollen, cytomegalic cell is typical of CMV infections. Cytology was used for diagnosis of the syndrome known as cytomegalic inclusion disease in newborns before the etiological agent was discovered. Before specific tests for rabies virus existed, rabies infections were identified by the cytoplasmic inclusion bodies known as Negri bodies. Observation of inflammation, inclusion bodies, or other histological changes can be an important aid in the diagnosis of the disease process and of a viral infection.

Electron Microscopy

EM provides a valuable adjunct to the other methods for direct detection *(7)*. The magnification achieved provides images of viruses that allow morphological identification of agents in original specimens. Diagnosis by EM is especially useful for agents that cannot be cultivated or are extremely fastidious, such as the agents causing human gastroenteritis and hepatitis. No *a priori* knowledge of which agents might be present in the specimen is required. A major disadvantage of EM is that, because of the great magnification, a minimum concentration of 10^5–10^6 virions per milliliter is necessary to have sufficient numbers of agents per field to view virions. For immune EM, the aggregation of a specific agent by antibodies can increase sensitivity but it is targeted to only one agent at a time. Agents of gastroenteritis such as rotavirus, astrovirus, and enteric adenovirus and of hepatitis such as hepatitis A virus were first identified by EM.

Immunological Methods

The immunological methods described using labeled antibodies to identify virus grown in cell culture are equally or more important for direct detection. Specific MAbs are especially useful, conferring both sensitivity and specificity to the reaction. MAbs are less likely to exhibit background staining because of nonspecific or irrelevant antibody binding, which occurs with hyperimmune polyclonal serum. The direct approach, which is more specific and less sensitive than the indirect, is generally favored.

Similar to viral culture, the specimen used for direct detection is a critical limiting factor. For direct detection of virus-infected cells, they must be collected and placed onto glass slides for staining. Specimens must include adequate numbers of target cells for tests to be valid. Swabs may be placed in phosphate-buffered saline and vortexed or vigorously rotated to release cells from the swab matrix, or the swab may be applied directly to the slide. When preparing cells from suspension, the suspension is centrifuged, resuspended in a small volume, and dropped onto a glass slide to air dry, and fixed. Skin and mucous membrane lesions are scraped vigorously, and the cells are deposited on the slide, air dried, and fixed. The slide is than stained with specific MAbs and observed for specific viral staining.

Fluorescent Labeled Antibodies

Commercially available FITC-labeled antibodies for direct detection of herpes I and II viruses, VZV, influenza A and B, RSV, adenoviruses, and others are available. Direct immunofluorescence assays (DFAs) is less sensitive for agents that grow well in culture, such as for herpes or influenza, and more sensitive for other viruses that do not grow as well, such as RSV *(8)*. DFA is the standard test for detection of rabies in brains of infected animals; there is close to 100% sensitivity *(9)*.

Solid-Phase Quantitative Assays

Direct procedures that provide rapid results are obtainable in the solid-phase quantitative format using antibodies labeled with horseradish peroxidase or alkaline phosphatase. Tests using this format are commercially available for adeno-, rota-, and astroviruses. The specimens are diarrheal stools. Antiviral-specific antibody is attached to a microwell or bead in a plate, and the specimen is added. Following washing and addition of an antiviral enzyme-labeled antibody, the enzyme substrate is added. Cleavage of the substrate results in the production of a colored compound that is soluble and can be read visually or by a plate reader. In a slightly different format used for influenza and RSV, the specimen is washed through a membrane that traps viral particles. In the case of a positive reaction, a color develops on the membrane.

Viral Nucleic Acids: Amplification and Detection

Because of their great potential to provide sensitive and specific diagnostic tests, methods for direct detection of viral nucleic acid have been of interest for many years. Nucleic acid detection has become more practical and prominent, particularly since the description and development of the PCR *(10,11)*.

Hybridization, Primers, and Probes

Detection of specific nucleic acid in a specimen depends on hybridization (i.e., specific binding) of a sequence of complementary bases between two single-stranded segments of nucleic acid. One strand of known sequence is used to bind to and detect the second strand, the target. The known strand may contain a radioisotope, enzyme, biotin, or another label and serve as a probe for the second strand, or it may bind and serve as the primer for enzyme-catalyzed synthesis of continuing sequences along the target strand. The specificity of the reaction derives from the uniqueness of the nucleic acid of each group of agents. The sensitivity derives from the number of hybridization reactions that occur and the nature of the probe label. Direct hybridization of labeled probes to extracted sample nucleic acid was attempted. However, this approach was not sufficiently sensitive for detection of specific nucleic acid.

The expanding databases recording viral nucleic acid sequences have made it possible to develop probes and primer sets that can be extremely specific or much broader in the range of viruses they detect. For instance, for the enteroviruses there are primers that detect all members of the group *(12,13)* and others specific for serotypes, such as primer sets specific for polioviruses *(14)*.

Specimen Preparation

For nucleic acid from clinical specimens to be accessible for hybridization, the specimen must undergo preparative steps to extract and expose the target. These extraction steps may be by a variety of protocols *(15)* that ultimately free the nucleic acid from the cellular matrix or from virions; alternatively, it may prepare cells or tissue for *in situ* hybridization. The extraction procedure depends on the type of specimen and whether the desired target is deoxyribonucleic acid (DNA), ribonucleic acid (RNA), or both. Although there are reliable in-house procedures for extraction, many laboratories rely on commercial preparations. One potential problem is that inhibitors of the enzymatic reactions involved in PCR primer extension or other enzymatic reactions may be present in stools, respiratory or other clinical specimens. The presence of inhibitors can be demonstrated by testing diluted specimen and observing a positive reaction in the diluted material and a negative one in the undiluted.

Polymerase Chain Reaction

The ability to amplify the target DNA by the PCR has made the detection of host nucleic acid both practical and the method of choice for many purposes. The method, first described in the middle 1980s, has many applications. Awarding the 1989 Nobel Prize for Medicine to the inventor of the method, Kerry Mullis, recognized the significance of the discovery.

PCR allows the number of DNA molecules to be increased twofold with each round of amplification, so that with 30 rounds of PCR a single molecule can be amplified to more than a billion. The obvious benefit is that a single molecule of DNA that would be extremely difficult or impossible to detect by molecular methods increases in number so that detection becomes practical. The mechanics and uses of PCR, by which specific fragments of DNA are amplified, have been described many times (for review, *see* ref. *16*). Briefly, two oligonucleotide primers, 15–30 bases each, complementary to opposite strands of DNA are designed so that extension of the oligonucleotides copies the DNA sequence between the primers from the opposite strands. Excess primers, temperature-stable DNA polymerase, salts, and nucleotides for DNA synthesis is added. The PCR is initiated by heating double-stranded DNA so that strand separation occurs, the temperature is lowered so that annealing occurs between primers and DNA template, and extension of the primers to copy the template is catalyzed by the polymerase. The temperature is again raised to melt the strands, and a second cycle is initiated. Each round doubles the number of amplified targets. The products of first-round PCR will include one of the primers; products amplified in subsequent rounds of PCR will have a primer at each end. These newly synthesized fragments, including primers and internal sequences, are called an *amplicon*.

Viral RNA or messenger RNA may also be amplified by PCR. However, first the RNA is copied into complementary DNA using the enzyme reverse transcriptase. Reverse transcriptase has been engineered into the temperature-resistant DNA polymerase enzyme so that production of complementary DNA and PCR can be done in a single reaction by changing the reaction conditions.

Analysis

Following the PCR, the reaction mix is analyzed for the presence of amplicons. Detection of products based on size, shape, and charge is done by gel electrophoresis.

Following electrophoresis, the gel is stained with ethidium bromide and viewed with a source of ultraviolet light to detect the location of bands. These bands are compared with the location of marker bands of known molecular weight to determine the size of fragments. In some cases, the size of the bands is used as the marker for the synthesis of specific fragments. However, nonspecific fragments having the same electrophoretic mobility as specific ones may be generated during the reaction; thus, the size of the fragment does not confer the specificity that can be gained by hybridization of a probe. The probe is selected to hybridize with the region of the amplicon between the primers. The amount of hybridization is proportional to the number of amplicons produced in the PCR reaction.

The hybridization reaction may be done in solution or on a solid support. However, most of the formats for detection of PCR products use solid-phase systems. In one variation of this format, the fragments from a gel are blotted unto a support matrix and fixed. A labeled probe is then added and reacted with the blot. If the probe hybridizes, the location of the amplican can be determined by autoradiography for radiolabeled probes and by the deposition of a colored precipitate using enzyme probes labeled systems.

An alternative solid-phase hybridization technique is to attach the unlabeled probe to the wells of a 96-well plate. An aliquot of the amplified product is added to the wells and allowed to hybridize. Controls include negative and low-positive samples. The amount of hybridization can be quantified by adding an MAb to double-stranded DNA conjugated to an enzyme. The substrate is then added, and the amount of enzymatic activity is determined. Another variation on this method is to use primers labeled with biotin. Amplified products that hybridize will include the biotin-labeled primers. Avidin conjugated with an enzyme is then added. Detection of the enzyme activity is as previously described.

Purified nucleic acids can be further characterized for genetic variation by restriction enzyme analysis. Restriction enzymes recognize unique sequences of four to six nucleotides and cut the DNA at the site of the sequences, producing new, smaller segments from the original piece. For instance, if a single DNA segment is cut once by a restriction enzyme, the result is two new segments with an aggregate molecular weight that equals that of the original segment. The number of cuts and the size of the products are determined by electrophoresis. Comparison of the REA fragments with the known pattern for the same enzyme with genetic variants provides a more complete description of the amplified DNA. For instance, this method can be used for strain typing. The restriction fragments of the amplified DNA are compared with the fragments from different strains to determine molecular relationships.

Sequencing of amplicans provides the most complete description of the fragment. A powerful technique called cycle sequencing, which allows sequencing of small quantities of amplicon, has been described *(17)*. Sequence information makes it possible to obtain information on strain variation that can be related to pathogenesis or molecular epidemiology and used in a variety of ways.

Real-Time PCR

Real-time detection of DNA amplification by PCR is possible using the TaqMan detection system from Roche and Perkin-Elmer. The oligonucleotide probe is designed with a reporter molecule at one end and a molecule that quenches the reporter molecule at the other. The quencher molecule interferes with the fluorescence of the reporter as long as the oligonucleotide is intact. When hybridized to the target, the probe is digested by the nuclease activity of the Taq polymerase. The reporter molecule fluoresces when separated from the quenching activity. With each round of PCR, the amount of fluorescence increases proportional to the amount of amplication that has occurred. The real-time progress of the PCR is measured by the increase of fluorescence, monitoring the progress of the PCR reaction without further analysis of the amplicon products. Thus, results are available without further product analysis.

Advantages of PCR are that PCR is a rapid method that is potentially highly sensitive and specific. PCR can amplify a single copy of nucleic acid that may represent a noninfectious virion or an agent that cannot be cultured under any conditions. PCR has not been fully standardized, so many laboratories have in-house procedures. Without standardized tests, it is difficult to compare results between laboratories. Also, PCR is subject to contamination, resulting in false-positive results and inhibition of the reaction, resulting in false negatives.

Interpretation

The significance of a positive result for direct detection of an agent depends on the sensitivity and specificity of the test, the relationship of the agent with the syndrome or disease in question, and the site from which the specimen was obtained. However, the value of a positive result is that when indicated it allows for immediate action to be taken.

REFERENCES

1. Enders JF, Weller TH, Robbins FC. Cultivation of Lansing strain of poliomyelitis virus in cultures of various human embryonic tissues. Science 1949;109:85.
2. Schnurr D. Enteroviruses. In: Lennette EH, Smith TH, eds. Laboratory Diagnosis of Viral Infections. New York: Dekker, 1999:376–383.
3. Hsiuing GD. Latent virus infections in primate tissues with special reference to simian viruses. Bacteriol Rev 1968;32:185–205.
4. Gleaves CA, Smith TF, Shuster EA, Pearson GR. Rapid detection of cytomegalovirus in MRC-5 cells inoculated with urine specimens by using low-speed centrifugation and monoclonal antibody to an early antigen. J Clin Microbiol 1984;19:917–919.
5. Forghani B, Hagens S. Diagnosis of viral infections by antigen detection. In: Lennette EH, Lennette DA, Lennette ET, eds. Diagnostic Procedures for Viral, Rickettsial and Chalmydial Infections, 7th ed. Washington, DC: Dekker, 1995:79–96.
6. Caruso JL, Howell DN. Surgical pathology and diagnostic cytology of viral infections. In: Lennette EH, Smith TF, eds. Laboratory Diagnosis of Viral Infections. New York: Dekker, 1999:21–43.
7. Miller SE. Electron microscopy of viral infections. In: Lennette EH, Smith TF, eds. Laboratory Diagnosis of Viral Infections. New York: Dekker, 1999:45–70.
8. Tristram DA, Welliver RC. Respiratory syncytial virus. In: Lennette EH, Smith TF, eds. Laboratory Diagnosis of Viral Infections. New York: Dekker, 1999:772–786.
9. Smith JS. Rabies virus. In: Murray PR, Baron EJ, Pfaller MA, Tenover FC, Yolken RH, eds. Manual of Clinical Microbiology, 7th ed. Washington, DC: American Society for Microbiology, 1999:1099–1106.
10. Mullis KB, Faloona FA. Specific synthesis of DNA in vitro via a polymerase-catalyzed chain reaction. Meth Enzymol 1987;155:335–350.
11. Persing DH, ed. PCR Protocols for Emerging Infectious Diseases. Washington, DC: ASM Press, 1996.

12. Chapman NM, Tracy S, Gauntt CJ, Fortmuller U. Molecular detection and identification of enteroviruses using enzymatic amplification and nucleic acid hybridization. J Clin Microbiol 1990;28:843–850.
13. Rotbart HA. Enzymatic RNA amplification of the enteroviruses. J Clin Microbiol 1990;28:438–442.
14. Kilpatrick DR, Nottay B, Yang C, et al. Group-specific identification of polioviruses by PCR using primers containing mixed-base or deoxyinosine residues at positions of codon degeneracy. J Clin Microbiol 1996;34:2990–2996.
15. Forghani B, Erdman DD. Amplification and detection of viral nucleic acids. In: Lennette EH, Lennette DA, Lennette ET, eds. Diagnostic Procedures for Viral, Rickettsial and Chlamydial Infections, 7th ed. Washington, DC: Dekker, 1995:98–99.
16. Persing DH. In vitro nucleic acid amplification techniques. In: Persing DH, Smith TF, Tenovir FC, White TJ, eds. Diagnostic Molecular Microbiology, Principles and Applications. Washington, DC: American Society of Microbiology, 1993:51–88.
17. Ruana G, Kidd KK. Coupled amplification and sequencing of genomic DNA. Proc Natl Acad Sci U S A 1991;88:2815–2819.

4

Placental Histopathology

Edwina J. Popek

INTRODUCTION

Excellent in-depth discussions of placental pathology in intrauterine infections are found in current placental pathology texts *(1–3)*. The integrity of the fetal-placental-maternal unit is key to the prevention of intrauterine infection. Infectious agents must traverse placental barriers to reach the fetus. In most instances, intrauterine infection leaves "footprints" in the placenta, either as direct evidence of infection (organisms) or indirect evidence of infection (inflammation or tissue injury). The placenta acts as a successful barrier to fetal infection. In most cases, despite placental infection, the fetus remains uninfected, although not necessarily unaffected by the infection. Other factors that affect the severity of intrauterine infection include the pathogen load, the virulence of the organism, immunocompetence of both mother and fetus, and gestational age at time of infection.

There are two basic modes of intrauterine infection, ascending and hematogenous. In addition, organisms harbored within the birth canal may infect an infant during the birthing process, often resulting in features similar to an ascending infection but with late onset of symptoms. Rarely, infection may reach the fetus through invasive procedures such as amniocentesis. Infection of the maternal endometrium or fallopian tube can also directly infect the chorion and amnion. Some infectious agents have a preferred mode of infection; others may be acquired by multiple modes (Table 1.)

The placenta demonstrates two relatively distinct patterns of inflammation in response to either an ascending (chorioamnionitis) or hematogenous (villitis) infection. Therefore, examination of the placenta may be very helpful in determining the mode of infection, the specific infectious agent, and even the potential for fetal/neonatal infection. In general, the severity of placental inflammation is reflected in fetal/neonatal disease, although as in all medicine, there are exceptions. For example, parvovirus can cause hydrops and intrauterine fetal demise without any maternal or fetal inflammation, but many intranuclear viral inclusions may be seen in circulating nucleated red blood cells. The human immunodeficiency virus (HIV) virus leaves no footprints of infection in the placenta, even in cases of documented intrauterine transmission.

Virtually nothing is actually known, as opposed to assumed, about the effects of ascending infection on placental function. Salafia et al. have reported abnormal fetal heart rate tracing (bradycardia, variable and late decelerations) in cases associated with

From: *Infectious Disease: Congenital and Perinatal Infections: A Concise Guide to Diagnosis*
Edited by: C. Hutto © Humana Press Inc., Totowa, NJ

Table 1
Modes of Perinatal Infection, Selected Agents, and Placental Pathology

	Bacteria	Viruses	Other	Placenta	Fetal
Hemato-genous	*Listeria*, syphilis, *E. coli* (rare)	CMV, HSV (rarely), HIV, parvovirus B19, rubella, enterovirus	*Toxoplasmosis, Trypanosoma*	Acute or chronic villitis, chronic vasculitis, necrotizing funisitis	Sepsis, viremia, disseminated infection, tissue necrosis
Ascending	Group B streptococcus, *E. coli*, *Listeria*	CMV, HSV, HIV	*Mycoplasma, Ureaplasma, Candida*	Acute chorioamnionitis, acute funisitis, rarely necrotizing funisitis	Cutaneous, pneumonia, gastroenteritis, sepsis
Intrapartum	Group B streptococcus, *Listeria, E. coli*	CMV, HSV, HIV, HBV	*Candida*	Chorioamnionitis	Cutaneous, eye, rarely systemic
Postnatal	Group B streptococcus, *E. coli*	CMV, HSV, HIV, enterovirus		Normal	Miscellaneous, agent specific

chorioamnionitis *(4)*, although Leo et al. report that clinical chorioamnionitis is not predictive of abnormal fetal heart rate tracing *(5)*. Hyde et al. attributed the abnormal heart rates to vasospasm *(6)*, but endothelial injury, sludging of fetal blood flow, and early thrombosis within inflamed vessels is a more likely explanation. Fetal and maternal inflammatory cytokines are now under investigation as potential mediators of fetal injury *(7,8)*. Fetal sepsis is associated with acidosis *(9)*.

More is known about the effects of villitis on placental function. Inflamed villi have reduced function. Thrombosis of villous capillaries and larger stem vessels may be caused by focal inflammation, resulting in the release of cytokines. Obliteration of fetal vessels may be a fetal response to the presence of inflammatory cells and may act to protect the fetus from any potentially infectious agents and perhaps even protect against inflammatory cytokines reaching the fetal circulation. Regardless of the type or etiology of the inflammation, the end point is avascular villi. These villi are no longer functional for nutrient and oxygen exchange. Decreased placental reserve capacity and intrauterine growth retardation (IUGR) occurs when significant numbers of villi become involved; the degree of IUGR is proportional to the amount of villitis.

PATHOGENESIS OF ASCENDING INFECTION

Most cases of ascending infection are bacterial in origin. Organisms colonizing the cervix, vagina, or perineum may infect the maternal endometrium or fetal membranes at the cervical os. Although it is true that ruptured membranes carry an increased risk for infection of the amniotic cavity, most cases of premature rupture of membranes (PROM) are secondary to the membranes already weakened by infection. Bacteria can cross intact membranes *(10)*. The structure of the fetal membranes is complex. Amnion and chorion completely surround the gestational sac. The chorion of the free membranes is in direct contact with the maternal decidualized endometrium, and the attached chorion is exposed to the maternal blood flow within the subchorionic intervillous space. The chorion has three layers and is thicker than the amnion, which has five thinner layers but greater tensile strength *(11)*.

Most infants born with a clinical or histological diagnosis of chorioamnionitis are not septic but may have localized infection in the lungs or within the gastrointestinal tract from aspirated or swallowed contaminated amniotic fluid. The more severe the inflammation within the membranes is, the more likely the infant will be septic. Even more predictive for fetal sepsis is the presence of a fetal inflammatory reaction within the umbilical cord (funisitis) or chorionic plate vessels (vasculitis) *(2,12)*. Necrotizing chorioamnionitis and three-vessel inflammation of the umbilical cord are associated with an increased incidence of preterm birth and perinatal death *(12,13)*. Only 20–33% of women with histologically important inflammation of the membranes are symptomatic *(12,13)*.

ACUTE CHORIOAMNIONITIS

Benirschke and Kaufmann feel that chorioamnionitis (which they use as synonymous with acute chorioamnionitis) is **always** (their bold) caused by infection *(3)*. Other forms of injury to the placenta, such as infarction, will also illicit an acute inflammatory reaction but will be localized to the area of injury. Acute chorioamnionitis is the most common diagnosis rendered on the placenta. Despite this, no universally accepted definition, grading, or staging system has been developed.

Acute Chorioamnionitis: Gross and Microscopic

The gross appearance of the membranes is a very poor indicator of inflammation (Fig. 1). The membranes are usually macroscopically normal. Infection may result in slight clouding (loss of translucency) of the membranes, granularity or a dull appearance, which may be obscured by formalin fixation. Only severe inflammation will result in grossly thickened, cloudy membranes that may be yellow or green because of the pyocyanin within the white blood cells obscuring the fetal vessels on the chorionic plate. Infection may result in membrane edema.

Grading of Acute Chorioamnionitis

The amount of inflammation used to define chorioamnionitis differs from publication to publication. It has been described generally as "locally dense or had necrosis" *(14)* or specifically as one focus of at least 5 neutrophils *(4)* or 10 or greater neutrophils in 10 nonadjacent fields at 400× magnification within free or attached membranes *(15,16)*. Defined criteria for examination of membranes in preterm premature rupture of membranes (PPROM) have been reported *(17)*. An attempt has been made to come to a consensus for the definition for both grade and stage of acute inflammation *(18)*.

Staging of Acute Chorioamnionitis

Naeye used three histological stages of chorioamnionitis (I, II, III) to indicate subchorionic inflammation, chorionic inflammation, and full-thickness inflammation of both chorion and amnion, respectively *(19)*. Early infection may be confined to the maternal decidua near the cervical os, exemplified by diffuse sprinkling of maternal neutrophils that is often associated with some decidual necrosis. Membrane rupture occurs overlying the cervical os, probably because of unequal stretch or unequal wall

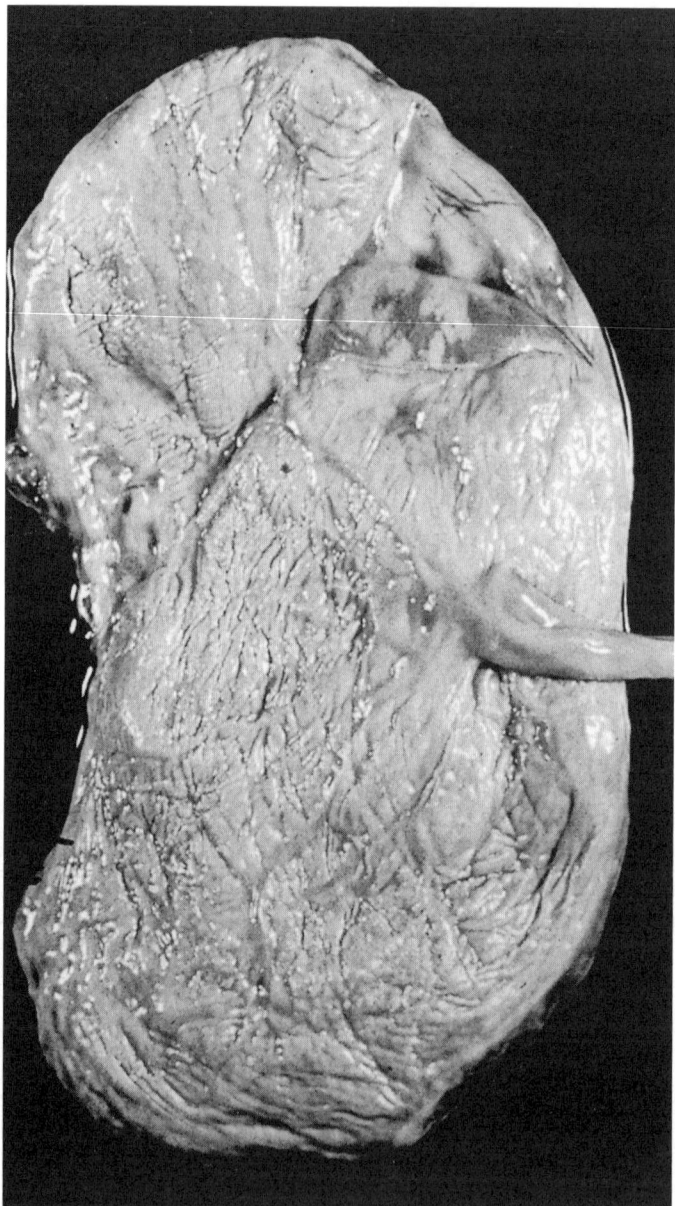

Fig. 1. Gross appearance of the severely inflamed placenta.

tension or possibly because of a loss of decidual blood supply in that area *(20)*. Some acute decidual inflammation is seen in 85% of term deliveries, especially near the zone of membrane rupture *(2)*. Inflammation marginated at the junction of the cellular and fibroblastic chorion indicates migration toward the amniotic cavity and is a feature of intra-amniotic fluid infection *(4)* (Fig. 2). Maternal neutrophils marginate within the subchorionic fibrinoid prior to migrating in the chorion and amnion on their way toward the amniotic fluid cavity (Fig. 3A). Chellam and Rushton suggested that this is equivalent to margination of inflammatory cells within a vascular space and therefore

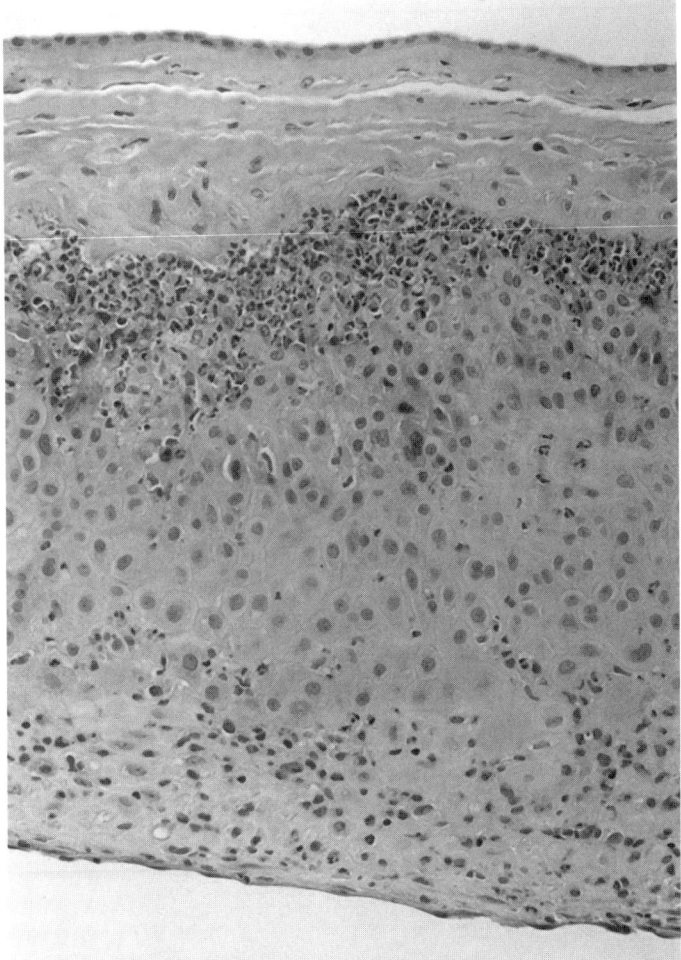

Fig. 2. Marginated acute chorionitis with very little neutrophil degeneration and no decidual necrosis, indicating maternal inflammatory response to bacteria or bacterial products in the amniotic fluid.

may represent the earliest maternal response to infection within the amniotic cavity *(21)*. The inflammatory infiltrate progresses through the chorion (chorionitis) and amnion (chorioamnionitis) (Fig. 3B) and eventually into the amniotic fluid. Because inflammation is chemotactically attracted to stimulus within the amniotic fluid, thickening of the membranes either by squamous metaplasia or placement of the chorionic plate vessels will focally interrupt this process.

Romero and Mazur proposed a four-stage clinical progression of ascending infection *(22)*. Stage I is an overgrowth of organisms in the vagina or cervix. Stage II is localized inflammation of the intrauterine cavity localized to the decidua. Stage III is intra-amniotic infection. Stage IV is infection of the fetus through breathing or swallowing the contaminated amniotic fluid or through cutaneous infection, including conjunctiva. It would be appropriate to add a stage V to this scheme to indicate systemic fetal infection (sepsis or meningitis).

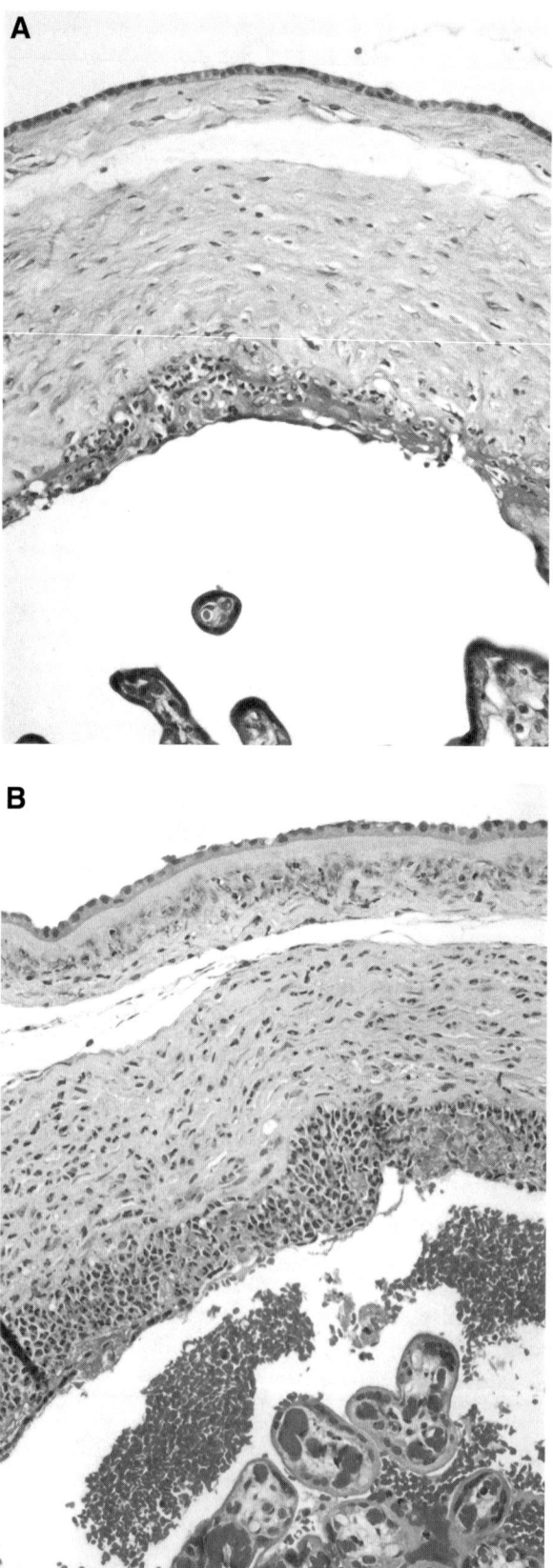

Duration of Infection

Location and appearance of the inflammation has led to assumptions about duration of infection. In general, the inflammatory response is neutrophilic regardless of the duration of infection. Intact neutrophils have led some to estimate infection of less than 24 hours because the average life span of neutrophils outside the vascular space is 24 hours *(23,24)*. The problem with this correlation is that the neutrophils that migrate into the avascular tissues of the amnion may not disintegrate as quickly as in ischemic tissues as studied in acute myocardial infarction. Naeye reported that maternal inflammation is subchorial intervillositis in the first 48 hours of an infection, and that only in the next few subsequent days do the neutrophils migrate into the chorionic plate *(19)*. The maternal inflammatory cells continue their progress toward the amniotic fluid cavity. The time necessary for complete progress from the maternal space to the intra-amniotic fluid space has been estimated at 5–7 days but may occur more quickly with highly virulent organisms *(19)*. Dating chorioamnionitis with any degree of precision is felt to be imprudent *(1)*.

Placental Cultures

Cultures of the placenta to assess intrauterine infection are of limited value, in part because of antibiotic use during labor and especially because of contamination with a vaginal delivery. There is no correlation between organisms isolated from the cervical canal or the placenta and fetal infection *(25)*. Micro-organisms were not isolated significantly more often from placentas in cases with chorioamnionitis than those without *(26)*. There was a correlation between increased severity of membrane inflammation and fetal vascular inflammation with increasing incidence of positive cultures *(26)*. In preterm labor, bacteria can be isolated from amniotic fluid with intact membranes or from placental cultures with variable success *(27)*. Approximately 70% of placental cultures are positive when there is histological chorioamnionitis *(27)*. Any cultures should be sent directly from labor and delivery. There is a decreased recovery of organisms with refrigeration and a prolonged interval between delivery and cultures. It has been proposed that cultures are most reliable when obtained from the space between the amnion and chorion because surface contamination is eliminated. Cultures for aerobes, anaerobes, *Mycoplasma*, and *Ureaplasma* will increase the yield.

Microscopic Identification of Bacteria Within the Placental Membranes

It is actually the exception rather than the rule to find the causative organism within the placental membranes. Group B streptococcus may show significant colonization of the umbilical cord and membranes with little or no maternal inflammation *(28)*. Fetal vasculitis is present in 0–58% *(29,30)*, may be more prolific than the maternal inflammation, and is frequently eosinophilic *(2)*. *Fusobacterium* sp. is a long, thin, filamentous, Gram-negative bacterium. The organisms have a "hair-on-end" appearance and characteristically cause necrotizing amnionitis. *Listeria monocytogenes* is a small, Gram-positive coccobacillus that frequently colonizes the subamniotic tissues and

---

Fig. 3. *(opposite page)* (**A**) Subchorionic margination of maternal neutrophils may be the earliest indication of actual infection within the amniotic fluid. (**B**) Acute chorioamnionitis, full-thickness inflammation, is caused by infection and not other forms of amnion stimulus.

amnion epithelium in large numbers. Special stains for organisms rarely are positive if they are not already apparent on the routine hematoxylin and eosin (H&E) stain.

PROM, PPROM, and Preterm Labor and Premature Delivery

Prematurity is strongly associated with chorioamnionitis, accounting for at least 50% of preterm deliveries. The incidence of clinical chorioamnionitis decreases with gestational age, is nearly 100% at 24 weeks, 73% prior to 30 weeks, and 3–4% of term deliveries *(2,31–33)*. The actual incidence of histological chorioamnionitis is unknown. Preterm birth occurs in 11% of all pregnancies in the United States, with 50% caused by premature onset of labor, 33% caused by PROM, and the remaining 20% caused by specific maternal or fetal considerations *(34)*. Prematurity is increasing, mostly because of the increased number of multiple fetal pregnancies from assisted reproductive technology. Prematurity is responsible for the majority of neonatal morbidity, mortality, and long-term neurological sequelae *(34)*. Histological chorioamnionitis is the most important predictor of infection in premature newborns *(35)*. More women with PROM have histological chorioamnionitis than those without PROM *(36)*, but positive amniotic fluid cultures occur in a significant number of women with premature labor and intact membranes *(37)*, indicating that rupture is not a prerequisite for intra-amniotic infection.

The histology of PPROM was not different between those who received antibiotics and those who did not, suggesting that the membrane changes preceded the antibiotics *(38)*. In preterm delivery, there is no increase in maternal inflammation from rupture of membranes to delivery, but fetal inflammation increases with a greater latency period *(39)*. PROM because of bacteria may be secondary to production of bacterial proteases and can degrade collagen and weaken membranes *(40)*, or the inflammatory response may produce cytokines or prostaglandins, which stimulate labor *(41)*. The release of steroids in response to inflammation paradoxically results in the amnion stimulating prostaglandin production *(11)*.

Bacterial vaginosis (BV) is characterized by changes in the microbiological flora of the vagina, where there is a transition from *Lactobacillus* sp to Gram-negative and anaerobic bacteria. The most characteristic organisms are *Gardnerella vaginalis, Chlamydia, Myocoplasma*, and anaerobes such as *Bacteroides* and *Mobiluncu*s *(42,43)*. There are no studies correlating the clinical diagnosis of BV and placental pathology. BV is associated with second trimester fetal loss and premature delivery *(44,45)*. Placental changes often include severe chorioamnionitis, which is frequently necrotizing and polymicrobial *(43)*.

Acute Chorioamnionitis and Meconium

Of meconium-stained placentas, 64% have significant inflammation of the fetal membranes, thought to be the etiology of the meconium spill *(19)*. Although several investigators have implied that the presence of meconium is a risk factor for infection, it is mostly likely the other way around *(46,47)*, possibly because of an alteration in the antimicrobial properties of the amniotic fluid *(48)*. Meconium may be passed because of postmaturity (6%); decreased uteroplacental blood flow; or decreased fetal-placental blood flow, usually because of cord compression (6%), birth asphyxia (1%), and unknown causes (25%) *(19)*. Kaspar et al. reported that 20% of their cases of meconium had associated chorioamnionitis, 25% had fetal vascular thrombosis, 38% had infarcts, and 14.5% had villitis *(48)*, suggesting a less-important role of ascending infection.

Most investigators agree that meconium itself does not cause inflammation of the membranes. It has been suggested that interleukin (IL)-8 within the meconium may be the etiology for neutrophilic inflammation in the lungs of babies with meconium aspiration syndrome *(33)*, as it does in in vitro studies *(49)*. No similar study has been associated with placental inflammation.

Acute Chorioamnionitis and Villous Edema

Villous edema is commonly seen in conjunction with chorioamnionitis, especially with preterm delivery; 25% occurs in preterm placentas vs 11% at term *(50)*. Edema may be focal or diffuse, mild or severe. It occurs as a fetal response rather rapidly after the "stress" and then disappears over the next 24 hours or so. Postedematous placentas may have residual Hofbauer cell hyperplasia. The associated increased morbidity with edematous villi may result from an increased diffusion distance between the maternal intervillous space and fetal capillaries. This must be considered in the context of the initial stressor, which is usually chorioamnionitis, and prematurity.

Acute Chorioamnionitis and Placental Abruption

The second most common etiology of placental abruption is chorioamnionitis; the first is maternal preeclampsia. Chorioamnionitis with abruption is especially well documented in preterm gestations *(51)*. This form of abruption is usually marginal, beginning at the placental edge nearest the cervix. Large areas of decidual necrosis and acute inflammation may be identified in this area and may or may not have features of abruption.

Subacute Chorioamnionitis and Chronic Lung Disease

Ohyama et al. described a specific form of membrane inflammation that was associated with prematurity and development of chronic lung disease and accounted for 54% of placentas with chorioamnionitis *(52)*. Subacute chorioamnionitis was defined as a mixed degenerative neutrophil and mononuclear cell infiltrate. Amnion necrosis was present in 40%. Subacute chorioamnionitis was felt to be an indicator of persistent intrauterine inflammation, possibly caused by organisms with low virulence. Rarely, an antibiotic-treated acute chorioamnionitis may have mixed acute and chronic inflammation.

Chronic Chorioamnionitis

Chronic inflammation of the fetal membranes has rarely been described in conjunction with viral infections including herpes simplex virus (HSV) *(53)*, rubella *(54)*, and toxoplasmosis *(55)*. Chronic chorioamnionitis tends to be most often associated with nonspecific chronic inflammation elsewhere within the placenta, such as villitis of undetermined etiology (VUE) *(56)*. It is usually focal, rarely involves the amnion connective tissue, and does not result in necrosis of the amnion epithelium *(57)*. Chronic chorioamnionitis is often associated with chronic inflammatory lesions elsewhere within the placental or decidual tissues but can occur as an isolated phenomenon.

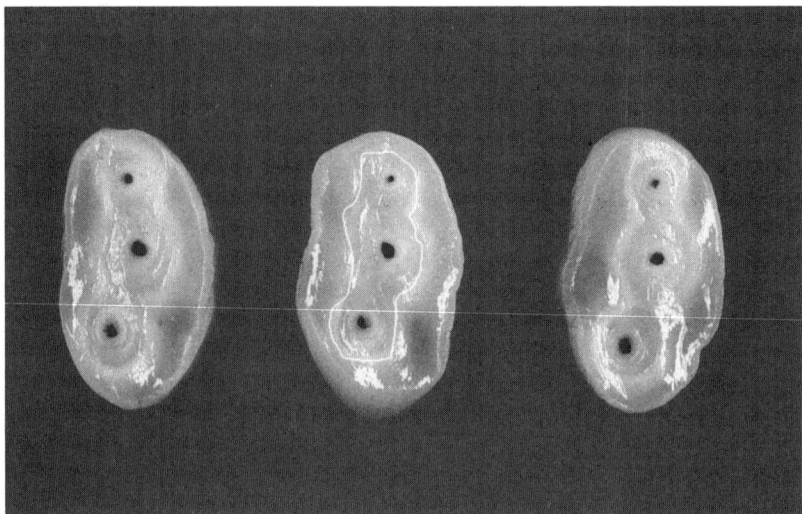

Fig. 4. Cross sections of premature umbilical cord showing an amniotropic distribution of white density representing neutrophils within the edematous stroma. White line outlines the inflammation in the center section.

FETAL INFLAMMATORY RESPONSE OF UMBILICAL AND CHORIONIC PLATE VESSELS

Fetal response to infection occurs after the maternal response and usually suggests a more well-established infection. It may be attenuated or absent in midgestation, although I have seen significant funisitis as early as 18 weeks of gestation.

Funisitis and Vasculitis: Gross and Microscopic

Funisitis can rarely be grossly identified. The umbilical cord may be quite edematous. Within the extra fluid within the cord substance, large accumulations of neutrophils may be visible as white rings incompletely around the fetal vessels (Fig. 4). The fetal response to infection within the amniotic fluid is toward the amnion surface (amniotropic), similar to an Ochterlony reaction. Concentric inflammation may be the result of cord injury. Funisitis may be segmental because of positioning of the cord within the uterus *(23)*; thus, the recommendation is for examination of two sections of umbilical cord.

An acute fetal inflammatory response is most often a response to ascending bacterial infection. Chronic vasculitis or funisitis is less common but may occur in cases of hematogenously acquired viral infection *(58)*. In severely macerated fetuses, caution should be used in diagnosing funisitis as degeneration of the vascular smooth muscle may falsely give the impression of inflammation.

Acute inflammation of the chorionic plate vessels may precede inflammation of the umbilical vessels. Gross examination rarely demonstrates an amniotropic intravascular density. Inflammation of the chorionic plate vessels is usually obscured by the associated chorioamnionitis. Chronic fetal vasculitis is most often a nonspecific response associated with VUE. Inflammation of the chorionic plate may therefore be a combination of maternal and fetal inflammation. The fetal inflammatory response frequently includes eosinophils as an acute reaction, not only in the preterm *(21)*, but also in the term baby. This may be caused by the small pool of neutrophils and the presence of large amounts of eosinophilic extramedullary hematopoiesis within the liver. The most severe consequence of inflammation of the chorionic plate vessels is thrombosis.

Grade of Fetal Vasculitis and Funisitis

As with chorioamnionitis, no uniform definition has been accepted, but van Hoeven defined funisitis as the presence of neutrophils within the vessel wall, with or without extension into the substance of Wharton's jelly. Simple margination of neutrophils was excluded from the definition *(14,16,18)*.

Stage of Fetal Vasculitis and Funisitis

The umbilical vein becomes inflamed first, maybe beginning at the placental end of the cord *(59)*. Inflammation begins as margination of neutrophils at the endothelium with progressive movement through the muscle into the cord substance (Fig. 5A–C).

Necrotizing or Sclerosing Funisitis

Necrotizing or sclerosing funisitis is evidence of a prolonged fetal inflammatory response. Fetal neutrophils that have migrated out of the umbilical vessels toward the amnion surface undergo degeneration, necrosis, and finally calcification (Fig. 6A). Lack of lymphatic drainage of the umbilical cord results in accumulation of debris (Fig. 6B). The etiology has been attributed to a number of organisms, which have in common the ability to result in prolonged infection without spontaneous uterine contractions. In many cases, no infectious cause is identified. The most common etiology is syphilis *(60)*, but it has also been reported in HSV *(61)*, and cultures have been positive with common organisms such as group B streptococcus and *Gardnerella (62)*. There was no statistically significant correlation between the degree of necrotizing funisitis and fetal outcome; however, poorer fetal outcome is suggested with severe necrotizing funisitis, including a high rate of IUGR, stillbirth, necrotizing enterocolitis, and chronic lung disease *(52,63)*.

Umbilical Cord Microabscesses (Candida Funisitis)

The most common congenital fungal infection is caused by *Candida* sp. Although *Candida* vaginitis is a very common complication of pregnancy, it rarely results in chorioamnionitis. The risk of *Candida* colonization is increased with cerclage or the presence of other foreign bodies and coexistent infection *(64)*. Term infants may be colonized but are usually asymptomatic. *Candida* funisitis is life-threatening in a preterm infant.

The diagnosis of *Candida* infection is often made on the gross examination of the umbilical cord. The cord surface is studded with 0.05- to 0.2-cm yellow-white plaques that seem to be just under the amnion (Fig. 7A). Histological confirmation may be difficult if the exact area from the cord is not submitted. Acute inflammation from the cord vessels extends to the basement membrane of the amnion epithelium and forms a microabscess. The yeast and pseudohyphae are very difficult to see on routine stains and usually require a silver stain (Fig. 7B). Although chorioamnionitis often accompanies *Candida* funisitis, rarely are organisms seen within the membranes *(65)*. *Candida*

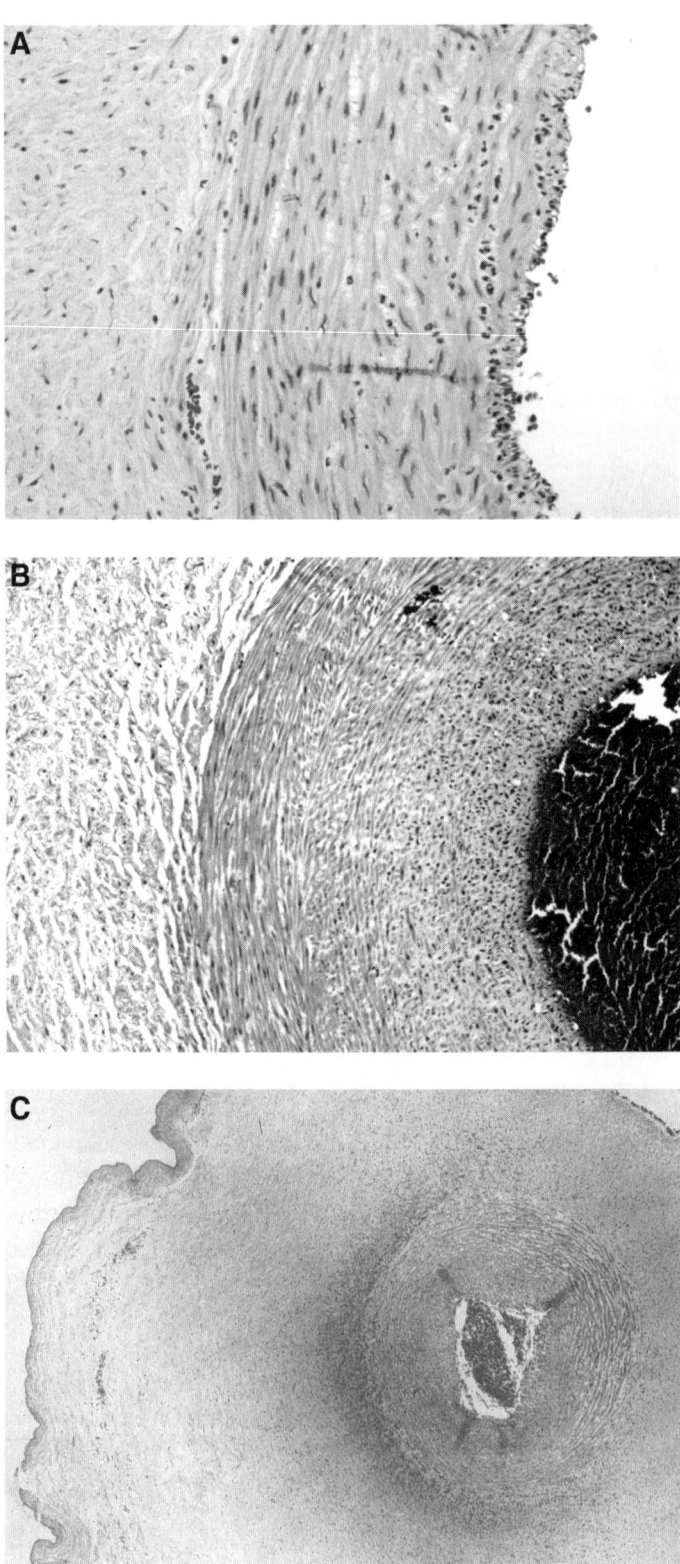

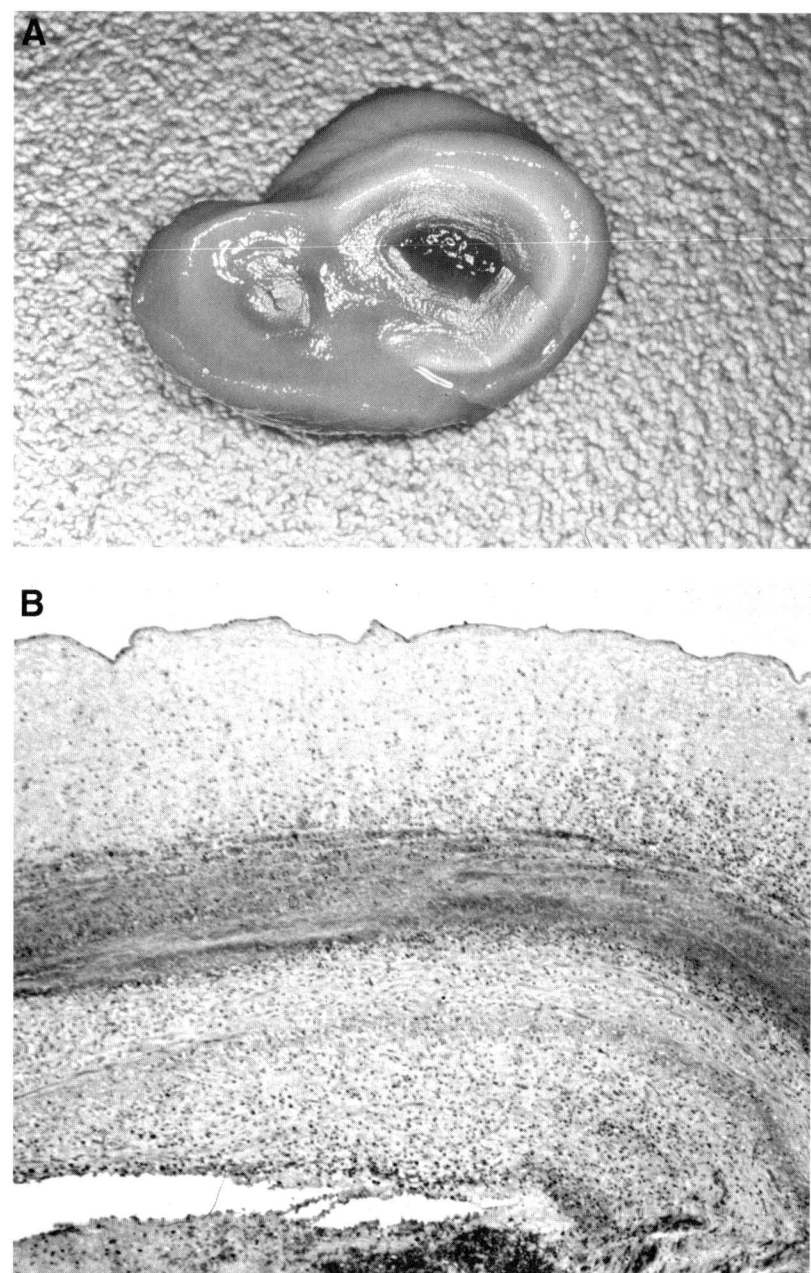

Fig. 6. (A) Cross section of umbilical cord with necrotizing funisitis. Note dense white band partially surrounding the umbilical vein. **(B)** Sclerosing funisitis with necrotic debris within the umbilical cord stroma caused by syphilis.

Fig. 5. *(opposite page)* **(A)** Umbilical vein with early phlebitis and margination of neutrophils. Neutrophils are seen beneath the endothelium and within the muscular wall. **(B)** Umbilical arteritis with extension of neutrophils into the muscular wall. **(C)** Funisitis with extension of neutrophils into Wharton's jelly in an amniotropic pattern around an umbilical artery.

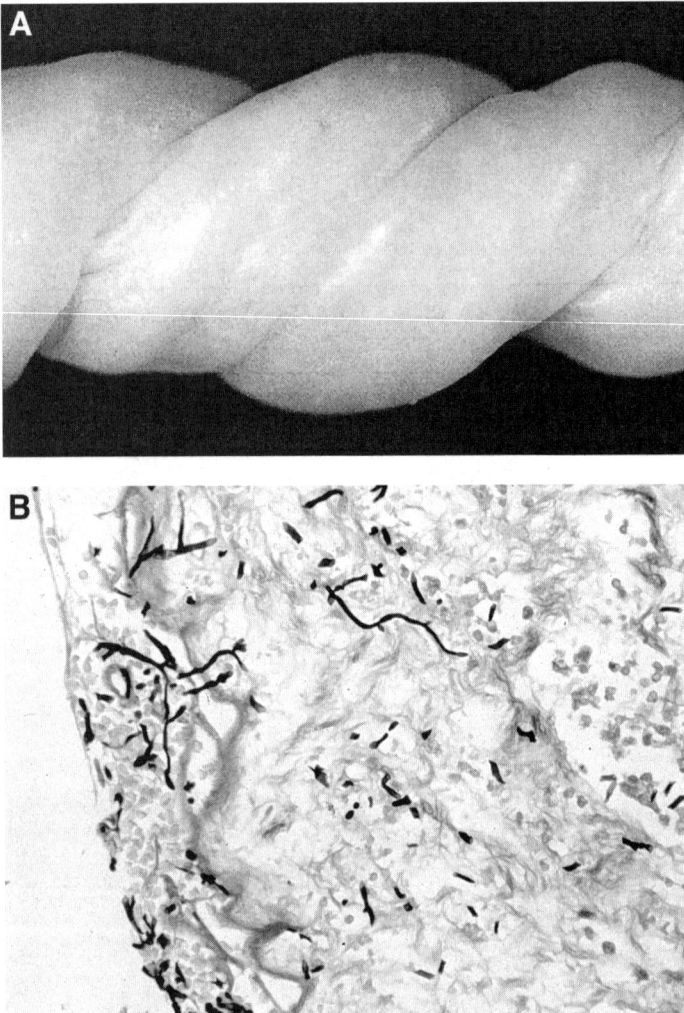

Fig. 7. (A) *Candida albicans* funisitis at term. Edema of umbilical cord, with 1- to 2-mm pinpoint yellow-white lesions on or just beneath the cord amnion epithelium. **(B)** *Candida albicans* pseudohyphae are very difficult to identify on H&E stains; all cases suspicious for *Candida* should be stained with a silver stain.

glabrata may also cause cord microabscesses but more often has widespread involvement of the membranes without production of pseudohyphae.

Funisitis Caused by Meconium Aspiration or Vascular Smooth Muscle Injury

Although acute chorioamnionitis is thought to be exclusively caused by infection, funisitis may be caused by other things. In the case of cord compression, inflammation may be secondary to tissue injury. Theoretically, the inflammatory cells should be evenly distributed around the injured vessel, not in the usual amniotropic pattern.

Meconium-laden macrophages have been identified within Wharton's jelly and are associated with smooth muscle injury and inflammation of the umbilical cord vessels *(66)*. Meconium-associated inflammation is usually more severe in the cord than the membranes. This may be because of direct injury of the cord vessels by meconium. It has been postulated that the muscle injury is secondary injury caused by vasoconstriction. The presence of meconium within the fetal lung may also set up an inflammatory response, which is then manifest within the cord vessels *(67)*.

MATERNAL DECIDUITIS

Decidua is the adapted endometrial stromal as a result of progesterone stimulation. Decidua surrounds the entire placenta. Decidua basalis is at the base of the placenta and includes the maternal spiral arteries and venous sinuses. Decidua parietalis or capsularis is present on the maternal surface of the free membranes. In nearly all cases of ascending infection, the maternal decidua is also inflamed. This can be quite severe and may result in decidual necrosis and abruption.

Small numbers of lymphocytes are normally present within the decidua. Increased numbers have been associated with pregnancy-induced hypertension and in idiopathic IUGR *(19)*. Chronic decidual inflammation may be associated with infection or maternal immune response *(68)*. A quantitative definition of chronic deciduitis has yet to be established. Deciduitis is usually reported as focal, multifocal, or diffuse; mild, moderate, or severe; with or without plasma cells. The diagnosis should also note if the inflammation is perivascular and whether it is within the decidua parietalis, decidua basalis, or both *(69)*.

PATHOGENESIS OF INTRAUTERINE-ACQUIRED MATERNAL HEMATOGENOUS INFECTION

Infectious agents within the maternal blood may infect the placental villi from the intervillous space. For this to happen, there must be maternal bacteremia, viremia, or parasitemia. Rarely, villitis may be seen as a late complication associated with chorioamnionitis as the result of fetal sepsis and reinfection of the placental villi. Most cases of villitis are idiopathic, referred to as VUE *(70)*. Infectious etiologies are most often viral. Infection may stay confined to the placental tissues or enter the fetal bloodstream through the villous capillaries.

There are several proposed mechanisms for how the infectious agents gain entrance to the fetal system. The two most commonly accepted theories include either the direct transport of infected maternal cells or free pathogen into the fetal circulation or contiguous infection of a placental cell with subsequent infection of fetal cell. Placental factors that control this include physical barriers (villus trophoblast epithelium) and immune mechanisms (probably related to both maternal and fetal immune competence), especially the phagocytic and killing capabilities of the Hofbauer cell.

Gross and Microscopic Appearance of Placental Villitis

The gross appearance of a placenta with villitis is usually normal. There may rarely be a granular, hydropic, or pale appearance of the parenchyma (Fig. 8A). In cases of abscess formation, white nodules may be visible on the basal plate or cut surface (Fig. 8B). Pallor or friability of the villi may be caused by widespread necrosis, atrophy, and fibrin deposition but is nonspecific and may be caused by prolonged retention after fetal demise or immaturity of the placenta *(70,71)*. Villitis is usually considered a microscopic diagnosis. Examination of four blocks of placenta is sufficient for detection of the majority of cases of villitis *(72)*.

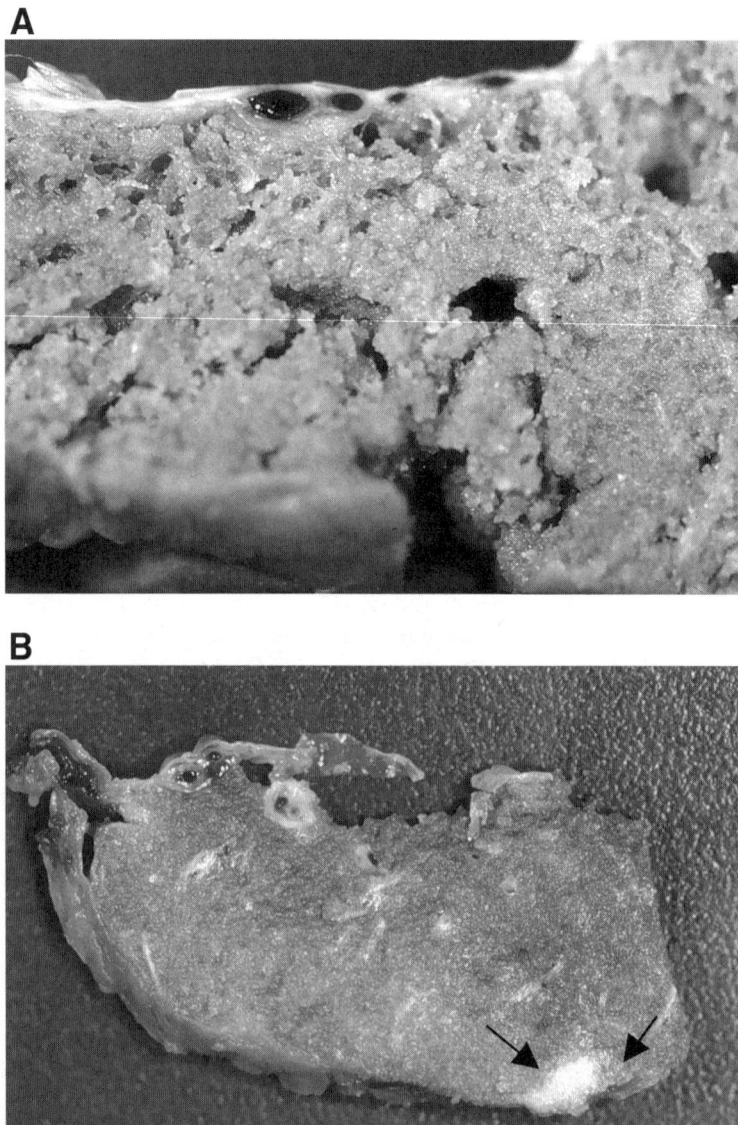

Fig. 8. (A) Cut surface of a formalin-fixed placenta showing a dense granularity caused by severe diffuse granulomatous villitis of undetermined etiology. **(B)** Cut surface of a placenta showing a small yellow nodule at the basal plate (arrows) that could be consistent with a large number of lesions but represents a microabscess caused by *Listeria monocytogenes*.

Classification of Villitis

Altshuler has described villitis based on tissue response as proliferative, necrotizing, reparative, and stromal fibrosis. It was proposed that these may be progressive stages of villitis, with necrosis as the initial acute stage and fibrosis the end point of the various forms *(73)*. Villitis can be described by the type of inflammation: acute (neutrophilic); chronic (lymphocytic, histiocytic, lymphohistiocytic plasmacytic, mixed);

or granulomatous (including Langhans-type giant cells). Categorizing the villitis based on the type of inflammation is more useful in determining the etiology. The villous inflammation is a combination of maternal and fetal inflammatory cells *(74)*. The number of inflammatory cells within the villus necessary to diagnose villitis has not been specified.

Villitis of Undetermined Etiology

Most cases of villitis are thought to be an immune reaction against fetal/placental antigens and are referred to as nonspecific villitis or VUE (Fig. 9A). The lymphocytes within the stroma are predominantly helper/inducer CD3[+] or CD4[+], T cells, with few suppressor, CD8[+] T cells, CD45/LCA positive, and CD68 macrophages *(75–78)* and no B cells or plasma cells. The placenta has a limited ability to respond specifically to various antigenic stimuli. The histology of villitis is sufficiently varied to suggest that the entity designated as VUE may well be a response to more than one antigen/organism. Anchoring villi at the placental base are intimately associated with maternal tissues and do not have a protective syncytiotrophoblast layer. In this way, the anchoring villi may be more susceptible to maternal immune stimulus *(76)*. Involvement of the stem villi occurs in about 10% of cases. This is usually associated with a higher grade of villous inflammation. Intercellular adhesion molecule 1 is not normally present on villous trophoblast but is in the inflamed villi. The intercellular adhesion molecule is involved in lymphocyte–endothelial interactions *(78)*.

VUE has been reported in 5–18% *(3,79)* of placentas. The lower incidence is from random placentas, and the higher incidence is from placentas that were selected for examination based on abnormal maternal or fetal features. The only consistent finding in infants is IUGR *(3)*. There was some correlation between severity of villitis and severity of IUGR *(61)*.

Specific Villitides

Villitis attributable to specific infectious agents is the exception, probably accounting for only 5% of all villitides *(2)*. Acute villitis is seen in maternal sepsis with organisms such as *Escherichia coli*, group B streptococcus, and *L. monocytogenes* (Fig. 9B). The inflammatory infiltrates in VUE and known infectious etiologies are similar *(77)* and have provided "circumstantial evidence that VUE is the result of chronic infection" *(80*, p. 261). Most investigators are less convinced of an underlying pathogen in most cases of VUE. The most significant difference in VUE and the specific villitides appears to be the presence of significant numbers of plasma cells, which should be a warning to rule out infectious agents, particularly cytomegalovirus (CMV) (Fig. 9C), syphilis, and HSV. Granulomatous villitis (Fig. 9D) may be seen in infection with organisms that cause granulomatous inflammation elsewhere and include mycobacterium, toxoplasmosis, herpes simplex virus, and varicella.

Maternal Intervillositis

Acute intervillositis is most often associated with severe chorioamnionitis and may be a feature of maternal sepsis. Chronic intervillositis may be a complication of any form of chronic villitis. It may also occur as an isolated abnormality; most are thought to be caused by maternal immune reaction. The maternal space has increased mononuclear cells, usually macrophages that are CD68 positive. There is usually some syncy-

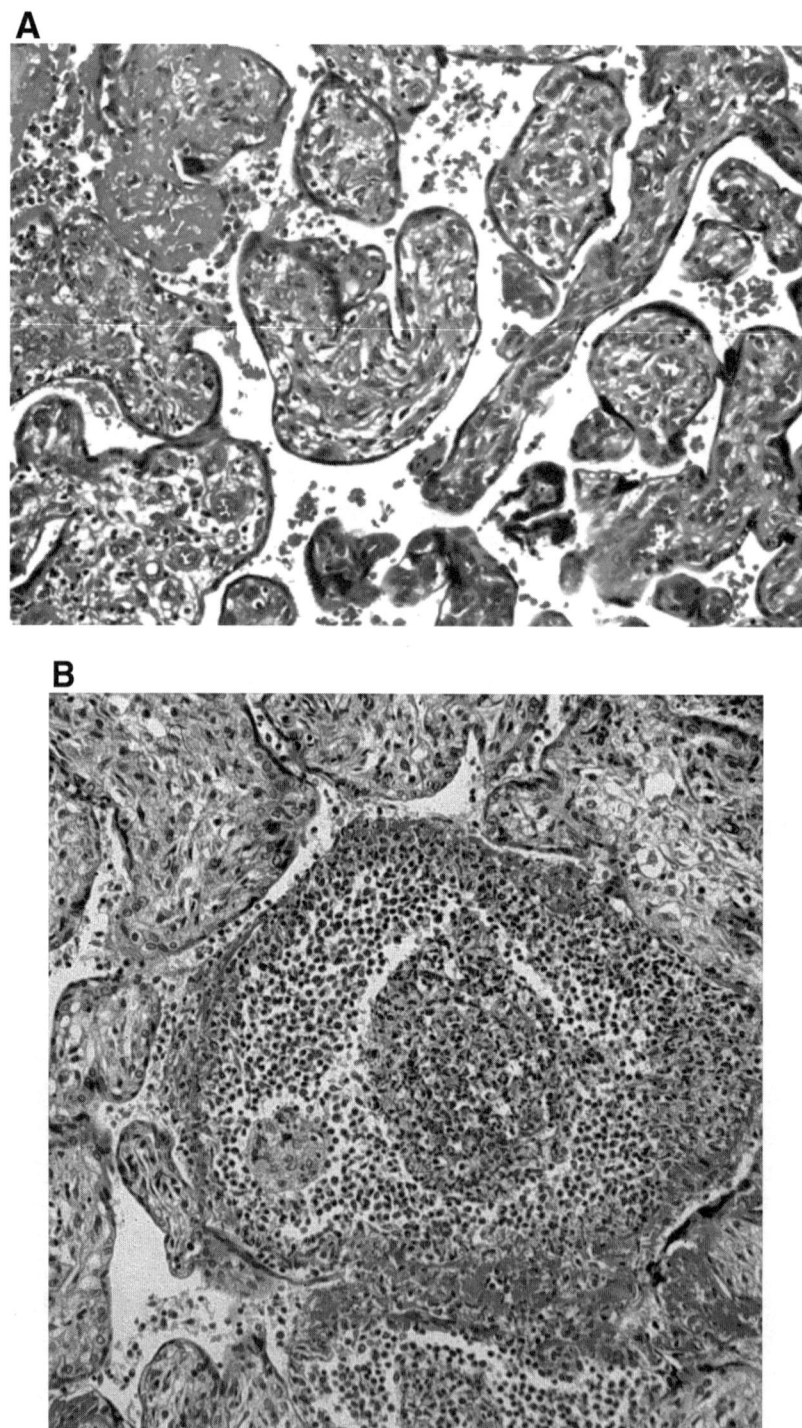

Fig. 9. (**A**) Villitis of undetermined etiology (VUE), lymphocytic or lymphohistiocytic in-flammation with the villous stroma. The inflamed villi are larger and hypovascular compared to the adjacent normal villi. (**B**) Acute villitis is classically associated with *Listeria*. Initially, the neutrophils are located beneath the syncytiotrophoblast basement membrane with

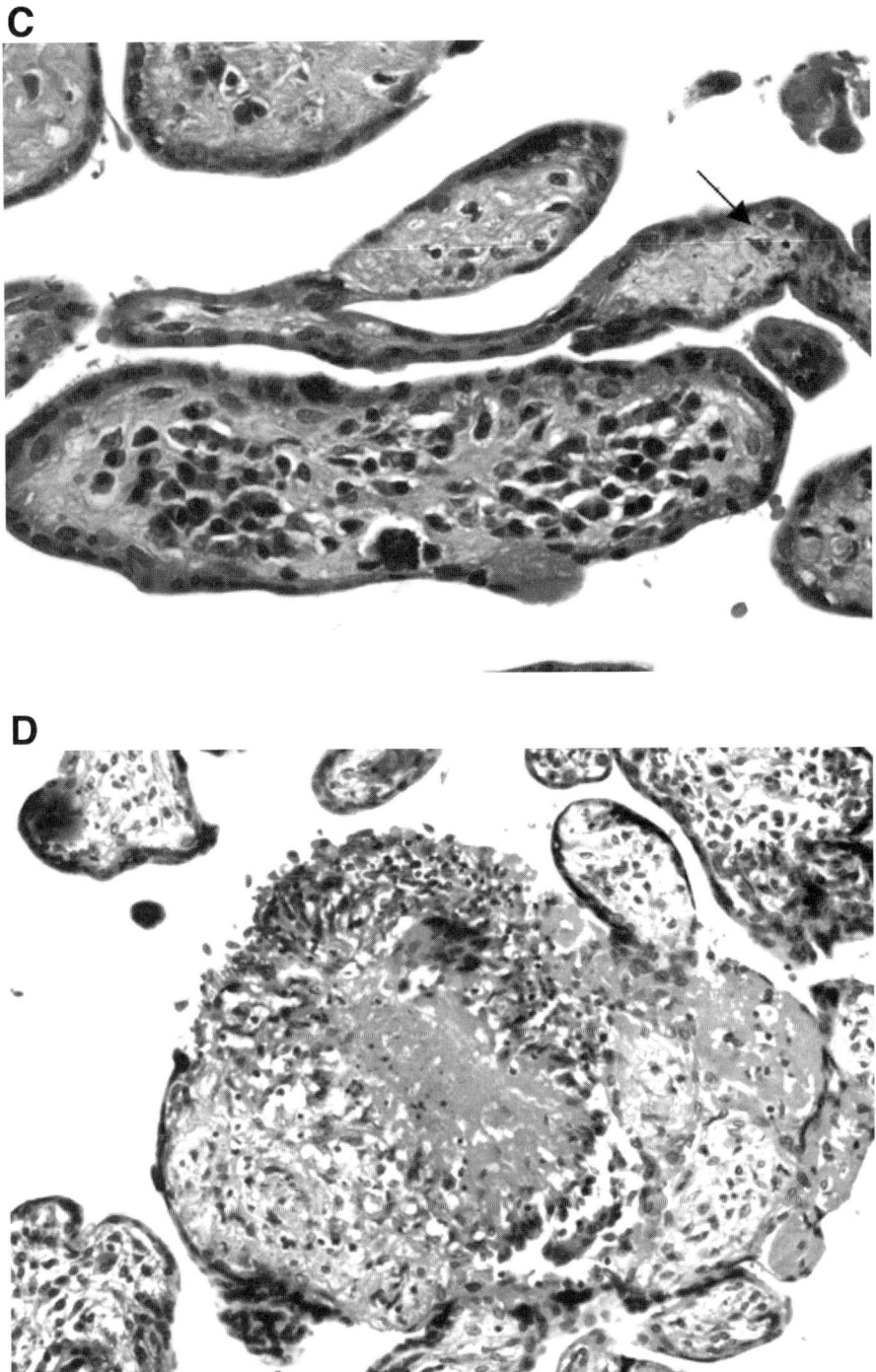

Fig. 9. *(continued)* subsequent destruction of the villous stroma. Organisms may be seen within these abscesses with Gram stain. (**C**) Symptomatic congenital CMV disease characteristically results in a lymphoplasmacytic villitis. The presence of hemosiderin within avascular villi is a feature of prior viral injury to the endothelium (arrow). (**D**) Granulomatous villitis with Langhans-type giant cells and central necrosis in a case of congenital toxoplasmosis.

tiotrophoblast injury *(80)*; increased fibrin and fibrinoid deposition occurs with coalescence of the villi into nodules. The placenta is usually grossly unremarkable unless there is sufficient fibrinoid deposited to result in a granular appearance. Intervillositis may be associated with features of low uteroplacental blood flow, atheromas, and IUGR and has been seen in preeclampsia and maternal autoimmune diseases. Intervillositis often has additional features of massive perivillous fibrinoid deposition, often referred to as the maternal floor infarct *(81,82)*. Malaria will produce a similar histiocytic response *(83)*.

SPECIAL STAINS AND MOLECULAR TECHNIQUES IN THE DIAGNOSIS OF INFECTIOUS AGENTS

There have been considerable advances in the use of molecular techniques for rapid detection of pathogens, especially those that are fastidious or nonculturable. Some of the rewards of diagnostic molecular techniques include rapid turnaround time, increased specificity, enhanced sensitivity, ability to identify esoteric micro-organisms, quantitation, genotyping, and monitoring of drug resistance. Qualitative assays determine presence or absence of a nucleic acid consistent with the presence of an infectious agent. Polymerase chain reaction (PCR) replaces the conventional process of biological amplification (growth in culture) with enzymatic amplification, allowing identification of as few as 100 copies of a particular deoxyribonucleic acid (DNA) sequence *(84)*. Reverse transcription PCR may be useful in detection of ribonucleic acid (RNA) virus infections, including hepatitis C virus, HIV, and enteroviruses *(85,86)*. Because of the sensitivity, contamination is a constant threat, and specimen integrity is very important. These techniques are labor intensive and expensive. Most of the newer techniques allow for extraction of DNA from fixed tissues, but it is still preferable in some cases to have −70°C frozen samples (which should be handled in a manner similar to tissue culture). It must be remembered that a positive PCR does not mean the same thing as a positive culture (viability) or a rise in antibody titer (response to recent infection). Sequence analysis can be used to subtype or detect drug resistance *(84)*.

More readily accessible to most laboratories is immunohistochemistry to identify specific antigens (CMV, parvovirus, toxoplasmosis, syphilis, group B streptoccus) within formalin-fixed, paraffin-embedded tissue samples *(87–91)*. I have found CMV and parvovirus immunohistochemistry to be the most useful, especially in identifying positive cells in autolyzed tissues.

Less-sophisticated methods may also be useful in identifying infectious agents. Many micro-organisms are readily identifiable on routine H&E stain. Tissue Gram stains such as Brown and Bren are useful for Gram-positive organisms, but Brown and Hopps or the Gram-Twort method is preferable for Gram-negative organisms. Silver impregnation methods (Steiner and Steiner, Warthin-Starry) will stain virtually all bacteria and most fungi. They are sensitive for identifying small numbers of bacteria. The advantage of silver is that very thin organisms are coated with the metal, making them visible with light microscopy, which is particularly applicable to *Fusobacterium* and syphilis. *Treponema* spirochetes are identified within the necrotic debris of the necrotizing funisitis of the umbilical cord, but organisms have also been identified within cord free of inflammation *(89)*. If the patient has been treated within a few hours of delivery, no organisms will be seen. Histological examination alone may be as specific and nearly as sensitive as the PCR performed on formalin-fixed, paraffin-embedded tissues. Steiner and Steiner stain and Warthin-Starry stains are difficult to perform and yield fewer positive results compared to PCR *(92)*.

REFERENCES

1. Fox H. Infections and inflammatory lesions of the placenta. In: Fox H, ed. Pathology of the Placenta, 2nd ed. Philadelphia: Saunders, 1997:294–343.
2. Hyde SR, Altshuler G. Infectious disorders of the placenta. In: Lewis SH, Perrin E, eds. Pathology of the Placenta, 2nd ed. New York: Churchill-Livingstone, 1999:317–342.
3. Benirschke K, Kaufmann P. Infectious diseases. In: Benirschke K, Kaufmann P, eds. Pathology of the Human Placenta, 4th ed. New York: Springer, 2000:591–684.
4. Salafia CM, Mangam HE, Weigl CA, Foye GJ, Silberman L. Abnormal fetal heart rate patterns and placental inflammation. Am J Obstet Gynecol 1989;160:140–147.
5. Leo MV, Skurnick JH, Ganesh VV, Adhate A, Apuzzio JJ. Clinical chorioamnionitis is not predicted by umbilical artery Doppler velocimetry in patients with premature rupture of the membranes. Obstet Gynecol 1991;79:916–918.
6. Hyde S, Smotherman J, Moore JI, Altshuler G. A model of bacterially induced umbilical vein spasm, relevant to fetal hypoperfusion. Obstet Gynecol 1989;73:966–970.
7. Gomez R, Romero R, Gabio G, Yoon BH, Mazor M, Stanley B. The fetal inflammatory response syndrome. Am J Obstet Gynecol 1998;179:194–202.
8. Baud O, Emile D, Pelletier E, et al. Amniotic fluid concentration of interleukin-1B, interleukin-6 and TNF-α in chorioamnionitis before 32 weeks of gestation: histologic associations and neonatal outcome. Br J Obstet Gynecol 1999;106:72–77.
9. Meyer BA, Dickinson JE, Chambers C, Parisi VM. The effect of fetal sepsis on umbilical cord gases. Am J Obstet Gynecol 1992;116:612–617.
10. Galask RP, Varner MW, Petzold CR, Wilbur SL. Bacterial attachment of the chorioamniotic membranes. Am J Obstet Gynecol 1984;148:915–928.
11. Epstein FH. Premature rupture of the fetal membranes. N Engl J Med 1998;338:663–670.
12. van Hoeven KH, Anyaegbunam A, Hochester H, et al. Clinical significance of increasing histologic severity of acute inflammation in the fetal membranes and umbilical cord. Ped Pathol Lab Med 1996;16:731–744.
13. de Araujo MC, Schultz R, Vaz FA, Massad E, Feferbaum R, Ramos JL. A case-control study of histological chorioamnionitis and neonatal infection. Early Human Dev 1994;16:51–58.
14. Stallmach T, Karolyi L. Augmentation of fetal granulopoiesis with chorioamnionitis during the second trimester of gestation. Hum Pathol 1994;25:244–247.
15. de Felice C, Toti P, Laurini RN, et al. Early neonatal brain injury in histologic chorioamnionitis. J Pediatr 2001;138:101–104.
16. Salafia CM, Weigl C, Silberman L. The prevalence and distribution of acute placental inflammation in uncomplicated term pregnancies. Obstet Gynecol 1984;73:282–289.
17. Bendon RW, Faye-Petersen O, Pavlova Z, et al. Histologic features of chorioamnion membrane rupture: development of methodology. Ped Pathol Lab Med 1997;17:27–42.
18. Redline RW, Faye-Petersen O, Heller D, et al. Amniotic infection syndrome: nosology and reproducibility of placental reaction patterns. Ped Dev Pathol 2003;6:435–448.
19. Naeye RL. Disorders of the placenta and decidua. In: Naeye RL, ed. Disorder of the Placenta, Fetus and Neonate: Diagnosis and Clinical Significance. St. Louis: Mosby, 1992:118–247.
20. Bendon RW. Histopathology of fetal membrane rupture: a review of the literature. Semin Perinatol 1996;20:381–388.
21. Chellam VG, Rushton DI. Chorioamnionitis and funiculitis in the placentas of 200 births weighing less than 2.5 kg. Br J Obstet Gynaecol 1985;92:808–814.
22. Romero R, Mazor M. Infection and preterm labor. Clin Obstet Gynecol 1988;31:553–584.
23. Salafia C. Chorioamnionitis. Path Case Rev 1997;2:250–255.

24. Egger G, Spendel S, Porta S. Characteristics of ingress and life span of neutrophils at a site of acute inflammation, determined with the Sephades model in rats. Exp Pathol 1988;35:209–281.
25. Svensson L, Ingemarsson I, Mardh PA. Chorioamnionitis and the isolation of microorganisms from the placenta. Obstet Gynecol 1986;67:403–409.
26. Romero R, Salafia CM, Athanassiadis AP, et al. The relationship between acute inflammatory lesions of the preterm placenta and amniotic fluid microbiology. Am J Obstet Gynecol 1992;166:1382–1388.
27. Hillier SL, Martius J, Krohn MJ, Kiviat N, Holmes KK, Eschenback DA. A case-control study of chorioamnionic infection and histologic chorioamnionitis in prematurity. N Engl J Med 1988;319:972–978.
28. Novak RW, Platt MS. Significance of placental findings in early-onset group B streptococcal neonatal sepsis. Clin Pediatr 1985;24:256–258.
29. Vollman JH, Smith WL, Ballard ET, et al. Early onset group B streptococcal disease: clinical, roentgenographic and pathologic features. J Pediatr 1976;89:199–204.
30. Craig JM. Group B β hemolytic streptococcal sepsis in the newborn. Perspect Pediatr Pathol 1981;6:139–151.
31. Cassell GH, Hauth JC, Andrews WW, et al. Chorioamnion colonization: correlation with gestational age in women following spontaneous vs induced delivery. Am J Obstet Gynecol 1993;168:425.
32. Salafia CM, Weigl C, Silberman L. The prevalence and distribution of acute placental inflammation in uncomplicated term pregnancies. Obstet Gynecol 1989;73:383–389.
33. Keski-Nisula L, Aalto M-L, Katila M-L, Kirkinen P. Intrauterine inflammation at term: a histopathologic study. Hum Pathol 2000;31:841–846.
34. Andrews WW, Hauth JC, Goldenberg RL. Infection and preterm birth. Am J Perinatol 2000;17:357–365.
35. de Araujo MC, Schultz R, Latorre RDO, Ramos JL, Vaz FA. A risk factor of early-onset infection in premature newborns: invasion of chorioamnionic tissues by leukocytes. Early Hum Dev 1999;56:1–15.
36. Naeye RL, Peters EC. Causes and consequences of premature rupture of fetal membranes. Lancet 1980;1:192–194.
37. Romero R, Sirouri M, Oyarzun E, et al. Prevalence, microbiology and clinical significance of intra amniotic infection in women with preterm labor and intact membranes. Am J Obstet Gynecol 1989;161:817–824.
38. Bendon RW, Faye-Petersen O, Pavlova Z, et al. Fetal membrane histology in preterm premature rupture of membranes: comparison to controls, and between antibiotic and placebo treatment. Pediatr Dev Pathol 1999;2:552–558.
39. Ghidini A, Salafia CM, Minior VK. Lack of relationship between histologic chorioamnionitis and duration of the latency period in preterm rupture of membranes. J Matern Fetal Med 1998;7:238–242.
40. McGregor JA, French JI, Lawellin D, Branco-Buff A, Smith C, Todd JK. Bacterial protease-induced reduction of chorioamnionic membrane strength and elasticity. Obstet Gynecol 1987;69:167–174.
41. Hillier SL, Witkin SS, Krohn MA, Watta DH, Kiviat NB, Eschenback DA. The relationship of amniotic fluid cytokines and preterm delivery, amniotic fluid infection, histologic chorioamnionitis and chorioamnion infection. Obstet Gynecol 1993;81:941–948.
42. Spiegel CA, Amsel R, Eschenbach D, Cshoenknecht F, Holmes KK. Anaerobic bacteria in nonspecific vaginitis. N Engl J Med 1980;303:601–607.
43. Martius J, Eschenbach DA. The role of bacterial vaginosis as a cause of amniotic fluid infection, chorioamnionitis and prematurity—a review. Arch Gynecol Obstet 1990;247:1–13.
44. Llahi-Camp JM, Rai R, Iscon C, Regan L, Taylor-Robinson D. Association of bacterial vaginosis with a history of second trimester miscarriage. Hum Reprod 1996;11:1575–1578.

45. Hauth JC, Goldenberg RL, Andrews WW, DuBard MB, Cooper RL. Reduced incidence of preterm delivery with metronidazole and erythromycin in women with bacterial vaginosis. N Engl J Med 1995;33:1732–1736.
46. Wen TS, Erikensen NL, Blanco JD, Graham JM, Oshiro BT, Prieto JA. Association of clinical intra-amniotic infection and meconium. Am J Perinatol 1993;10:438–440.
47. Romero R, Hanaoka S, Mazor M, et al. Meconium-stained amniotic fluid: a risk factor for microbial invasion of the amniotic cavity. Am J Obstet Gynecol 1991;164:859–862.
48. Kaspar HG, Abu-Musa A, Hannoun A, Seoud M, Shammas M, Usta I, Khalili A. The placenta in meconium staining: lesions and early neonatal outcome. Clin Exp Obstet Gynecol 2000;27:63–66.
49. de Beaufort AJ, Pelikan DMV, Elferink JG, Berger HM. Effect of interleukin 8 in meconium on in-vitro neutrophil chemotaxis. Lancet 1998;352:102–105.
50. Shen-Schwarz S, Ruchelli E, Brown D. Villous oedema of the placenta: a clinicopathological study. Placenta 1989;10:297–307.
51. Darby MJ, Caritis SN, Shen-Schwarz S. Placental abruption in the preterm gestation: an association with chorioamnionitis. Obstet Gynecol 1989;74:88–92.
52. Ohyama M, Itani Y, Yamanaha M, et al. Re-evaluation of chorioamnionitis and funisitis with a special reference to subacute chorioamnionitis. Hum Pathol 2003;33:183–190.
53. Altshuler G. Pathogenesis of congenital herpes virus infection: case report including a description of the placenta. Am J Dis Child 1974;127:427–429.
54. Garcia AGP, Marques RLS, Lobato YY, Fonseca ME, Wigg MD. Placental pathology in congenital rubella. Placenta 1985;6:281–295.
55. Garcia AGP. Congenital toxoplasmosis in two successive sibs. Arch Dis Child 1968;43:705–710.
56. Jacques SM, Qureshi F. Chronic chorioamnionitis: a clinicopathologic and immunohistochemical study. Hum Pathol 1998;29:1457–1461.
57. Gersell DJ, Phillips NJ, Beckerman K. Chronic chorioamnionitis: a clinicopathologic study of 17 cases. Int J Gynecol Pathol 1991;10:217–229.
58. Navarro C, Blanc WA. Chronic viral funisitis. J Pediatr 1977;91:967–973.
59. Reyes C, Popek E. Funisitis: where does it begin? [abstract]. Pediatr Dev Pathol 2000;3:311.
60. Fojaco RM, Hensley GT, Moskowitz L. Congenital syphilis and necrotizing funisitis. JAMA 1989;261:1788–1790.
61. Heifetz SA, Bauman M. Necrotizing funisitis and herpes simplex infection of placental and decidual tissues: study of four cases. Hum Pathol 1994;25:715–722.
62. Jacques SM, Quershi F. Necrotizing funisitis. A study of 45 cases. Hum Pathol 1992;23:1278–1283.
63. Craver RD, Baldwin VJ. Necrotizing funisitis. Obstet Gynecol 1992;79:64–70.
64. Hood IC, DeSa DJ, Whyte RK. The inflammatory response in candidal chorioamnionitis. Hum Pathol 1983;14:984–990.
65. Schwartz DA, Reef S. *Candida albicans* placentitis and funisitis: early diagnosis of congenital candidemia by histopathologic examination of the umbilical cord vessel. Pediatr Infect Dis J 1990;9:661–665.
66. Altshuler G, Hyde S. Meconium-induced vasoconstriction: a potential cause of cerebral and other fetal hypoperfusion and of poor pregnancy outcome. Child Neurol 1989;4:137–142.
67. Burgess AM, Hutchins GM. Inflammation of the lungs, umbilical cord and placenta associated with meconium passage in utero, a review of 123 autopsied cases. Pathol Res Pract 1996;192;1121–1128.
68. Bendon RW, Miller M. Letter to the editor: plasma cells in the decidua. Placenta 1990;11:369–370.
69. Khong TY, Bendon RW, Qureshi F, et al. Chronic deciduitis in the placental basal plate: definition and interobserver reliability. Hum Pathol 2000;31:292–295.

70. Russell P. Inflammatory lesions of the human placenta. III: the histopathology of villitis of unknown aetiology. Placenta 1980;1:227–244.
71. Kaplan C. The placenta and viral infection. Semin Diagn Pathol 1993;10:232–250.
72. Knox WF, Fox H. Villitis of unknown aetiology: its incidence and significance in placentae from a British population. Placenta 1984;5:395–402.
73. Altshuler G, Russell P. The human placental villitides, a review of chronic intrauterine infection. In: Münster EG, Kirsten WH, eds. Current Topics in Pathology. New York: Springer-Verlag, 1975:64–112.
74. Redline R, Patterson P. Chronic villitis is associated with major infiltration of fetal tissues by maternal calls [abstract]. Mod Pathol 1993;6:7P
75. Schwartz DA, Khan R, Stoll B. Characterization of the fetal inflammatory response to cytomegalovirus placentitis. An immunohistochemical study. Arch Pathol Lab Med 1992;116:21–27.
76. Labarrere CA, McIntyre JA, Faulk WP. Immunohistologic evidence that villitis in human normal term placenta is an immunologic lesion. Am J Obstet Gynecol 1990;162:515–522.
77. Greco MA, Wieczorek RM, Sachdev R, Kaplan C, Nuovo GJ, Demopoulos RI. Phenotype of villous stromal cells in placentas with cytomegalovirus, syphilis and nonspecific villitis. Am J Pathol 1992;141:835–842.
78. Xiao J, Garcia-Lloret M, Winkler-Lowen B, Miller R, Simpson K, Guilbert LJ. ICMA-1 mediated adhesion of peripheral blood monocytes to the maternal surface of placental syncytiotrophoblasts. Implications for placental villitis. Am J Pathol 1997;150:1845–1860.
79. Salafia CM, Silberman L, Herrera NE, Mahoney MJ. Placental pathology at term associated with elevated mid-trimester maternal serum α-fetoprotein concentration. Am J Obstet Gynecol 1988;158:1064–1066.
80. Gersell DJ. Chronic villitis, chronic chorioamniontis and maternal floor infarction. Semin Diagn Pathol 1993;10:251–266.
81. Doss BJ, Greene MF, Hill J, Heffner LJ, Bieber FR, Genest DR. Massive chronic intervillositis associated with recurrent abortion. Hum Pathol 1995;26:1245–1251.
82. Jacques SM, Qureshi F. Chronic intervillositis of the placental. Arch Pathol Lab Med 1993;17:1032–1035.
83. Ismail MR, Ordi J, Menendez C, et al. Placental pathology in malaria: histological, immunohistochemical and quantitative study. Hum Pathol 2000;31:85–93.
84. Mitchell PS, Persing DH. Current trends in molecular microbiology. Lab Med 1999;30:263–270.
85. Euscher E, Davis J, Holtzman I, Nuovo GJ. Coxsackie virus infection of the placenta associated with neurodevelopmental delays in the newborn. Obstet Gynecol 2001;98:1019–1026.
86. Sheikh AU, Polliotti BM, Miller RK. Human immunodeficiency virus infection: in situ polymerase chain reaction localization in human placentas after in utero and in vitro infection. Am J Obstet Gynecol 2000;182:207–213.
87. Ozono K, Mushiake S, Takeshima T, Nakayama M. Diagnosis of congenital cytomegalovirus infection by examination of placenta: application of polymerase chain reaction and *in situ* hybridization. Pediatr Path Lab Med 1997;17:249–258.
88. Muhlemann K, Miller RK, Metlay L, Menegus MA. CMV infection of the human placenta: an immunocytochemical study. Hum Pathol 1992;23:1234–1237.
89. Schwarz TF, Nerlich A, Hottentrager B, et al. Parvovirus B19 infection of the fetus histology and in situ hybridization. Am J Clin Pathol 1991;96:121–126.
90. Tsai MM, O'Leary TJ. Identification of *Toxoplasma gondii* in formalin-fixed, paraffin-embedded tissue by polymerase chain reaction. Mod Pathol 1993;6:185–188.
91. Guarner J, Greer PW, Bartlett J, et al. Congenital syphilis in a newborn: an immunopathologic study. Mod Pathol 1999;12:82–87.
92. Genest DR, Choi-Hong SR, Tate JE, Qureshi F, Jacques SM, Crum C. Diagnosis of congenital syphilis from placental examination: comparison of histopathology, Steiner stain, and polymerase chain reaction for *Treponema pallidum* DNA. Hum Pathol 1996;27:366–372.

Diagnosis of Specific Infections   II

5

Herpes Simplex Virus

David W. Kimberlin

THE VIRUS

Herpes simplex virus type 1 (HSV-1) and herpes simplex virus type 2 (HSV-2) are two of the eight known viruses that make up the human herpesvirus family. As with all herpesviruses, they are large, enveloped virions with an icosahedral nucleocapsid consisting of 162 capsomeres arranged around a linear, double-stranded deoxyribonucleic acid (DNA) core. The DNAs of HSV-1 and HSV-2 are largely colinear, and considerable homology exists between the HSV-1 and HSV-2 genomes. These homologous sequences are distributed over the entire genomic map, and most of the polypeptides specified by one viral type are antigenically related to polypeptides of the other viral type. This results in considerable cross-reactivity between the HSV-1 and HSV-2 glycoproteins, although unique antigenic determinants exist for each virus.

Two biological properties of HSV that directly influence human disease are neurovirulence and latency. *Neurovirulence* refers to the affinity with which HSV is drawn to and propagated in neuronal tissue. This can result in profound disease with severe neurological sequelae, as is the case with HSV encephalitis. *Latency* is the process by which the HSV genome infects neuronal cells and is then maintained in the cell in a repressed (or latent) state. From this latent state, the viral genome may subsequently become activated, resulting in viral replication and, in some cases, the redevelopment of herpetic lesions.

The mechanisms by which HSV establishes latency are under intense investigation, but they remain unknown at this time. It is accepted that, following primary infection, replication of the virus at the portal of entry, usually oral or genital mucosal tissue, results in infection of sensory nerve endings. HSV virions are then transported to central axons by the sensory nerves, and from there are transported to the dorsal root ganglia via retrograde axonal flow. After transport is complete, virus replicates for several days in the sensory ganglia that innervate the sites of inoculation. Once replication in the sensory ganglia is complete, latency is established. Use of antiviral agents after the establishment of latency will not result in elimination of the virus.

Recurrences appear in the presence of both cell-mediated and humoral immunity. Recurrences can occur spontaneously, or they can be associated with physical or emotional stress, fever, exposure to ultraviolet light, tissue damage, and immune suppression. Infectious virus can be cultured from the mucocutaneous lesions of recurrent HSV

From: *Infectious Disease: Congenital and Perinatal Infections: A Concise Guide to Diagnosis*
Edited by: C. Hutto © Humana Press Inc., Totowa, NJ

Table 1
Summary of 71 Patients Reported With Intrauterine HSV Infection

	Number of cases (%) (N = 71)
Sex	
Male	17 (24)
Female	26 (37)
Not reported	28 (39)
Virus	
HSV-1	5 (7)
HSV-2	43 (61)
Not reported	23 (32)
Findings	
Prematurity	42 (59)
Small for gestational age	17 (24)
Spectrum of disease	
Cutaneous lesions/scarring alone	5 (7)
Ocular + CNS lesions	4 (6)
Cutaneous + ocular lesions	10 (14)
Cutaneous + CNS lesions	24 (34)
Cutaneous + ocular + CNS lesions	28 (39)
Hepatitis	10 (14)
Associated dysmorphic abnormalities	6 (8)

From ref. *1*.

infection. As with the establishment of latency, the mechanisms involved in reactivating the latent viral genome remain to be elucidated.

TIMING, ROUTE OF TRANSMISSION, AND CLINICAL MANIFESTATIONS OF NEONATAL HERPES SIMPLEX VIRUS

HSV disease of the newborn is acquired in one of three distinct time intervals: intrauterine (*in utero*), peripartum (perinatal), and postpartum (postnatal). Among infected infants, the time of transmission for the overwhelming majority (~85%) of neonates is in the peripartum period. An additional 10% of infected neonates acquire the virus postnatally, and the final 5% are infected with HSV *in utero*.

Intrauterine HSV disease occurs in approx 1 in 300,000 deliveries (*1*). Although rare, *in utero* disease is unlikely to be missed because of the degree of involvement of affected babies. Infants acquiring HSV *in utero* typically have a triad of clinical findings consisting of cutaneous manifestations (scarring, active lesions, hypo- and hyperpigmentation, aplasia cutis, or an erythematous macular exanthem), ophthalmological findings (micro-opthalmia, retinal dysplasia, optic atrophy, or chorioretinitis), and neurological involvement (microcephaly, encephalomalacia, hydranencephaly, or intracranial calcification) (*2–5*). A summary of 71 infants with intrauterine HSV infection and disease is presented in Table 1.

HSV infections acquired either peripartum or postpartum can be further classified as (1) encephalitis, with or without skin, eye, or mouth (SEM) involvement (central ner-

Table 2
Signs and Symptoms of Neonatal HSV Disease Prior to Initiation of Antiviral Therapy

	Disease classification			
	SEM ($n = 64$)	CNS ($n = 63$)	Disseminated ($n = 59$)	Total ($N = 186$)
Skin vesicles				
Number of patients	53 (83%)	40 (63%)	34 (58%)	127 (68%)
Duration of symptoms (days ± SE)	3.8 ± 0.5	6.1 ± 1.0	3.7 ± 0.6	4.5 ± 0.4
Lethargy				
Number of patients	12 (19%)	31 (49%)	28 (47%)	71 (38%)
Duration of symptoms (days ± SE)	3.3 ± 0.7	4.6 ± 0.7	3.4 ± 0.7	3.9 ± 0.4
Fever				
Number of patients	11 (17%)	28 (44%)	33 (56%)	72 (39%)
Duration of symptoms (days ± SE)	4.6 ± 1.5	3.1 ± 0.4	4.6 ± 0.6	4.0 ± 0.4
Conjunctivitis				
Number of patients	16 (25%)	10 (16%)	10 (17%)	36 (19%)
Duration of symptoms (days ± SE)	6.5 ± 1.5	4.1 ± 1.3	5.9 ± 1.9	5.7 ± 0.9
Seizure				
Number of patients	1 (2%)	36 (57%)	13 (22%)	50 (27%)
Duration of symptoms (days ± SE)	7.0	2.9 ± 0.5	2.5 ± 0.7	2.9 ± 0.4
DIC				
Number of patients	0 (0%)	0 (0%)	20 (34%)	20 (11%)
Duration of symptoms (days ± SE)	—	—	1.5 ± 0.3	1.5 ± 0.3
Pneumonia				
Number of patients	0 (0%)	2 (3%)	22 (37%)	24 (13%)
Duration of symptoms (days ± SE)	—	9.0 ± 6.0	4.0 ± 0.8	4.5 ± 0.9

From ref. *12*.

vous system [CNS] disease); (2) disseminated infection involving multiple organs, including the CNS, lung, liver, adrenal glands, skin, eye, or mouth (disseminated disease); and (3) disease localized to the skin, eyes, or mouth (SEM disease). This classification system is predictive of both morbidity and mortality *(6–9)*.

One-third of all neonates with HSV infection are categorized as having CNS disease (with or without SEM involvement) *(10)*. Clinical manifestations of encephalitis, either alone or in association with disseminated disease, include seizures (both focal and generalized), lethargy, irritability, tremors, poor feeding, temperature instability, and bulging fontanelle. Of those infants with CNS disease without visceral dissemination, between 60 and 70% have associated skin vesicles at any point in the disease course *(11,12)*. Table 2 lists the frequency and duration of signs and symptoms present prior to initiation of acyclovir therapy for 186 neonates treated in clinical studies conducted between 1981 and 1997 by the National Institute of Allergy and Infectious Diseases Collaborative Antiviral Study Group.

Historically, disseminated HSV infections have accounted for approx 50–66% of all children with neonatal HSV disease. However, this figure has been reduced to about 23% since the development and utilization of antiviral therapy, likely the consequence of recognizing and treating SEM infection before its progression to more severe disease *(10)*. Encephalitis is a common component of this category of infection, occurring in about 60–75% of infants with disseminated disease *(13)*. Although the presence of a vesicular rash can greatly facilitate the diagnosis of HSV infection, over 20% of neonates with disseminated HSV disease will not develop cutaneous vesicles during the course of their illness *(10,11,12,14)*.

Infection localized to SEM disease has historically accounted for approx 18% of all cases of neonatal HSV disease. With the introduction of early antiviral therapy, this frequency has increased to 43% *(10)*. Patients with SEM or disseminated disease generally present to medical attention at 10–12 days of life; patients with CNS disease on average present somewhat later, at 16–19 days of life *(12)*.

RISK OF MATERNAL INFECTION DURING PREGNANCY

Genital herpes occurs with a frequency of about 1% at any time during gestation *(15,16)*. Recurrent genital herpes infections are the most common form of genital HSV during gestation *(13)*. However, as discussed below, it is the woman with primary HSV disease who is at highest risk of transmitting the virus to her baby. About 10% of HSV-2-seronegative pregnant women have an HSV-2-seropositive sexual partner and thus are at risk of contracting a primary HSV-2 infection *(17)*. Among such discordant couples, women who are seronegative for both HSV-1 and HSV-2 have an estimated chance of seroconversion for either virus of 3.7%; those women who are already seropositive for HSV-1 have an estimated chance of HSV-2 seroconversion of 1.7% *(18)*. Approximately two-thirds of women who acquire genital herpes during pregnancy have no symptoms to suggest a genital HSV infection *(18)*.

Several prospective studies have evaluated the frequency and nature of viral shedding throughout pregnancy in women with a known history of genital herpes. In a predominantly white, middle-class population, recurrent infection was documented in 84% of pregnant women with a history of recurrent disease *(19)*. Moreover, at least 12% of the recurrent episodes involved asymptomatic viral shedding. In the same report, viral shedding occurred in 0.56% of cervical cultures obtained during clinical episodes of infections and in 0.66% of cervical cultures obtained during intercurrent periods (periods between clinical episodes). These data are similar to those obtained from other populations *(20–22)*.

Overall, the observed rate of shedding among pregnant women with asymptomatic infection has varied more than that among nonpregnant women (from 0.2 to 7.4%), depending on the study population and trial design *(20,21,23,24)*. These data indicate that the frequency of cervical shedding is low, rendering the risk of transmission of virus to the infant even lower when the maternal infection is recurrent. The frequency of viral shedding in gravid women with recurrent infection does not appear to vary significantly by trimester *(19,23)*. Likewise, the frequency of recurrences has not been shown to vary from one pregnancy to the next *(24)*.

For neonatal transmission to occur in the peripartum period, the gravid woman must be shedding virus, either symptomatically or asymptomatically, at the time of delivery. The incidence of viral excretion proximate to delivery ranges from 0.20 to 0.39% for all pregnant women, irrespective of past history *(21,25–27)*. Among pregnant women with a known history of recurrent genital HSV, the rate of excretion may be as high as 0.77–1.4% *(22)*.

Of women who deliver an HSV-infected infant, 60–80% have no evidence of genital HSV infection at the time of delivery and have neither a past history of genital herpes nor a sexual partner reporting a history of genital HSV *(10,28,29)*. For significant improvement in the prevention of neonatal HSV to occur, the means of identifying women who are seropositive but have no known history of genital herpes, as well as of identifying seronegative women at risk for acquiring infection from a seropositive sexual partner, must be greatly improved. The development of type-specific, commercially available serologic assays with high sensitivity and specificity may provide the means to accomplish this, as discussed below.

RISK OF NEONATAL INFECTION

Factors that influence transmission from mother to neonate include type of maternal infection (primary vs recurrent), maternal antibody status, duration of rupture of membranes, and integrity of mucocutaneous barriers (e.g., use of fetal scalp electrodes). Several studies have demonstrated that infants born to mothers who have a first episode of genital HSV infection near term are at much greater risk of developing neonatal herpes than are those whose mothers have recurrent genital herpes. In three separate studies, 3 of 6, 2 of 6, and 6 of 18 infants born to mothers with first episode (primary or initial) genital HSV infections at delivery developed neonatal infection, for an overall attack rate of 36.7% (11 of 30 infants) *(16,25,30)*. In contrast, among infants delivered to mothers with recurrent HSV infection and documented viral shedding at the time of delivery, the rate of neonatal infection has been reported to be between 3 *(25)* and 4.3% *(16)*.

These findings are strengthened by data from an ongoing study in Seattle, Washington, of women with subclinical shedding of HSV proximate to the time of delivery (Fig. 1) *(31)*. Almost 32,000 women have been cultured within 48 hours of delivery. Of these, there were 116 women who both were shedding HSV and for whom sera was available for serologic analysis. In this large trial, 67% of babies delivered to women with first-episode primary infection (no preexisting HSV-1 or HSV-2 antibody) developed neonatal HSV disease, compared with 29% of babies delivered to women with first-episode nonprimary infection (preexisting antibody to the other HSV serotype) and 1% of babies delivered to women with recurrent HSV disease *(31)*.

The pregnant woman's antibody status at delivery also influences the severity of infection and the likelihood of viral transmission. Transplacentally acquired maternal neutralizing antibodies have a protective effect on both the acquisition of and the outcome from infection following neonatal exposure to HSV during delivery *(29,32,33)*. Complete neutralization of virus by antibody may occur in some infants, and prolongation of the incubation period and modification of the infection may occur in others.

The duration of membrane rupture appears to have an impact on the risk for acquisition of neonatal infection. Cesarean delivery in a woman with active genital lesions can reduce the infant's risk of acquiring HSV if performed within 4 hours of rupture of membrane *(34)*. Based on this observation, it is currently recommended that women with active genital lesions at the time of onset of labor be delivered by cesarean section, although the potential benefits of such delivery when membranes have been ruptured beyond 4 hours has not been proven. Importantly, neonatal infection has occurred in spite of cesarean delivery performed prior to the rupture of membranes *(10)*.

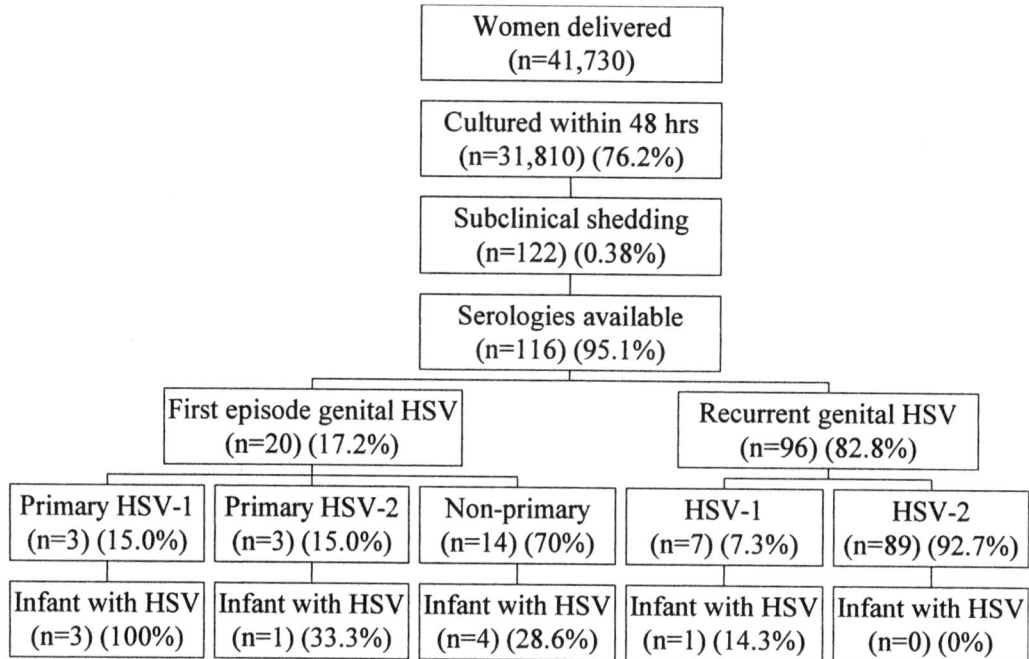

Fig. 1. Neonatal transmission as a function of maternal infection. (Adapted from ref. *31*.)

Last, the application of fetal scalp monitors around the time of delivery may increase the risk of neonatal HSV infection by providing a potential site of inoculation for the virus *(35,36)*. The risks and benefits of such devices should be considered carefully for women with a history of recurrent genital HSV infections.

PRENATAL EVALUATION OF THE PREGNANT WOMAN

As indicated in the preceding section, it is the woman with primary genital HSV infection who is at highest risk of transmitting HSV to her newborn baby during birth. Despite this fact, considerable attention is focused clinically on the woman with a history of genital HSV that preceded her current pregnancy. Prenatal cultures of the vaginal tract do not predict whether a woman with a history of genital HSV will be shedding virus at the time of delivery *(27)* and as such have no role in the evaluation of such women. There is active debate in the obstetrical community regarding whether, for women with known recurrent HSV disease and active lesions at delivery, the surgical risks of cesarean delivery outweigh the small (<2%) risk of the baby contracting neonatal HSV. At the current time, however, women with active lesions noted at the time of labor are delivered by cesarean section to minimize risk of transmission to the baby, regardless of whether they have recurrent infection or primary infection.

Until recently, the commercially available serologic assays were unable to distinguish between HSV-1 and HSV-2 antibodies. This severely limited their utility in the obstetrical population. In the past few years, type-specific antibody assays manufactured by Focus Technologies have been approved by the Food and Drug Administration *(37)*. Several additional tests that claim to distinguish between HSV-1 and HSV-2 antibody are commercially available, but high cross-reactivity rates negate their utility

(37a). At the current time, the optimal application of these type-specific assays has not been determined. Ongoing studies conducted through the Centers for Disease Control and Prevention ultimately may answer these important questions within the next few years.

CLINICAL EVALUATION OF THE INFANT

Many different conditions may mimic HSV disease. In the infant with disseminated infection and its associated multiorgan involvement, other conditions that must be considered include hyaline membrane disease, intraventricular hemorrhage, necrotizing enterocolitis, and overwhelming bacterial sepsis caused by, among others, group B streptococcus, *Staphylococcus aureus*, *Listeria monocytogenes*, and Gram-negative bacteria.

The vesicular rash that occurs with HSV infection may be confused with the cutaneous manifestations of other infectious diseases, such as varicella-zoster virus infection, postnatally acquired enteroviral disease, and disseminated cytomegalovirus infection. Such distinctions are especially difficult when HSV assumes an atypical cutaneous presentation. Definitive confirmation of HSV disease can be achieved by culture of the skin vesicles. Noninfectious cutaneous conditions such as incontinentia pigmenti, acrodermatitis enteropathica, erythema toxicum, and neonatal melanosis should also be considered. Lesions associated with these diseases can often be distinguished rapidly from those caused by HSV by the presence of eosinophils on staining of a tissue scraping, by peripheral eosinophilia, and by appropriate viral cultures.

The most difficult clinical diagnosis to make is that of HSV encephalitis, in large part because nearly 40% of infants with CNS infection do not have skin lesions at the time of clinical presentation *(11,12)*. Clinical diagnosis under these conditions is based on a high index of suspicion. This is especially true if the patient's bacterial cultures are negative at 48–72 hours. Infection of the CNS should be suspected in the neonate who has evidence of acute neurological deterioration with the onset of seizures, especially when this occurs in the absence of intraventricular hemorrhage or metabolic imbalances. Serial increases in cerebrospinal fluid (CSF) cell counts and protein concentrations also suggest the possibility of HSV disease. An electroencephalogram, and to a lesser degree a computed tomographic scan of the head, may be of benefit in this situation *(12)*.

LABORATORY ASSAYS FOR THE DIAGNOSIS OF NEONATAL HERPES SIMPLEX VIRUS DISEASE

Isolation of HSV by culture remains the definitive diagnostic method of establishing HSV disease. If skin lesions are present, a scraping of the vesicles should be transferred in appropriate viral transport media on ice to a diagnostic virology laboratory. Such specimens are inoculated into cell culture systems, which are then monitored for cytopathic effects characteristic of HSV replication. Other sites from which virus may be isolated include the CSF, urine, blood, stool or rectum, oropharynx, and conjunctivae *(38)*. Duodenal aspirates for HSV isolation may be indicated in infants with hepatitis, necrotizing enterocolitis, or other gastrointestinal manifestations of disease. Typing of an HSV isolate may be done by one of several techniques but is not generally available outside research laboratories.

Cytological examination of cells from the maternal cervix or from the infant's skin, mouth, conjunctivae, or corneal lesions may be useful in making a presumptive diagnosis of HSV infection. Because these methods have a sensitivity of only 60–70%, they should not be the sole diagnostic determinant for HSV infection in the newborn *(39)*. For neonatal lesions, material from the vesicle should be obtained by scraping the periphery of the base of the lesion, smearing this on a glass slide, and promptly fixing it in cold ethanol. Following staining, the preparation should be viewed by a trained cytologist. The presence of intranuclear inclusions and multinucleated giant cells are indicative of, but not diagnostic for, HSV infection.

In contrast to other congenital and neonatal infections, serologic diagnosis of HSV infection is not of great clinical value. With the licensure of reliable type-specific assays, one barrier to interpreting serologic results in babies with suspected HSV disease has been removed. However, the presence of transplacentally acquired maternal immunoglobulin G still confounds the assessment of the neonatal antibody status during acute infection, especially given the large proportions of the adult American population who are HSV-1 and HSV-2 seropositive. Serial antibody assessment may be useful in the very specific circumstance of a mother who has a primary infection late in gestation and transfers very little or no antibody to the fetus. In general, however, serologic studies play no role in the diagnosis of neonatal HSV disease.

The diagnosis of neonatal HSV infections has been revolutionized by the application of polymerase chain reaction (PCR) technology to clinical specimens, including CSF *(40–43)* and blood *(41,43–45)*. The reported sensitivity of PCR in the diagnosis of CNS disease has ranged from 75 to 100% *(40–43)*. Although this broad range can be explained at least partly by differences in the methodologies of the individual studies, many of which involved retrospective PCR analysis of stored biological specimens, the variability in performance of PCR between laboratories warrants consideration. Interlaboratory standards that ensure identical specimens processed in two different laboratories will yield identical results are largely nonexistent. Furthermore, the performance of PCR is highly dependent on the manner in which the specimen was collected and maintained prior to reaching the laboratory for PCR analysis. Given these caveats, interpretation of PCR results must be correlated with the patient's clinical presentation and disease course.

CONCLUSION

Tremendous advances have occurred over the past three decades in our knowledge of the natural history of neonatal HSV infection and disease. Although diagnostic advances have included such tools as PCR, prompt diagnosis of neonatal HSV disease will continue to rely primarily on a high index of suspicion. An understanding of the biology and natural history of HSV in the gravid woman and the neonate provides the foundation of such an index.

REFERENCES

1. Baldwin S, Whitley RJ. Intrauterine herpes simplex virus infection. Teratology 1989;39:1–10.
2. Florman AL, Gershon AA, Blackett PR, Nahmias AJ. Intrauterine infection with herpes simplex virus: resultant congenital malformations. JAMA 1973;225:129–132.
3. Karesh JW, Kapur S, MacDonald M. Herpes simplex virus and congenital malformations. South Med J 1983;76:1561–1563.
4. Monif GR, Kellner KR, Donnelly WH Jr. Congenital herpes simplex type II infection. Am J Obstet Gynecol 1985;152:1000–1002.

5. Hutto C, Arvin A, Jacobs R, et al. Intrauterine herpes simplex virus infections. J Pediatr 1987;110:97–101.
6. Whitley RJ, Nahmias AJ, Soong S-J, et al. Vidarabine therapy of neonatal herpes simplex virus infection. Pediatrics 1980;66:495–501.
7. Whitley R, Arvin A, Prober C, et al. A controlled trial comparing vidarabine with acyclovir in neonatal herpes simplex virus infection. N Engl J Med 1991;324:444–449.
8. Kimberlin DW, Lin C-Y, Jacobs RF, et al. Safety and efficacy of high-dose intravenous acyclovir in the management of neonatal herpes simplex virus infections. Pediatrics 2001;108:230–238.
9. Whitley R, Arvin A, Prober C, et al. Predictors of morbidity and mortality in neonates with herpes simplex virus infections. N Engl J Med 1991;324:450–454.
10. Whitley RJ, Corey L, Arvin A, et al. Changing presentation of neonatal herpes simplex virus infection. J Infect Dis 1988;158:109–116.
11. Sullivan-Bolyai JZ, Hull HF, Wilson C, Smith AL, Corey L. Presentation of neonatal herpes simplex virus infections: implications for a change in therapeutic strategy. Pediatr Infect Dis 1986;5:309–314.
12. Kimberlin DW, Lin C-Y, Jacobs RF, et al. The natural history of neonatal herpes simplex virus infections in the acyclovir era. Pediatrics 2001;108:223–229.
13. Whitley RJ. Herpes simplex virus infections. In: Remington JS, Klein JO, eds. Infectious Diseases of the Fetus and Newborn Infants, 3rd ed. Philadelphia: Saunders, 1990:282–305.
14. Arvin AM, Yeager AS, Bruhn FW, Grossman M. Neonatal herpes simplex infection in the absence of mucocutaneous lesions. J Pediatr 1982;100:715–721.
15. Nahmias AJ, Keyserling HL, Kerrick GM. Herpes simplex. In: Remington JS, Klein JO, eds. Infectious Diseases of the Fetus and Newborn Infants, 2nd ed. Philadelphia: Saunders, 1983:636–678.
16. Nahmias AJ, Josey WE, Naib ZM, Freeman MG, Fernandez RJ, Wheeler JH. Perinatal risk associated with maternal genital herpes simplex virus infection. Am J Obstet Gynecol 1971;110:825–837.
17. Kulhanjian JA, Soroush V, Au DS, et al. Identification of women at unsuspected risk of primary infection with herpes simplex virus type 2 during pregnancy. N Engl J Med 1992;326:916–920.
18. Brown ZA, Selke S, Zeh J, et al. The acquisition of herpes simplex virus during pregnancy. N Engl J Med 1997;337:509–515.
19. Vontver LA, Hickok DE, Brown Z, Reid L, Corey L. Recurrent genital herpes simplex virus infection in pregnancy: infant outcome and frequency of asymptomatic recurrences. Am J Obstet Gynecol 1982;143:75–84.
20. Rattray MC, Corey L, Reeves WC, Vontver LA, Holmes KK. Recurrent genital herpes among women: symptomatic vs asymptomatic viral shedding. Br J Vener Dis 1978;54:262–265.
21. Bolognese RJ, Corson SL, Fuccillo DA, Traub R, Moder F, Sever JL. Herpesvirus hominis type II infections in asymptomatic pregnant women. Obstet Gynecol 1976;48:507–510.
22. Arvin AM, Hensleigh PA, Prober CG, et al. Failure of antepartum maternal cultures to predict the infant's risk of exposure to herpes simplex virus at delivery. N Engl J Med 1986;315:796–800.
23. Harger JH, Pazin GJ, Armstrong JA, Breinig MC, Ho M. Characteristics and management of pregnancy in women with genital herpes simplex virus infection. Am J Obstet Gynecol 1983;145:784–791.
24. Harger JH, Meyer MP, Amortegui AJ. Changes in the frequency of genital herpes recurrences as a function of time. Obstet Gynecol 1986;67:637–642.
25. Brown ZA, Benedetti J, Ashley R, et al. Neonatal herpes simplex virus infection in relation to asymptomatic maternal infection at the time of labor. N Engl J Med 1991;324:1247–1252.
26. Tejani N, Klein SW, Kaplan M. Subclinical herpes simplex genitalis infections in the perinatal period. Am J Obstet Gynecol 1979;135:547.

27. Prober CG, Hensleigh PA, Boucher FD, Yasukawa LL, Au DS, Arvin AM. Use of routine viral cultures at delivery to identify neonates exposed to herpes simplex virus. N Engl J Med 1988;318:887–891.
28. Whitley RJ, Nahmias AJ, Visitine AM, Fleming CL, Alford CA Jr, NIAID Collaborative Antiviral Study Group. The natural history of herpes simplex virus infection of mother and newborn. Pediatrics 1980;66:489–494.
29. Yeager AS, Arvin AM. Reasons for the absence of a history of recurrent genital infections in mothers of neonates infected with herpes simplex virus. Pediatrics 1984;73:188–193.
30. Brown ZA, Vontver LA, Benedetti J, et al. Effects on infants of a first episode of genital herpes during pregnancy. N Engl J Med 1987;317:1246–1251.
31. Corey L, Wald A. Genital herpes. In: Holmes KK, Sparling PF, Mardh PA, et al., Sexually Transmitted Diseases, 3rd ed. New York: McGraw-Hill, 1999:285–312.
32. Prober CG, Sullender WM, Yasukawa LL, Au DS, Yeager AS, Arvin AM. Low risk of herpes simplex virus infections in neonates exposed to the virus at the time of vaginal delivery to mothers with recurrent genital herpes simplex virus infections. N Engl J Med 1987;316:240–244.
33. Yeager AS, Arvin AM, Urbani LJ, Kemp JA III. Relationship of antibody to outcome in neonatal herpes simplex virus infections. Infect Immun 1980;29:532–538.
34. Nahmias AJ, Josey WE, Naib ZM, Freeman MG, Fernandez RJ, Wheeler JH. Perinatal risk associated with maternal genital herpes simplex virus infection. Am J Obstet Gynecol 1971;110:825–837.
35. Parvey LS, Ch'ien LT. Neonatal herpes simplex virus infection introduced by fetal-monitor scalp electrodes. Pediatrics 1980;65:1150–1153.
36. Kaye EM, Dooling EC. Neonatal herpes simplex meningoencephalitis associated with fetal monitor scalp electrodes. Neurology 1981;31:1045–1047.
37. Prince HE, Ernst CE, Hogrefe WR. Evaluation of an enzyme immunoassay system for measuring herpes simplex virus (HSV) type 1-specific and HSV type 2-specific IgG antibodies. J Clin Lab Anal 2000;14:13–16.
37a. Ashley RL. Sorting out the new HSV type specific antibody tests. Sex Transm Infect 2001;77:232–237.
38. American Academy of Pediatrics. Herpes simplex. In: Pickering LK, ed. 2000 Red Book: Report of the Committee on Infectious Diseases, 25th ed. Elk Grove Village, IL: American Academy of Pediatrics, 2000:309–318.
39. Boehm FH, Estes W, Wright PF, Growdon JF Jr. Management of genital herpes simplex virus infection occurring during pregnancy. Am J Obstet Gynecol 1981;141:735–740.
40. Kimberlin DW, Lakeman FD, Arvin AM, et al. Application of the polymerase chain reaction to the diagnosis and management of neonatal herpes simplex virus disease. J Infect Dis 1996;174:1162–1167.
41. Kimura H, Futamura M, Kito H, et al. Detection of viral DNA in neonatal herpes simplex virus infections: frequent and prolonged presence in serum and cerebrospinal fluid. J Infect Dis 1991;164:289–293.
42. Troendle-Atkins J, Demmler GJ, Buffone GJ. Rapid diagnosis of herpes simplex virus encephalitis by using the polymerase chain reaction. J Pediatr 1993;123:376–380.
43. Malm G, Forsgren M. Neonatal herpes simplex virus infections: HSV DNA in cerebrospinal fluid and serum. Arch Dis Child Fetal Neonatal Ed 1999;81:F24–F29.
44. Barbi M, Binda S, Primache V, Tettamanti A, Negri C, Brambilla C. Use of Guthrie cards for the early diagnosis of neonatal herpes simplex virus disease. Pediatr Infect Dis J 1998;17:251–252.
45. Diamond C, Mohan K, Hobson A, Frenkel L, Corey L. Viremia in neonatal herpes simplex virus infections. Pediatr Infect Dis J 1999;18:487–489.

6

Cytomegalovirus

Suresh B. Boppana

INTRODUCTION

Cytomegaloviruses (CMVs) belong to the betaherpesviruses subfamily of herpesviruses and are ubiquitous but highly species-specific viruses that infect many animals, including humans *(1)*. Infection with CMV is common in all populations and rarely associated with symptomatic infection in normal hosts. In contrast, it is a major cause of multiorgan disease in immunocompromised patients. CMV is also a leading cause of congenital infection and a leading infectious cause of brain disease and hearing loss in children in the United States and western Europe. As with other herpesviruses, primary infection with CMV is followed by a persistent infection.

VIRUS CHARACTERISTICS

CMV is morphologically similar to other herpesviruses and is the largest member of the family *(2)*. The virus consists of a 64-nm core enclosed by a 110-nm icosahedral capsid. The capsid is surrounded by a poorly defined amorphous tegument that itself is surrounded by a loosely applied, lipid-containing tegument *(2)*. The genome of CMV consists of linear double-stranded deoxyribonucleic acid (DNA) molecule approx 240 kb *(3,4)*. The genome of CMV is similar to that of herpes simplex virus in that it has long and short unique segments, both of which are bounded by homologous repetitive sequences. The CMV genome is approx 50% larger than herpes simplex virus and encodes for at least 35 structural proteins and an undefined number of nonstructural proteins *(5)*. Although the replication of CMV is very similar to that described for herpes simplex virus, the replicative cycle is much slower than for herpes simplex *(6)*.

PUBLIC HEALTH IMPORTANCE

The public health importance of congenital CMV infection is attributed to its frequency and the occurrence of central nervous system (CNS) impairments in a significant proportion of infected children. Studies that have screened large numbers of newborns for prenatal CMV infection have reported rates of 0.3–1.4% *(7–11)*. In the United States, the overall rate of congenital CMV infection is often estimated at 1% of all live births, a rate that equates to about 40,000 new cases per year *(11,12)*. Although most infants with congenital CMV infection will not suffer any neurological impairment, studies in Sweden and the United States have shown that congenital CMV infec-

From: *Infectious Disease: Congenital and Perinatal Infections: A Concise Guide to Diagnosis*
Edited by: C. Hutto © Humana Press Inc., Totowa, NJ

Table 1
**Rates of Maternal CMV Seroprevalence and Congenital
CMV Infection in Various Populations**

Location	% Mothers seropositive	% Congenital CMV infection	Reference
Aarhus-Viborg, Denmark	52	0.4	*15*
Abidjan, Ivory Coast	100	1.4	*7*
Birmingham, AL			*17*
Low-income group	77	1.25	
Middle-income group	36	0.53	
Hamilton, Ontario, Canada	44	0.42	*9*
London, UK	56	0.3	*16*
Sao Paulo, Brazil			*18*
Low-income group	84	0.98	
Middle-income group	67	0.46	
Seoul, South Korea	96	1.2	*10*

tion is a leading cause of hearing loss in children *(13,14)*. Considering auditory, visual, cognitive, and motor deficits, congenital CMV infection is probably the leading infectious cause of CNS damage in children in the United States. It is estimated that between 4000 and 6000 children born each year in the United States will develop permanent neurological deficits *(11)*.

EPIDEMIOLOGY OF CYTOMEGALOVIRUS INFECTION IN MOTHERS

Numerous cross-sectional, serological studies, dating to the 1960s, have demonstrated that CMV infection is ubiquitous in humans. Table 1 compares the CMV seroprevalence rates in women of childbearing age from various populations. Higher rates of CMV seroprevalence have been demonstrated in non-white and low-income populations in both developed and developing countries *(7,15–18)*. The prevalence of maternal CMV infection is an important determinant of the frequency and significance of vertical transmission of CMV in a population. The rates of congenital CMV infection are directly proportional to the rates of maternal seropositivity in the population. In addition, the rates of intrapartum and breast milk transmission vary directly with the rate of maternal seroprevalence.

INCIDENCE AND SOURCES OF CYTOMEGALOVIRUS INFECTION

The overall incidence of CMV infection in adults estimated from large studies of blood donors, hospital workers, and pregnant women is around 1–2% per year *(17,19,20)*. Higher rates of primary CMV infection have been documented in women of lower socioeconomic status. In developing countries, most people acquire CMV during early childhood. Studies have clearly shown the importance of both sexual activity and close contact with CMV-infected children as sources of maternal CMV infection *(11)*. Evidence for sexual transmission of CMV is provided by studies that showed higher rates of CMV seropositivity in young women with other indicators of sexual activity, such as sexually transmitted diseases, greater number of sex partners, or young age at sexual debut *(21,22)*. The results of a case-control study showed that history of sexually transmitted disease in the mother was an independent risk factor for the birth of a newborn with congenital CMV infection *(23)*.

A dramatic rise in age-related prevalence of CMV infection in children attending child care centers compared with those kept at home has been demonstrated. Furthermore, the transmission of CMV strains among children in this setting has been documented by molecular epidemiology *(24)*. Studies of parents of children attending day care centers and child care workers demonstrated a high rate of seroconversion and a strong association between care of younger CMV-shedding children and seroconversion *(25–27)*. Molecular analysis of the isolates provided further evidence for transmission of CMV strains from child to caregiver *(26–28)*.

Vertical Transmission

CMV can be transmitted from mother to child transplacentally, during birth, and in the postpartum period via breast milk. Congenital CMV infection rates are directly related to maternal seroprevalence rates. Rates of congenital CMV infection are higher in developing countries and higher for low-income groups in developed countries *(7,10,29)*. The mechanisms for this increased rate of congenital CMV in populations with high seroprevalence rates are not clear. Studies of risk factors for congenital CMV infection have also documented an association between young maternal age and increased rates of congenital CMV infection *(30)*. Preece at al. also found that non-white race and single marital status were independently associated with increased risk of congenital CMV infection *(31)*. Fowler et al. reported an increased risk of congenital CMV infection in women with sexually transmitted diseases, single mothers, and those younger than 20 years *(32)*.

Intrapartum Transmission

Intrapartum transmission of CMV occurs in around 50% of infants born to mothers shedding CMV from the cervix or vagina at the time of delivery *(33)*. Genital tract shedding of CMV is more common in younger women, declining from around 15% in young teenagers to less than 1% in women over 30 years of age *(34,35)*. Rates of CMV excretion from the cervix and vagina also change during gestation, with low rates early in gestation increasing to rates that equal or exceed those in nonpregnant women late in gestation. Cervical shedding of CMV has also been associated with other sexually transmitted diseases and with a greater number of sexual partners *(36)*. In the United States, approx 10% of women shed CMV at the time of delivery; rates as high as 40% have been reported in Taiwanese women *(36,37)*.

Postnatal Transmission

Breast milk is a principal route of transmission of CMV from mother to the child during infancy. Between 27 and 70% of seropositive women shed CMV in breast milk *(38,39)*. It was reported that transmission of CMV to nursing infants of seropositive mothers was related to duration of breastfeeding and detection of CMV in milk by virus isolation *(40)*. The proportion of infants acquiring CMV is directly related to maternal seroprevalence rates and the frequency of breastfeeding.

Vertical transmission of CMV plays an important role in the epidemiology of human CMV infection. In countries where a high proportion of infants acquire CMV from a maternal source, the majority of children are infected in early childhood. Aside from the medical significance of congenital CMV infection, infants who acquire CMV *in utero*, during delivery, or from mother's milk shed virus for years and serve as a source of the virus for other children and caregivers with whom they have close contact.

Nosocomial Transmission

Blood products and transplanted organs are the most important vehicles of transmission of CMV in the hospital setting; the latter are unlikely to be of concern during pregnancy. Transmission of CMV through packed red blood cell, leukocyte, and platelet transfusions poses a risk of severe disease for seronegative small premature infants and immunocompromised patients *(41)*. The risk of transmission of CMV with blood products increases with the number of units transfused, the presence of white blood cells, and the lack of serum antibody in the recipient *(42)*. Prevention of blood product transmission of CMV can be achieved by using seronegative donors or by special filters that remove white blood cells *(41,43,44)*. Another potential source of nosocomial CMV infection of particular concern to those in reproductive medicine is semen donated for artificial insemination *(45,46)*. Although no cases of congenital CMV infection attributed to donor insemination have been reported, the fact that sexual activity is clearly a risk for CMV infection and that virus can commonly be recovered from semen suggests a need for caution. The American Fertility Society has recommended serological screening of semen donors for antibody to CMV *(47)*. Person-to-person transmission of CMV requires contact with infected body fluids and therefore should be prevented by routine hospital infection control precautions. Studies in health care settings found no evidence of increased risk of CMV infection in settings in which patients shedding CMV are encountered *(19,48)*.

CONSEQUENCES OF MATERNAL CYTOMEGALOVIRUS INFECTION

The natural history of CMV infection during pregnancy is complex and has not been defined completely. A schematic representation of the consequences of CMV infections during pregnancy is shown in Fig. 1. Unlike rubella and toxoplasmosis, for which intrauterine transmission occurs only as a result of primary infection acquired during pregnancy, congenital CMV infection has been shown to occur in children born to mothers who have had CMV infection prior to pregnancy (nonprimary infection) *(16,49–51)*. In fact, congenital CMV infection following a nonprimary maternal infection has been shown to be common, especially in highly immune populations *(7,16,49,51)*.

Although the pathogenesis of intrauterine transmission of CMV has not been clearly defined, maternal immune response has been shown to be a crucial determinant of the transplacental transmission of CMV. The importance of maternal immune responses is evident by the substantial protection that preconceptional immunity to CMV provides against intrauterine transmission and damaging fetal infection. Although this protection is not complete, the transmission rates decrease by about 25-fold in mothers with preconceptional immunity compared to those with primary infection *(17,20,52)*. *Primary maternal infection* is defined as an initial acquisition of CMV during pregnancy and is identified by conversion from serum antibody-negative to antibody-positive status or by the detection of circulating immunoglobulin (Ig) M antibody to CMV. However, one should be cautious with this definition because the presence of CMV IgM antibodies against CMV has been demonstrated in women with evidence of past infec-

Maternal CMV infection

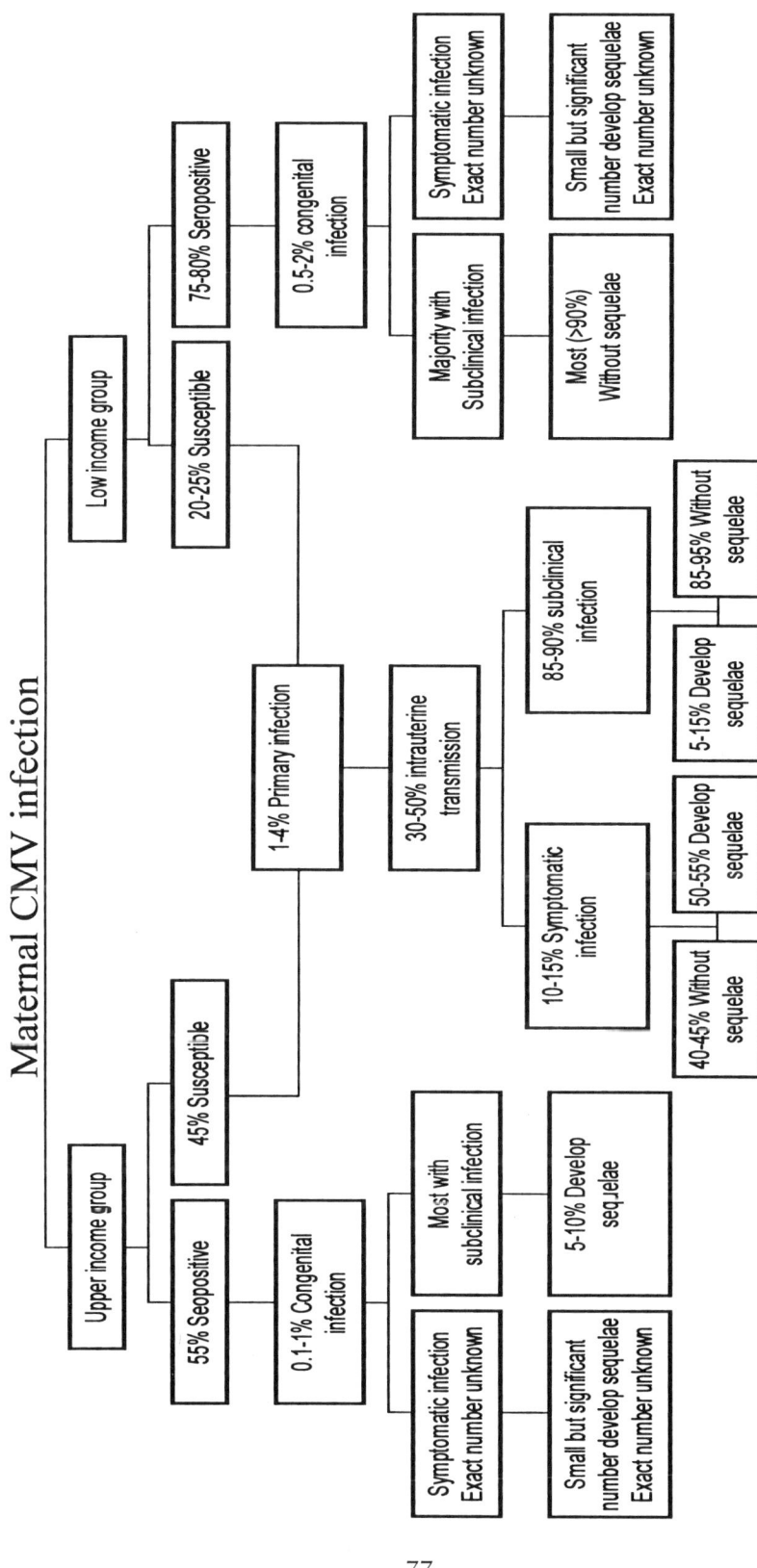

Fig. 1. Schematic representation of the consequences of CMV infection during pregnancy. (Adapted from ref. *11*.)

tion *(53,54)*. Although the occurrence of congenital CMV infection in children born to immune mothers (nonprimary maternal infection) was clearly documented, it was thought that congenitally infected children who were born to mothers with a nonprimary maternal infection rarely if ever develop long-term sequelae *(49,55)*. However, more recent data from the natural history studies of congenital CMV infection in the United States and Europe showed that a significant proportion of these children are also at risk for an adverse outcome *(56–58)*.

The mechanisms of transplacental transmission of CMV in immune women are not clearly defined. A nonprimary maternal infection could be caused by reactivation of endogenous latent CMV or reinfection with a new virus strain. The results of a study demonstrated that acquisition of a new CMV strain between pregnancies in women who were CMV seropositive at the time of the first pregnancy was associated with an increased risk of intrauterine transmission and severe fetal infection *(59)*. The results of that study also showed that the virus isolated from the infected infants was similar to the new CMV strain acquired by the mother. These women had serologic evidence of reinfection between pregnancies.

LABORATORY DIAGNOSIS OF MATERNAL INFECTION

Suspicion of CMV infection during pregnancy usually arises as a result of a mononucleosis-like illness or maternal exposure to CMV. Evaluation of these patients focuses on determination of whether the mother has primary CMV infection because the primary maternal infection is associated with intrauterine transmission in about a third to half of such cases *(17)*. Serologic tests that measure IgG antibodies against CMV are readily available. If the serologic tests for both IgG and IgM antibody are negative, the individual does not have CMV infection or has not yet seroconverted, and serology should be repeated 1–2 weeks later. If IgG antibody is positive and IgM antibody is negative, it suggests past (nonprimary) maternal CMV infection.

However, assays for IgG antibody vary in sensitivity, and the duration of IgM antibody persistence after a primary infection also varies with individual patients *(60,61)*. If both IgG and IgM antibody are positive, it is likely but not certain that the patient has experienced a recent CMV infection. However, the detection of CMV-specific IgM antibodies to diagnose primary CMV infection is somewhat difficult as the currently available assays are relatively insensitive. Most commercially available methods for the detection of CMV-IgM antibodies employ an enzyme immunoassay (EIA) format, and the estimated sensitivity varies in IgM assays, ranging between 50 and 90% in immunocompetent adults. Many different CMV antibody assays that have considerable variability in sensitivity and specificity for detection of IgM antibody are in use by diagnostic laboratories. Thus, it is essential that clinicians understand the limitations of serological diagnosis of primary maternal CMV infection.

For virus isolation, although CMV excretion is a relatively common event during and after pregnancy, studies have shown that virus isolation from urine or the cervix or both during pregnancy is not predictive of intrauterine transmission *(35,36)*.

PRENATAL DIAGNOSIS

Prenatal serological screening of pregnant women for CMV infection is not performed on a routine basis at this time because of false-positive results with IgM antibody assays. In addition, erroneous assumptions about the significance of IgG and IgM antibody levels could lead to provision of incorrect information regarding risk to the fetus. Even when a prenatal diagnosis of congenital CMV infection is accomplished, the only possible clinical recourse involves the decision of whether to terminate the pregnancy. Although CMV is a leading cause of brain disease and hearing loss in the United States, the outcome of congenital CMV infection is highly variable, thus limiting the value of prenatal diagnosis.

Studies using ultrasonography, amniocentesis, and fetal blood sampling have demonstrated that it is possible to make a prenatal diagnosis of congenital CMV infection *(62–67)*. Although the culture and PCR of the amniotic fluid for the detection of CMV or CMV DNA allows for prenatal identification of the majority of infected infants, the specificity of the PCR assay is only between 50 and 80% *(68–70)*. In addition, the sensitivity of the amniotic fluid culture or PCR is lower when the procedure is carried out before 21 weeks of gestation *(71)*. Moreover, the presence of CMV or CMV DNA in amniotic fluid and fetal blood samples does not appear to correlate with the symptomatic congenital infection or an adverse long-term outcome in infected children *(68,69)*.

Until reliable means of prenatal identification of infants at significantly increased risk for an adverse outcome are available, the value of prenatal diagnosis remains limited. To address this issue, studies have focused on the identification of the primary maternal CMV infection. This approach is based on the observation that transplacental transmission occurs about 25-fold more frequently in primary CMV infection during pregnancy than that occurring after a nonprimary maternal CMV infection. In addition, it was thought that symptomatic congenital CMV infection occurs almost exclusively following a primary maternal CMV infection *(55)*. This finding together with observations demonstrating that the majority of children with symptomatic congenital CMV infection will develop neurological sequelae has led to current vaccine development strategy aimed at preventing the primary CMV infection during pregnancy. However, more recent studies have shown that symptomatic congenital CMV infection and permanent sequelae can occur in children born to women with a nonprimary CMV infection. The exact incidence of intrauterine transmission and damaging congenital CMV infection following a nonprimary maternal infection has not yet been defined *(56,57,59)*.

Demonstration of IgG seroconversion would provide conclusive evidence for primary maternal CMV infection. However, it is not usually possible to verify seroconversion because serial serum specimens are not available in the majority of instances. As discussed in the section on maternal consequences of CMV infection, the value of IgM antibodies against CMV as a marker of primary infection is limited because of the persistence of IgM antiviral antibodies for prolonged periods after primary infection and the lack of sensitivity of commercial CMV-IgM antibody assays.

It has been suggested that determination of IgG avidity could discriminate between primary and nonprimary maternal infection. Several studies have examined the utility of antibody avidity determination in differentiation of primary from nonprimary maternal infections. These studies are based on the observation that affinity maturation of IgG antiviral antibodies is not complete until 4–5 months after the initial acquisition of CMV, and the IgG antibodies produced during the first few weeks to months following a primary infection are usually of low avidity *(72,73)*. However, the IgG avidity testing may not permit a clear identification of a primary infection in about 15% of the cases *(65)*. In addition, at the current time there are no reliable commercial IgG avidity assays available in the United States.

An enzyme immunoassay to determine antibodies against the antigenic domain 2 of the major glycoprotein B of CMV is under development and testing in Europe, and the early results are promising *(74,75)*. Several publications from the group of Italian investigators led by Landini proposed a series of prenatal diagnostic steps to identify infants with symptomatic congenital CMV infection. These investigators utilized a commercial EIA kit to determine the avidity of CMV-IgG antibodies (cytomegalovirus IgG avidity EIA WELL; Radim, Rome, Italy) to categorize maternal infection in IgG antibody-positive women as primary or nonprimary *(69)*. Women who were classified as having a primary maternal infection were offered amniocentesis between 21 and 25 weeks of gestation. The amniotic fluid was subjected to virus isolation by cell culture and the presence of viral DNA by PCR. The samples that were PCR positive were further analyzed for the amount of CMV DNA using a commercial quantitative PCR kit. Of the 110 women identified to have a primary infection, 57 underwent amniocentesis. The qualitative PCR had a sensitivity of 100% and specificity of 73%. The positive predictive value of a positive PCR was only 50%. The results of the quantitative PCR revealed that the presence of at least 10^3 genomic equivalents (ge) per milliliter of amniotic fluid had a sensitivity of 75% and specificity of 100%. It was also reported that a threshold of at least 10^5 ge/mL identified all but one of eight fetuses likely to have symptomatic infection. However, the exact sensitivity and specificity of the quantitative PCR for the prenatal identification of symptomatic congenital CMV infection was difficult to determine because the authors included both uninfected infants and those with asymptomatic infection in the comparison group *(69)*. Furthermore, one should be cautious about generalizing the results of the study because of the smaller number of infected children with a congenital CMV infection.

Amniotic fluid examination for the presence of CMV has been shown to be unreliable prior to 21–22 weeks of gestation *(71,76)*. Currently, there are very few options for intervention even if an accurate prenatal diagnosis of symptomatic congenital CMV infection is made when the determination is made after 24 weeks of gestation. Although the intrauterine transmission rate following a primary CMV infection during pregnancy is between 30 and 50%, the majority of infected infants develop normally. Furthermore, studies have demonstrated that symptomatic infection can occur in children born to women who were CMV seropositive prior to pregnancy, and these infected children of immune mothers are also at risk for developing neurological damage. In addition, amniocentesis between 21 and 25 weeks of gestation and the option of pregnancy termination may not be practical in the United States.

CONGENITAL INFECTION

Clinical Findings

Of the estimated 40,000 children born each year in the United States with congenital CMV infection, about 10–15% exhibit clinical findings suggestive of congenital infection at birth (symptomatic infection) *(11,12)*. It was thought that clinically apparent or symptomatic congenital CMV occurs almost exclusively following a primary CMV

Table 2
**Clinical and Laboratory Findings in Infants
With Symptomatic Congenital CMV Infection**

Finding	% With abnormality
Clinical abnormality	
Petechiae	76
Jaundice	67
Hepatosplenomegaly	60
Microcephaly	53
Small for gestational age	50
Chorioretinitis/optic atrophy	20
Purpura	13
Seizures	7
Laboratory abnormality	
Elevated transaminases (serum aspartate aminotransferase >80 U/L)	83
Conjugated hyperbilirubinemia (>2 mg/dL)	81
Thrombocytopenia ($<100 \times 10^3/mm^3$)	77
Elevated CSF protein (<120 mg/dL)	46

Modified from ref. *77*.

infection *(11,55)*. However, more recent data from natural history studies of congenital CMV infection from the United States and Europe have documented that symptomatic infection occurs in children born to immune mothers more frequently than has previously been recognized *(56,57)*. The typical findings that have been associated with generalized cytomegalic inclusion disease are characterized by multiorgan disease with prominent involvement of the reticuloendothelial system and CNS; however, around half of symptomatic infants have mild or atypical findings.

The frequency of various clinical and laboratory findings in 106 neonates with symptomatic congenital CMV infection is shown in Table 2. Petechiae, jaundice, and hepatosplenomegaly are the most frequently noted abnormalities and are present in approx 75% of symptomatic neonates *(77)*. In addition, half the infants are microcephalic and small for gestational age, and about a third are born prematurely, suggestive of significant prenatal insult. About two-thirds of symptomatic infants have clinical neurological abnormalities such as microcephaly, lethargy/hypotonia, poor suck, or seizures. Of the neonates who had ophthalmologic and audiologic assessments, chorioretinitis or optic atrophy was noted in 20% and an abnormal hearing screen in about half the children *(77)*. Other less-frequent findings include hydrocephalus, pneumonitis, and hemolytic anemia. About 10% of infants with symptomatic congenital CMV infection die during early infancy because of multiorgan disease with severe hepatic dysfunction, bleeding diathesis, and secondary bacterial infections *(77)*.

Laboratory Findings

The laboratory abnormalities seen in infants with symptomatic congenital CMV infection include (in decreasing order of frequency) elevated serum aspartate aminotransferase (>80 IU/L), conjugated hyperbilirubinemia (direct bilirubin >2 mg/dL), thrombocytopenia (<100,000/mm^3), atypical lymphocytosis, hemolytic anemia, and elevated cerebrospinal (CSF) fluid protein (>120 mg/dL). Elevations of serum transaminases and direct bilirubin are present in the immediate newborn period and peak during the second week of life *(77)*. However, hyperbilirubinemia and liver function abnormalities often persist beyond the neonatal period, resolving over a few months *(77)*. Thus, invasive procedures such as liver biopsy are not justified on the basis of persistent liver function abnormalities in infants with symptomatic congenital CMV infection. Thrombocytopenia is noted in the first few days of life in the majority of infants. The platelet count nadir occurs in the second week of life and normalizes in most patients by the third week of life. CSF abnormalities, especially elevated protein (>120 mg/dL) appear to correlate with clinical indicators of CNS damage *(78)*. About 70% of infants with symptomatic congenital CMV infection have an abnormal neonatal cranial computed tomographic scan; intracerebral calcifications are the most frequent finding *(78)*. Other less frequently noted computed tomographic scan findings include ventricular dilation, cortical atrophy, white matter abnormalities, and migration abnormalities.

Diagnosis of Congenital Infection

Congenital CMV infection is proven by isolation of virus from body fluids during the first 3 weeks of life. Urine and saliva (mouth swab) are equally useful for this purpose, although the latter is more easily collected. As newborns shed large amounts of virus, the detection of CMV in saliva and urine of newborns can be readily accomplished. Traditional virus isolation in tissue culture is the standard against which other methods are evaluated. Centrifugation-enhanced, rapid techniques (shell vial or Detection of Early Antigen Fluorescent Foci) are similar in sensitivity and specificity to standard viral isolation procedures; however, the rapid methods use monoclonal antibody to CMV immediate early antigens to detect infected tissue culture cells and provide results in 24 hours compared with several days to 2 weeks for tissue culture *(79–81)*.

The detection of CMV DNA in urine or saliva by PCR and other methods can also be used, but there is less experience with these methods and less certainty about their sensitivity and specificity *(82)*. Viremia is not present in all newborn infants with congenital CMV infection; therefore detection of virus in peripheral blood should not be relied upon to diagnose congenital infection *(83)*. Detection of IgM antibody to CMV is not as reliable as viral isolation and is not recommended for the diagnosis of congenital infection.

The age of the patient at the time of sample collection for detection of CMV is of some importance. Neonates who acquire CMV during birth or from breast milk shed virus after 3 weeks of age. Thus, detection of CMV in urine or saliva after 3 weeks of age is not unequivocal proof of CMV acquisition *in utero*.

REFERENCES

1. Weller TH. The cytomegaloviruses: ubiquitous agents with protean clinical manifestations. N Engl J Med 1971;285:203–214.
2. Smith J, DeHavern E. Herpes simplex and human cytomegalovirus replication in WI-38 cells. I. Sequence of viral replication. J Virol 1978;12:919–930.
3. Kilpatrick BA, Huang ES. Human cytomegalovirus genome: partial denaturation map and organization of genome sequences. J Virol 1977;24:261–276.

4. Lakeman A, Osborn JE. Size and infectivity of DNA from human and murine cytomegalovirus. J Virol 1979;30:414–416.
5. Sarov I, Abady I. The morphogenesis of human cytomegalovirus. Isolation and polypeptide characterization of cytomegalovirus and dense bodies. Virology 1975;66:464–473.
6. Honess RW, Roizman B. Regulation of herpesvirus macromolecular synthesis. I. Cascade regulation of the synthesis of three groups of viral proteins. J Virol 1974;14:8–19.
7. Schopfer K, Lauber E, Krech U. Congenital cytomegalovirus infection in newborn infants of mothers infected before pregnancy. Arch Dis Child 1978;53:536–539.
8. Fowler KB, Pass RF. Cytomegalovirus infection as a cause of hearing loss among children. Am J Public Health 1995;85:734.
9. Larke RBP, Wheatley E, saigal S, Chemesky MA. Congenital cytomegalovirus infection in an urban Canadian community. J Infect Dis 1980;142:647–653.
10. Sohn YM, Park KI, Lee C, Han DG, Lee WY. Congenital cytomegalovirus infection in Korean population with very high prevalence of maternal immunity. J Kor Med Sci 1992;7:47–51.
11. Stagno S. Cytomegalovirus. In: Remington JS, Klein JO, eds. Infectious Diseases of the Fetus and Newborn Infant, 4th ed. Philadelphia: Saunders, 1995:312–353.
12. Demmler GJ. Infectious Diseases Society of America and Centers for Disease Control. Summary of a workshop on surveillance for congenital cytomegalovirus disease. Rev Infect Dis 1991;13:315–329.
13. Harris S, Ahlfors K, Ivarsson S, Lemmark B, Svanberg L. Congenital cytomegalovirus infection and sensorineural hearing loss. Ear Hear 1984;5:352–355.
14. Hicks T, Fowler K, Richardson M, Dahle A, Adams L, Pass R. Congenital cytomegalovirus infection and neonatal auditory screening. J Pediatr 1993;123:779–782.
15. Andersen H, Brostrom K, Hansen HB, et al. A prospective study on the incidence and significance of congenital cytomegalovirus infection. Acta Paediatr Scand 1979;68(3):329–336.
16. Peckham CS, Chin KS, Coleman JC, Henderson K, Hurley R, Preece PM. Cytomegalovirus infection in pregnancy: preliminary findings from a prospective study. Lancet 1983;1:1352–1355.
17. Stagno S, Pass RF, Cloud G, et al. Primary cytomegalovirus infection in pregnancy. Incidence, transmission to fetus, and clinical outcome. JAMA 1986;256:1904–1908.
18. Pannuti CS, Vilas Boas LS, Angelo MJ, et al. Cytomegalovirus mononucleosis in children and adults: differences in clinical presentation. Scand J Infect Dis 1985;17:153–156.
19. Balcarek KB, Bagley R, Cloud GA, Pass RF. Cytomegalovirus infection among employees of a children's hospital; no evidence for increased risk associated with patient care. JAMA 1990;263:840–844.
20. Griffiths PD, Baboonian C. A prospective study of primary cytomegalovirus infection during pregnancy: final report. Br J Obstet Gynaecol 1984;91:307–315.
21. Chandler SH, Holmes KK, Wentworth BB, et al. The epidemiology of cytomegaloviral infection in women attending a sexually transmitted disease clinic. J Infect Dis 1985;152:597–605.
22. Sohn YM, Oh MK, Balcarek KB, Cloud GA, Pass RF. Cytomegalovirus infection in sexually active adolescents. J Infect Dis 1991;163:460–463.
23. Fowler KB, Pass RF. Sexually transmitted diseases in mothers of neonates with congenital cytomegalovirus infection. J Infect Dis 1991;164:259–264.
24. Hutto SC, Ricks R, Gravie M, Pass RF. Epidemiology of cytomegalovirus infections in young children: day care vs home care. Pediatr Infect Dis 1985;4:149–152.
25. Pass RF, Hutto C, Lyon MD, Cloud G. Increased rate of cytomegalovirus infection among day care center workers. Pediatr Infect Dis J 1990; 9:465–470.
26. Adler SP. Cytomegalovirus and child day care. Evidence for an increased infection rate among day-care workers. N Engl J Med 1989;321:1290–1296.
27. Pass RF, Little EA, Stagno S, Britt WJ, Alford CA. Young children as a probable source of maternal and congenital cytomegalovirus infection. N Engl J Med 1987;316:1366–1370.

28. Murph JR, Bale JF Jr, Murray JC, stinski MF, Perlman S. Cytomegalovirus transmission in a midwest day care center: possible relationship to child care practices. J Pediatr 1986;109:35–39.

29. Stagno S, Pass RF, Dworsky ME, et al. Congenital cytomegalovirus infection: the relative importance of primary and recurrent maternal infection. N Engl J Med 1982;306:945–949.

30. Fowler KB, Stagno S, Pass RF. Maternal age and congenital cytomegalovirus infection: screening of two diverse newborn populations, 1980–1990. J Infect Dis 1993;168:552–556.

31. Preece PM, Tookey P, Ades A, Peckham CS. Congenital cytomegalovirus infection: predisposing maternal factors. J Epidemiol Community Health 1986;40:205–209.

32. Fowler KB, Stagno S, Pass RF. Rates of congenital cytomegalovirus infection based on newborn screening in two populations over an 11 year interval. Pediatr Res 1991;29:90A.

33. Reynolds DW, Stagno S, Hosty TS, Tiller M, Alford CA Jr. Maternal cytomegalovirus excretion and perinatal infection. N Engl J Med 1973;289:1–5.

34. Knox GE, Pass RF, Reynolds DW, Stagno S, Alford CA. Comparative prevalence of subclinical cytomegalovirus and herpes simplex virus infections in the genital and urinary tracts of low income, urban females. J Infect Dis 1979;140:419–422.

35. Pass RF, Stagno S, Dworsky ME, Smith RJ, Alford CA. Excretion of cytomegalovirus in mothers: observation after delivery of congenitally infected and normal infants. J Infect Dis 1982;146:1–6.

36. Shen CY, Chang SF, Yen MS, Ng HT, Huang ES, Wu CW. Cytomegalovirus excretion in pregnant and nonpregnant women. J Clin Microbiol 1993;31:1635–1636.

37. Stagno S, Reynolds D, Tsiantos A, et al. Cervical cytomegalovirus excretion in pregnant and nonpregnant women: suppression in early gestation. J Infect Dis 1975;131:522–527.

38. Stagno S, Reynolds D, Pass RF, Alford CA. Breast milk and the risk of cytomegalovirus infection. N Engl J Med 1980;302:1073–1076.

39. Ahlfors K, Ivarsson SA. Cytomegalovirus in breast milk of Swedish milk donors. Scand J Infect Dis 1985;17:11.

40. Dworsky M, Yow M, Stagno S, Pass RF, Alford CA. Cytomegalovirus infection of breast milk and transmission in infancy. Pediatrics 1983;72:295–299.

41. Yeager AS, Grumet FC, Hafleigh EB, Arvin AM, Bradley JS, Prober CG. Prevention of transfusion-acquired cytomegalovirus infections in newborn infants. J Pediatr 1981;98:281–287.

42. Ho M., ed. Cytomegalovirus Biology and Infection. New York: Plenum Press, 1991.

43. de Graan-Hentzen YC, Gratama JW, Mudde GC, et al. Prevention of primary cytomegalovirus infection in patients with hematologic malignancies by intensive white cell depletion of blood products. Transfusion 1989;29:757–760.

44. Gilbert GL, Hayes K, Hudson IL, James J. Prevention of transfusion-acquired cytomegalovirus infection in infants by blood filtration to remove leucocytes. Lancet 1989;1:1228–1231.

45. Lang DJ, Kummer JF. Cytomegalovirus in semen: observations in selected populations. J Infect Dis 1975;132:472–473.

46. Collier AC, Meyers JD, Corey L, Murphy VL, Roberts PL, Handsfield HH. Cytomegalovirus infection in homosexual men. Relationship to sexual practices, antibody to human immunodeficiency virus, and cell-mediated immunity. Am J Med 1987;23:593–601.

47. American Fertility Society. New guidelines for the use of semen donor insemination. Fertil Steril 1990;53(S1):1–7.

48. Balfour CL, Balfour HH. Cytomegalovirus is not an occupational risk for nurses in renal transplant and neonatal units. JAMA 1986;256:1909–1914.

49. Stagno S, Reynolds DW, Huang ES, Thames SC, Smith RJ, Alford CA. Congenital cytomegalovirus infection: occurrence in an immune population. N Engl J Med 1977;296:1254–1258.

50. Morris DJ, Sims D, Chiswick M, Das VK, Newton VE. Symptomatic congenital cytomegalovirus infection after maternal recurrent infection. Pediatr Infect Dis J 1994;13:61–64.

51. Ahlfors K, Ivarsson SA, Harris S, et al. Congenital cytomegalovirus infection and disease in Sweden and the relative importance of primary and secondary maternal infections. Scand J Infect Dis 1984;16:129–137.
52. Medearis DN. CMV immunity: imperfect but protective. N Engl J Med 1982;306:985–986.
53. Griffiths PD, Stagno S, Pass RF, Smith RJ, Alford CA Jr. Infection with cytomegalovirus during pregnancy: specific IgM antibodies as a marker of recent primary infection. J Infect Dis 1982;145:647–653.
54. McVoy MA, Adler SP. Immunologic evidence for frequent age-related cytomegalovirus reactivation in seropositive immunocompetent individuals. J Infect Dis 1989;160:1–10.
55. Fowler KB, Stagno S, Pass RF, Britt WJ, Boll TJ, Alford CA. The outcome of congenital cytomegalovirus infection in relation to maternal antibody status. N Engl J Med 1992;326:663–667.
56. Boppana SB, Fowler KB, Britt WJ, Stagno S, Pass RF. Symptomatic congenital cytomegalovirus infection in infants born to mothers with preexisting immunity to cytomegalovirus. Pediatrics 1999;104:55–60.
57. Ahlfors K, Ivarsson SA, Harris S. Report on a long-term study of maternal and congenital cytomegalovirus infection in Sweden. Review of prospective studies available in the literature. Scand J Infect Dis 1999;31:443–457.
58. Casteels A, Naessens A, Gordts F, De Catte L, Bougatef A, Foulon W. Neonatal screening for congenital cytomegalovirus infections. J Perinat Med 1999;27:116–121.
59. Boppana S, Rivera LB, Fowler KB, Mach M, Britt WJ. Intrauterine transmission of cytomegalovirus to infants of women with preconceptional immunity. N Engl J Med 2001;344:1366–1371.
60. Stagno S, Tinker MK, Elrod C, Fuccillo DA, Cloud G, O'Beirne AJ. Immunoglobulin M antibodies detected by enzyme-linked immunosorbent assay and radioimmunoassay in the diagnosis of cytomegalovirus infections in pregnant women and newborn infants. J Clin Microbiol 1985;21:930–935.
61. Kangro HO, Booth JC, Bakir TM, Tryhom Y, Sutherland S. Detection of IgM antibodies against cytomegalovirus: comparison of two radioimmunoassays, enzyme-linked immunosorbent assay and immunofluorescent antibody test. J Med Virol 1984;14:73–80.
62. Hohlfeld P, Vial Y, Maillard-Brignon C, Vaudaux B, Fawer CL. Cytomegalovirus fetal infection: Prenatal diagnosis. Obstet Gynecol 1991;78:615–618.
63. Lamy ME, Mulongo KN, Gadisseux JF, Lyon G, Gaudy V, Van Lierde M. Prenatal diagnosis of fetal cytomegalovirus infection. Am J Obstet Gynecol 1992;166:91–94.
64. Donner C, Liesnard C, Content J, Busine A, Aderca J, Rodesch F. Prenatal diagnosis of 52 pregnancies at risk for congenital cytomegalovirus infection. Obstet Gynecol 1993;82:481–486.
65. Lazzarotto T, Spezzacatena P, Varani S, et al. Anticytomegalovirus (anti-CMV) immunoglobulin G avidity in identification of pregnant women at risk of transmitting congenital CMV infection. Clin Diag Lab Immunol 1999;6:127–129.
66. Bodeus M, Hubinont C, Bernard P, Bouckaert A, Thomas K, Goubau P. Prenatal diagnosis of human cytomegalovirus by culture and polymerase chain reaction: 98 pregnancies leading to congenital infection. Prenatal Diagn 1999;19:314–317.
67. Liesnard C, Donner C, Brancart F, Gosselin F, Delforge ML, Rodesch F. Prenatal diagnosis of congenital cytomegalovirus infection: prospective study of 237 pregnancies at risk. Obstet Gynecol 2000;95:881–888.
68. Lipitz S, Yagel S, Shalev E, Achiron R, Mashiach S, Schiff E. Prenatal diagnosis of fetal primary infection. Obstet Gynecol, 1997;89:763–767.
69. Lazzarotto T, Varani S, Guerra B, Nicolosi A, Lanari M, Landini MP. Prenatal indicators of congenital cytomegalovirus infection. J Pediatr 2000;137:90–95.
70. Revello MG, Zavattoni M, Furione M, Baldanti F, Gerna G. Quantification of human cytomegalovirus DNA in amniotic fluid of mothers of congenitally infected fetuses. J Clin Microbiol 1999;37:3350–3352.

71. Donner C, Liesnard C, Brancart F, Rodesch F. Accuracy of amniotic fluid testing before 21 weeks' gestation in prenatal diagnosis of congenital cytomegalovirus infection. Prenatal Diagn 1994;14:1055–1059.
72. Grangeot-Keros L, Simon B, Audibert F, Vial M. Should we routinely screen for cytomegalovirus antibody during pregnancy? Intervirology 1998;41:158–162.
73. Lazzarotto T, Varani S, Spezzacatena P, et al. Delayed acquisition of high-avidity anticytomegalovirus antibody is correlated with prolonged antigenemia in solid organ transplant recipients. J Infect Dis 1998;178:1145–1149.
74. Schoppel K, Kropff B, Schmidt C, Vornhagen R, Mach M. The humoral immune response against human cytomegalovirus is characterized by a delayed synthesis of glycoprotein-specific antibodies. J Infect Dis 1997;175:533–544.
75. Rothe M, Hemprecht K, Lang D, et al. Diagnostic differentiation of primary versus secondary/recurrent infection of human cytomegalovirus by using a recombinant gB ELISA. Biotest Bull 2000;6:147–158.
76. Mulongo K, Lamy M, Van Lierde M. Requirements for diagnosis of prenatal cytomegalovirus infection by amniotic fluid culture. Clin Diagn Lab Immunol 1995;4:231–238.
77. Boppana SB, Fowler KB, Pass RF, Britt WJ, Stagno S, Alford CA. Newborn findings and outcome in children with symptomatic congenital CMV infection. Pediatr Res 1992;31:158A.
78. Boppana SB, Fowler KB, Vaid Y, et al. Neuroradiographic findings in the newborn period and long-term outcome in children with symptomatic congenital cytomegalovirus infection. Pediatrics 1997;99:409–414.
79. Balcarek KB, Warren W, Smith RJ, Lyon MD, Pass RF. Neonatal screening for congenital cytomegalovirus infection by detection of virus in saliva. J Infect Dis 1993;167:1433–1436.
80. Gleaves CA, Smith TF, Shuster EA, Pearson GR. Rapid detection of cytomegalovirus in MRC-5 cells inoculated with urine specimens by using low-speed centrifugation and monoclonal antibody to an early antigen. J Clin Microbiol 1984;19:917–919.
81. Boppana SB, Smith RJ, Stagno S, Britt WJ. Evaluation of a microtiter plate fluorescent antibody assay for rapid detection of human cytomegalovirus infections. J Clin Microbiol 1992;30:721–723.
82. Pass RF. Epidemiology and transmission of cytomegalovirus infection. J Infect Dis 1985;152:243–248.
83. Balcarek KB, Oh MK, Pass RF. Maternal viremia and congenital CMV infection. In: Michelson S, Plotkin SA, eds. Multidisciplinary Approach to Understanding Cytomegalovirus Disease. New York: Excerpta Medica, 1993:169–173.

7

Epstein-Barr Virus

Suresh B. Boppana

INTRODUCTION

Epstein-Barr virus (EBV) is a ubiquitous human herpesvirus. Infection with EBV is common, worldwide in distribution, and largely subclinical in early childhood. EBV has been established as the causative agent of heterophile-positive mononucleosis, which occurs most frequently in late adolescence or early adulthood. In addition, seroepidemologic data have suggested that EBV also plays an etiological role in African Burkitt's lymphoma and nasopharyngeal carcinoma.

Laboratory diagnosis of EBV infections is based primarily on serology. The detection of heterophile antibodies in patients with infectious mononucleosis is considered diagnostic of a primary EBV infection. EBV-specific serology can be used in those with a negative heterophile antibody test. Antibodies against several EBV antigens are produced at different times during the course of an infection. Typically, antibodies to EBV viral capsid antigen (VCA) and early antigen (EA) appear during the acute phase of the infection; those against EBV nuclear antigen develop weeks to months later (1). Primary infections can be diagnosed by detecting immunoglobulin (Ig) M antibodies against VCA. If no IgM antibodies are detected, then the presence of IgG antibodies to VCA and EA in the absence of antibodies against EBV nuclear antigen is strongly suggestive of either a primary or postacute infection. Although standard tissue culture methods are not helpful in recovering EBV, the virus can be detected by its ability to transform B lymphocytes into persistent lymphoblastoid cell lines. However, these methods are not routinely available in most clinical laboratories. Rapid diagnostic methods based on deoxyribonucleic acid (DNA) hybridization, monoclonal antibody techniques, or polymerase chain reaction (PCR) have also been developed.

MATERNAL INFECTION

EBV infections are very common during childhood. Seroepidemiologic studies of pregnant women have shown that 95% or more have evidence of prior EBV infection (2,3). Primary EBV infection during pregnancy is uncommon. Of the more than 12,000 pregnant women evaluated, EBV seroconversion was documented in only 3 women (4). Prospective follow-up studies involving fewer women failed to observe seroconversion during pregnancy (3,5). In a study of more than 2600 seropositive preg-

From: *Infectious Disease: Congenital and Perinatal Infections: A Concise Guide to Diagnosis*
Edited by: C. Hutto © Humana Press Inc., Totowa, NJ

nant women tested during the first trimester, Icart and Didier noted a serologic profile of primary EBV infection in 6 (0.2%) women *(6)*. The seroconversion estimate is higher when only seronegative susceptible women were considered *(7)*. Reactivation of latent EBV infection during pregnancy as suggested by changes in anti-EBV antibody profiles and oropharyngeal virus shedding appears to be more common than seroconversion *(8,9)*. It has been suggested that reactivation of EBV infection during pregnancy does not pose any risks to the fetus.

CONGENITAL AND PERINATAL INFECTION

Anecdotal reports have suggested that embryopathy may occur in very rare cases of primary maternal EBV infection in early gestation *(9,10)*. However, the exact risk of congenital infection with EBV is not known. Various congenital defects have been described in the few reported infants with documented congenital EBV infection or whose mothers had infectious mononucleosis during pregnancy *(11)*. No specific pattern has been recognized. Reported abnormalities include micrognathia, congenital heart disease, cataract, microphthalmia, hip dysplasia, biliary atresia, and central nervous system abnormalities. Other studies of women with infectious mononucleosis or primary asymptomatic EBV infection in early pregnancy failed to document serologic or virologic evidence of EBV infection in their offspring *(7)*. Although intrauterine transmission of EBV has been documented in a study using PCR, none of infants with positive PCR had clinical abnormalities *(12)*. Maternal human immunodeficiency virus infection was not shown to increase the risk of intrauterine transmission of EBV.

The possibility of EBV acquisition by neonates during passage through the birth canal has been raised by the results of a study in which cervical shedding of EBV was demonstrated in 5 out of 28 (18%) seropositive women *(13)*. However, no clear data are available regarding the incidence of perinatal transmission of EBV.

The diagnosis of congenital EBV infection can be established serologically or by attempting virus identification using lymphocyte transformation assays. PCR has been used for the detection of EBV DNA in infants, and this technique could become more useful in the diagnosis of congenital EBV infection. However, the sensitivity and specificity of the PCR assay for the diagnosis of intrauterine transmission of EBV has not been well defined. In addition, the PCR assay has not yet been standardized and thus is not available for routine use in clinical laboratories.

REFERENCES

1. Sumaya C. Epstein-Barr virus serologic testing: diagnostic indications and interpretations. Pediatr Infect Dis 1986;5:337–342.
2. Fleisher G, Bolognese R. Seroepidemiology of Epstein-Barr virus in pregnant women. J Infect Dis 1982;145:537–541.
3. Hunter K, Stagno S, Capps E, Smith RJ. Prenatal screening of pregnant women for infections caused by cytomegalovirus, Epstein-Barr virus, herpesvirus, rubella, *Toxoplasma gondii*. Am J Obstet Gynecol 1983;145:269–273.
4. Stagno S, Whitley R. Herpesvirus infection of pregnancy. Part I. Cytomegalovirus and Epstein-Barr virus infections. N Engl J Med 1985;313:1270–1240.
5. Le C, Chang S, Lipson M. Epstein-Barr virus infections during pregnancy: A prospective study and review of the literature. Am J Dis Child 1983;137:466–468.

6. Icart J, Didier J. Infections due to Epstein-Barr virus during pregnancy. J Infect Dis 1981;143:499–500.

7. Fleisher G, Bolognese R. Epstein-Barr virus infections in pregnancy: a prospective study. J Pediatr 1984;104:374–379.

8. Fleisher G, Bolognese R. Persistent Epstein-Barr virus infections and pregnancy. J Infect Dis 1983;147:982.

9. Costa S, Barrasso R, Terzano P, Zerbini M, Carpi C, Musiani M. Detection of active Epstein-Barr infection in pregnant women. Eur J Clin Microbiol 1985;4:335–336.

10. Joncas J, Alfieri C, Leyritz-Wills M, et al. Simultaneous congenital infection with Epstein-Barr virus and cytomegalovirus. N Engl J Med 1981;204:1399–1403.

11. Ornoy A, Dudai M, Sadovsky E. Placental and fetal pathology in infectious mononucleosis. A possible indicator of Epstein-Barr virus teratogenicity. Diagn Gynecol Obstet 1982;4:11–16.

12. Meyohas MC, Marechal V, Desire N, Bouillie J, Frotter J, Nicolas JC. Study of mother-to-child Epstein-Barr virus transmission by means of nested PCRs. J Virol 1996;70:6816–6819.

13. Sixbey J, Lemon S, Pagano J. A second site for Epstein-Barr virus shedding: the uterine cervix. Lancet 1986;2:1122–1124.

8

Varicella-Zoster Virus

Anne A. Gershon

INTRODUCTION

Varicella-zoster virus (VZV) is one of the eight herpesviruses that infects humans. The virus causes two diseases, varicella (chickenpox) and zoster (shingles) *(1)*. Varicella is primarily an illness of children, although as many as 5% of adults in the United States may be susceptible. Zoster is caused by reactivation of latent VZV infection in sensory ganglia, which resulted during the attack of varicella, usually years to decades previously. VZV is able to cause a persistent infection in sensory ganglia without harm, expressing only 5 of its 70 gene products *(2)*. In the setting of a low cell-mediated immune response to VZV, however, full gene expression can occur, and infectious virus may be formed within ganglia and transferred down the axon to the skin *(1)*. Zoster occurs in about 15% of people over their lifetime. It characteristically occurs despite the presence of high titers of antibodies to VZV. Little more is understood about reactivation of VZV; it occurs most commonly in elderly and immunocompromised populations. Reasons for its development in otherwise healthy young persons are not fully understood, but fortunately it is a rather uncommon occurrence.

Varicella

VZV is an enveloped deoxyribonucleic acid (DNA) virus that is closely related to herpes simplex viruses, although immunity to one virus does not confer immunity to the other. The primary infection, varicella, is an illness that typically presents with generalized skin rash and fever *(1)*. Subclinical infection occurs in about 5% of individuals. Children usually have no prodromal symptoms, although a prodrome of malaise and fever often occurs in adults. The skin rash is vesicular, with most lesions on the face, scalp, and trunk. Fewer lesions are present on the extremities. The rash is characteristically pruritic. The rash rapidly progresses from maculopapular lesions to vesicles, pustules, and crusts. The illness normally evolves over about 5 days, with a decrease in fever beginning to occur after several days. Following onset of rash, specific antibodies and cellular immunity develop. The antibodies persist for the lifetime of the individual, but the cell-mediated immune response falls off during middle age. The diagnosis of varicella can usually be made on clinical grounds because of the characteristic rash. Although there may have been a known exposure to someone with varicella or zoster, it is not uncommon for an individual to develop varicella with no

From: *Infectious Disease: Congenital and Perinatal Infections: A Concise Guide to Diagnosis*
Edited by: C. Hutto © Humana Press Inc., Totowa, NJ

recognized history of exposure. Although varicella is usually a mild infection in children, it may be severe or fatal in adults.

Zoster

Zoster is caused by reactivation of latent VZV *(1)*. It is associated with a unilateral rash, usually localized to the trunk or face, although the rash may involve an extremity. The lesions are vesicular and full of infectious virus, and they tend to coalesce. The individual is considered contagious to varicella susceptibles until the skin lesions have dried. Moist lesions may be present for days to weeks in immunocompromised patients with zoster. Pain is often a major complaint rather than itching. Zoster seems to increase in severity with increasing age; young individuals rarely have a severe form of the illness. Zoster is essentially not a fatal illness in otherwise healthy individuals.

Varicella Vaccine and Its Impact

Because of the licensure and widespread use of a live attenuated varicella vaccine (Oka strain) in 1995, in the United States there is now evidence for a decrease in incidence of clinical varicella in our country *(3)*. Approximately half of the states now require evidence of varicella immunization before a child can enter day care or primary school. The goal of the Centers for Disease Control and Prevention (CDC) is that, by the year 2010, more than 90% of children between the ages of 1 and 3 years will have received varicella vaccine. Based on computer modeling, it is also anticipated that, although the age when varicella is most frequent may become during adolescence and young adulthood, there will be fewer cases in these age groups than currently occur as long as high levels of immunization are achieved *(4)*.

Varicella vaccine is recommended for all healthy susceptible individuals in the United States and Canada who are older than 1 year old. Children younger than age 13 years are given one dose of vaccine, and those who are older than 13 years are given two doses 4–8 weeks apart *(1)*. The vaccine has proven to be safe and well tolerated in prelicensure and postlicensure studies *(5,6)*. Although about 5% of healthy vaccinees develop a mild vaccine-associated rash, transmission of the vaccine virus to others from healthy vaccinees has been recorded only three times. Transmission only occurs when the vaccinee manifests a rash. Varicella vaccine is not recommended for pregnant women or immunocompromised persons. It is currently recommended, however, that susceptible contacts of such individuals who are also susceptible to varicella be immunized. This is based on the very low probability of transmission of vaccine virus to others, lack of evidence that the vaccine virus can cause the congenital varicella syndrome (*see* Congenital Varicella Syndrome section), and the current continued circulation of the wild-type virus, particularly in schools, hospitals, and other institutions where susceptibles regularly gather.

TIMING AND ROUTES OF TRANSMISSION

The usual incubation period for varicella is 14 days, with extremes of 10–28 days *(1)*. The virus is transmitted by the airborne route; its source is thought to be the respiratory tract and skin of an infected individual. Although the virus spreads within the body mainly by cell-to-cell contact, cell-free virus is required for transmission from one patient to another. The skin blisters of varicella and zoster are full of cell-free infectious virus. Fortunately, the virus is rather labile, so it is not spread on clothing or other fomites. Transmission requires direct contact with an infected individual in the early stages of illness. Persons with zoster are capable of transmitting VZV to varicella susceptibles, although zoster patients are thought to be less infectious than varicella patients. Persons who have had varicella who are exposed to patients with VZV infections may have a boost in immunity to VZV; in one study, about one-third of parents exposed to their children with varicella had evidence of an increase in immunity. Because VZV spreads within the individual as an intracellular pathogen, the cell-mediated immune response is critical in recovery from the disease.

RISK OF MATERNAL INFECTION DURING PREGNANCY

Varicella can be an extremely serious disease in pregnant women. Fortunately, widespread use of vaccine is likely to decrease the overall incidence of varicella, including during pregnancy, because of individual and herd immunity. Eventually, it is hoped that widespread immunization of children will lead to only rare susceptibility during the childbearing years, as well as little circulation of the wild-type virus. This situation would be projected to make varicella in pregnancy extremely rare, as has occurred with rubella in pregnant women because of routine administration of rubella vaccine.

In the prevaccine era in the United States, it was estimated that there were 240–2400 annual cases of varicella in pregnant women (7). This is only an estimate because varicella is not a reportable disease nationally. The usual scenario is that if a pregnant woman contracts varicella, it is usually transmitted from her children, who were exposed to other children with chickenpox at school or day care. In the prevaccine era, the annual rate of varicella in children under the age of 10 years was 10% per year. Varicella is highly contagious, with an attack rate approaching 90% following a household exposure to the illness. Because varicella is so contagious in families, it makes the likelihood of contracting varicella for a susceptible woman with a young child attending school on the order of 5% during her pregnancy. The literature is replete with cases of severe varicella in pregnant women that proved fatal or near-fatal. Varicella is estimated to be 25 times more likely to be severe in adults than in children. There is thought to be an even greater risk associated with pregnancy, particularly during the third trimester. Presumably, this is caused by maternal immunosuppression, which is most intense during this period (7).

Most adults born in the continental United States are immune to varicella, even if they believe themselves to be susceptible. Individuals born in countries with tropical climates, however, are often susceptible to varicella, particularly if they moved into an area with a temperate climate as an adult (8). Therefore, it is likely that women who were born in the Caribbean, the Philippines, or Southeast Asia are likely to be varicella susceptible if they have no history of the illness. Ideally, such young women should have antibody testing before they become pregnant so that they can be immunized before pregnancy.

There is little information on the risk of developing zoster during pregnancy. A few studies have suggested that the incidence is about the same as that of varicella in pregnancy (7). The course of illness is not more severe in pregnant women, and as is discussed next, there is little if any risk to the fetus and newborn infant.

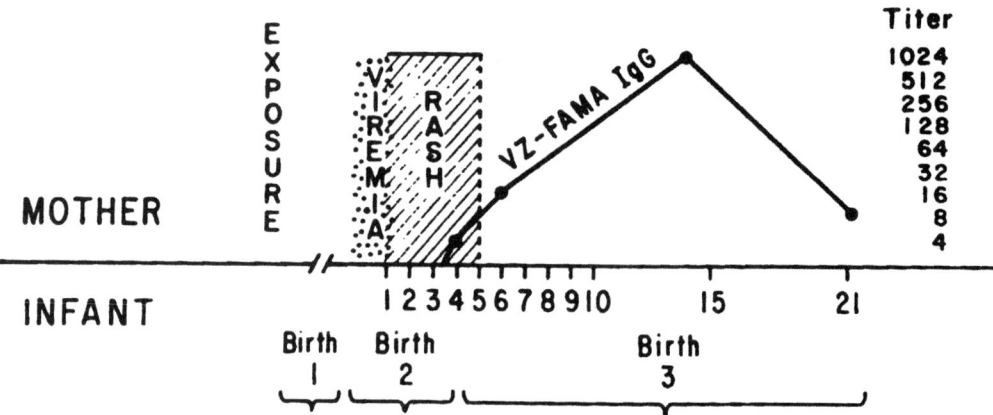

Fig. 1. Diagrammatic representation of transmission of varicella-zoster virus (VZV) and VZV antibody to the fetus in maternal varicella near term. (1) When the infant is born during the maternal incubation period, no varicella occurs unless the infant is exposed postnatally to the infection. (2) When the infant is born 0–4 days after onset of maternal varicella, disseminated varicella may develop because the infection will not be modified by maternal antibody. The onset of the varicella occurs between 5 and 10 days of age. (3) Infants born 5 days or more after maternal varicella receive maternal antibody, which leads to mild infection. This diagram is based on 50 newborn infants with varicella. (From ref. *15* with permission.)

RISK OF FETAL/NEONATAL INFECTION

In addition to postnatal spread by the airborne route, varicella may spread by the transplacental route from mother to infant. The transmission rate by this route is thought to be 25–50%; this is lower than the rate of transmission following household exposure, which is closer to 90% *(7)*. Women with active varicella at term are at risk of infecting their infants by the transplacental route as well as from exposure to external lesions following the baby's birth. It appears, however, that infants infected transplacentally are most at risk to develop severe varicella (*see* below). Fortunately, the immune response of the mother can have an impact in mitigating the course of varicella in the infant. Administration of varicella-zoster immune globulin (VZIG) can also compensate for this response in the infant.

The risk of infection of the offspring if the mother has gestational zoster appears to be minimal. This probably reflects the fact that individuals with zoster usually have high titers of antibodies to VZV. These high levels of antibodies are transferred from the mother to the fetus or infant and serve to protect against or modify the infection with VZV. In contrast, women who develop varicella have no detectable VZV antibodies during the period when they are viremic. Thus, transfer of the virus to the fetus at a high multiplicity of infection is likely to occur in varicella (*see* Fig. 1).

Fetal risks associated with maternal varicella include development of the congenital varicella syndrome, severe varicella in the infant, and the occurrence of zoster in infancy or early childhood *(7)*. The chances of developing these complications are related to the timing of maternal varicella regarding gestation.

Table 1
Manifestations of the Congenital Varicella Syndrome in Infants
With Developmental Defects Born to Women With VZV Infections
in Pregnancy (1947–1998) (N = 77)

Defect	%
Skin scars[a]	61
Eye abnormalities	56
Chorioretinitis	27
Horner's/anisocoria	16
Microphthalmia	19
Cataract	19
Nystagmus	13
Abnormal limb[b]	47
Hypoplasia	36
Equinovarus	14
Abnormal/absent digits	10
Cortical atrophy/mental retardation	40
Prematurity/low birth weight	36
Early death	26
Dysphagia/aspiration	19
Gastrointestinal tract abnormalities	12
Urinary tract abnormalities	10

[a]Cicatricial in 79%.
[b]11/28 (39%) with hypoplastic limb had mental retardation or early death. (Modified from ref. *14*, p. 698.)

Congenital Varicella Syndrome

Congenital varicella syndrome was first described in 1947 but seems to have been forgotten until 1974, when a newly recognized case was described in Canada *(9)*. Following this case report and review of the literature, many other reports of infants with a similar constellation of birth and developmental defects after maternal varicella followed *(7,10)*. Eventually, it became possible to specifically implicate VZV causally in these "classic" birth defects by the use of polymerase chain reaction (PCR). Unlike infants with the congenital rubella syndrome, babies with the congenital varicella syndrome do not asymptomatically shed virus at birth or afterward. If they develop zoster, and about 18% will do so, then it is possible to demonstrate VZV by culture or other specific means. Using PCR, moreover, it has been possible to demonstrate VZV DNA in affected tissues, such as the skin scars typical of the syndrome. Approximately 75 affected infants have now been reported *(7)*. Only a few classic cases have been virologically proven, leading to the definition of the syndrome. Most of the cases were diagnosed on clinical grounds only, but the signs and symptoms are so similar that there is little question about the existence of this syndrome.

The most frequently observed abnormalities are listed in Table 1. Cicatricial skin scars are the most common abnormality, observed in more than 50% of reported affected infants *(7)*. Eye damage of various types and limb abnormalities are extremely

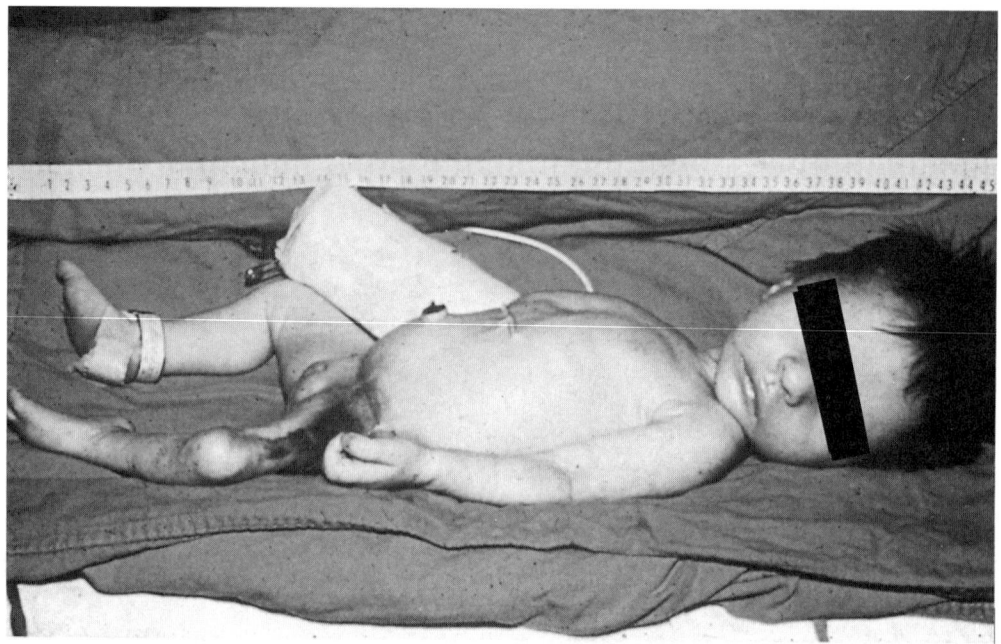

Fig. 2. This infant, whose mother had varicella during the 13th to 15th weeks of pregnancy, had bilateral microphthalmia with cataracts and an atrophic left leg. The infant died of bronchopneumonia at age 6.5 months. (From ref. *9* with permission.)

striking. The eyes may be hypoplastic, and there may be chorioretinitis, cataract, Horner's syndrome, and nystagmus. The typical limb deformity is hypoplasia, which is thought to be related to failure of the normal development of the nervous system of the extremity, which prohibits normal growth. In terms of pathogenesis of the syndrome, it has been proposed that these infants not only experience varicella *in utero*, but also experience zoster, which leads to the neurological damage. The skin scarring is frequently observed in a dermatomal distribution. Various degrees of involvement of the central nervous system have been described, with resultant motor and mental retardation. Many infants with severe forms of this syndrome have died in infancy or early childhood (Fig. 2).

Zoster during the first year of postnatal life, which is normally exceedingly rare, is extremely common in children with the congenital varicella syndrome; 18% of reported cases have manifested zoster *(7)*. This occurrence probably also relates to an increased incidence of latent infection when varicella develops in fetal life. By analogy, in animal models of latent infection with herpes simplex virus, the incidence of viral reactivation is directly related to the extent of latent infection in ganglia *(11)*.

Although it was once thought that the fetal risk from the congenital varicella syndrome was confined to maternal varicella in the first trimester, it is clear from the many published cases that the risk extends into the second trimester (Table 2). About half the reported cases have occurred after maternal varicella in the second trimester *(7)*.

It appears that maternal varicella does not increase the incidence of spontaneous abortion *(7)*. It is hoped that one effect of widespread use of varicella vaccine will be

Table 2
Risks to Pregnant Women and Their Offspring From VZV

Varicella	
Maternal	Bacterial superinfection (skin, soft tissue)
	Disseminated varicella with primary viral pneumonia
	Death
Fetus/neonate	Congenital varicella syndrome (2% after maternal varicella in first or second trimester)
	Disseminated varicella (born 4 days before or 2 days after maternal onset of rash)
	Development of zoster in early childhood
Zoster	
Maternal	Rash with pain
Fetus/neonate	Little or no risk

the virtual elimination of the congenital varicella syndrome, analogous to that which has occurred with congenital rubella. There is no evidence that the varicella vaccine virus causes the congenital syndrome, but vaccination is contraindicated during pregnancy. As it did for the rubella vaccine, the CDC has established a registry for outcomes of women inadvertently vaccinated during pregnancy *(12)*. To date, only about 50 such women have been followed to term. Before firm conclusions can be made, observation and follow-up of several hundred vaccinated susceptible women will be necessary. At present, there is no evidence of teratogenicity of the vaccine virus.

Severe Varicella in the Newborn Infant

Despite the potential severity and striking appearance of babies with the congenital syndrome, its occurrence is rare, developing in only an estimated 2% of offspring of women with varicella in the first or second trimester. Thus, the usual outcome of the fetus from maternal varicella is that the baby is well at birth and subsequently. However, if the mother has the onset of her varicella just prior to delivery, the outcome can be severe disseminated varicella in the baby. In this case, the pathogenesis is thought to relate to the immunosuppression of the mother, the immaturity of cell-mediated immunity in the young infant, and the absence of maternal antibodies in the fetus when the mother's onset of rash is between 4 days before and 2 days after delivery *(7)* (Fig. 1).

Since the institution, about 30 years ago, of the recommendation for passive immunization of exposed newborns with VZIG as soon as possible after birth, it is rare for a newborn infant to die of disseminated varicella. Before VZIG became available, one study suggested a 20% fatality rate when the mother had onset of rash less than 4 days and up to 2 days after onset of rash at delivery *(13)*. Infants in whom varicella is fatal often have a disseminated infection with pneumonia, extensive hemorrhagic skin vesicles, hepatitis, and thrombocytopenia. Mothers whose onset of rash is more than 48 hours after delivery may transmit varicella to their babies, but the disease is usually not severe because they transfer antibodies as well *(7)*.

Nursery outbreaks of varicella are rare, although exposure of infants in the nursery is not uncommon. It is hypothesized that most newborns are somewhat protected from varicella because of the presence of maternally derived antibodies to VZV. It is known that the presence of maternal antibodies may not fully protect very young infants from clinical varicella, but they usually develop a mild, modified form of chickenpox if they become ill *(7)*.

Zoster

Another outcome of maternal varicella is zoster in the young infant with no history of varicella in postnatal life. In general, zoster in young children is extremely rare. Zoster is increased in frequency, however, in infants whose mothers had gestational varicella, but it does not appear to be as frequent as zoster in babies with the congenital varicella syndrome. Zoster in these infants is often mild and not particularly painful. The rate of zoster in these babies is probably on the order of 3%, which is significantly higher than would normally be seen but obviously is not a serious health threat.

PRENATAL EVALUATION OF MOTHER

Women planning to become pregnant should be questioned about whether (and when) they had varicella. Those with a history of disease need no further evaluation, but those with a negative history should be tested for the presence of VZV antibodies. This is most practically done by enzyme-linked immunosorbent assay (ELISA) tests that are commercially available. Although in general these tests lack sensitivity, they are useful for determining natural immunity *(7,12)*. Women who have no history of varicella and who have no detectable VZV antibodies by ELISA should ideally be vaccinated before becoming pregnant. As has been mentioned, women reared in countries with a tropical climate are highly likely to be susceptible if they have no history of varicella. Immunization of adults requires two doses of vaccine administered 4–8 weeks apart. If the woman is already pregnant, she should not be immunized, but the CDC recommends immunization of close susceptible contacts, such as young children attending day care *(7,12)*. As noted, the vaccine virus is rarely transmitted from one person to another. It is unfortunate that one of the three instances of transmission of the vaccine virus to others occurred when an immunized child developed a vaccine-related rash, and 2 weeks later his pregnant mother developed mild varicella. The pregnancy was terminated, and the products of conception proved negative for VZV infection when tested by PCR. This unfortunate case is obviously one of extreme rarity, given that only three instances of transmission occurred after distribution of more than 20 million doses by the manufacturer (Merck) in the United States *(6)*. Therefore, the CDC continues to recommend vaccination of susceptible contacts of susceptible pregnant women. The risk of a varicella-susceptible pregnant woman acquiring fully virulent VZV during pregnancy, especially if there is already a young child in the family, would appear to outweigh the theoretical risks from infection by contact with a vaccinee by the Oka strain.

Women who have varicella while pregnant bear close medical attention. They should be carefully observed for development of disseminated VZV infection. Severe varicella may be manifested by high fever, chest or abdominal pain, shortness of breath, and cough. In severe cases, there may be hundreds to thousands of skin vesicles, which may become hemorrhagic and continue to erupt for many days. For best results, treatment should be started before this stage has been reached. As has been noted, the risk is greatest in the last trimester of pregnancy. Women who appear to be developing severe varicella should receive prompt treatment with intravenous acyclovir.

CLINICAL EVALUATION OF INFANT

The appearance of infants born to women with active varicella at term is dependent in large part on the length of time that the rash has been present. Infants born to women who had varicella 10–14 days previously may have lesions at birth, but these infants are not at risk to develop severe disease (Fig. 1). They are thought to be protected by maternally transmitted antibodies to VZV *(1)*. They do not need an extensive workup or antiviral therapy.

Babies whose mothers have the onset of rash in the high-risk period (4 days before to 2 days after delivery) do not need any particular diagnostic workup, but they should be given VZIG as soon as possible after birth. About 50% will nevertheless develop varicella, which is usually mild. A small percentage, however, may develop more severe varicella and require antiviral therapy. Treatment for these infants must be individualized carefully with close follow-up. It is preferable to overtreat in the sense of administering intravenous acyclovir to babies who may not turn out to need it rather than to withhold medication until an infant has developed full-blown disseminated varicella, which may be rapidly fatal. Infants with possible severe varicella should have a complete blood cell count, liver chemistries, and a chest x-ray at the bare minimum. A lumbar puncture is usually not indicated. Skin lesions that appear to be caused by varicella may be cultured for virus, tested for VZV antigens by immunofluorescence, or tested by PCR if available to make a laboratory diagnosis in atypical cases.

DIAGNOSTIC ASSAYS FOR EVALUATION OF INFANT AND MOTHER

As mentioned in the preceding section, it is possible to make a diagnosis of VZV infection by laboratory means if the illness seems atypical. Usually, however, the clinical presentation is characteristic enough to make laboratory confirmation of chickenpox or zoster unnecessary. PCR is the best means for documenting the congenital varicella syndrome *(7)*. This might be performed on a skin biopsy of an affected area or cerebrebrospinal fluid. It is also possible to detect VZV antigens when children thought to have this syndrome develop zoster *(7)*. Some of these infants may develop very mild manifestations of zoster, consisting of only a few vesicular lesions. Laboratory confirmation of VZV infection may be very useful in such situations.

Unfortunately, there are no reliable means to screen a woman to determine if her fetus has the congenital varicella syndrome *(7)*. Although some fetuses have been shown to have abnormalities on ultrasound, diagnosis has never been subjected to careful study because the number of cases is extremely small. Moreover, some fetuses have been found to demonstrate calcification in the liver but have been normal at birth. It does seem from the literature, however, that a fetus identified to have a hypoplastic limb by ultrasound is highly likely to have the syndrome, and with the limb abnormality, there is a 40% chance that the infant will have either brain damage or early death. In such instances, if it is not too late in gestation, termination of the pregnancy should be strongly considered *(7)*.

Most experts do not recommend termination when a woman has varicella during pregnancy unless obvious birth defects are present on ultrasound, as noted in this section *(7)*. The risk to the fetus of being born with a serious birth defect due to varicella is on the order of about 2%, which is not much greater than the overall risk of 4% without varicella. Obviously, however, the caregiver needs to provide a great deal of counseling in this situation because of its uncertainties.

REFERENCES

1. Arvin A, Gershon A. Live attenuated varicella vaccine. Annu Rev Microbiol 1996;50:59–100.
2. Lungu O, Panagiotidis C, Annunziato P, Gershon A, Silverstein S. Aberrant intracellular localization of varicella-zoster virus regulatory proteins during latency. Proc Natl Acad Sci U S A 1998;95:7080–7085.
3. Seward J, Peterson C, Mascola L, et al. Decline of Varicella Disease: Evidence of Vaccine Impact, Vol. 1629. Boston: Society for Pediatric Research, Boston, 2000.
4. Wharton M. The epidemiology of varicella-zoster virus infections. Infect Dis Clin North Am 1996;10:571–581.
5. Krause P, Klinman DM. Efficacy, immunogenicity, safety, and use of live attenuated chickenpox vaccine. J Pediatr 1995;127:518–525.
6. Sharrar RG, LaRussa P, Galea S, et al. The postmarketing safety profile of varicella vaccine. Vaccine 2000;19:916–923.
7. Gershon A. Chickenpox, measles, and mumps. In: Remington J, Klein J, eds. Infections of the Fetus and Newborn Infant, 5th ed. Philadelphia: Saunders, 2001:683–732.
8. LaRussa P, Steinberg S, Seeman MD, Gershon AA. Determination of immunity to varicella by means of an intradermal skin test. J Infect Dis 1985;152:869–875.
9. Srabstein JC, Morris N, Larke B, deSa D, Oxon DP, Castelino BB, Sum E. Is there a congenital varicella syndrome? J Pediatr 1974;84:239–243.
10. Enders G, Miller E, Cradock-Watson J, Bolley I, Ridehalgh M. Consequences of varicella and herpes zoster in pregnancy: prospective study of 1739 cases. Lancet 1994;343:1548–1551.
11. Lekstrom-Himes JA, Pesnicak L, Straus SE. The quantity of latent viral DNA correlates with the relative rates at which herpes simplex virus types 1 and 2 cause recurrent genital herpes outbreaks. J Virol 1998;72:2760–2764.
12. Centers for Disease Control and Prevention. Prevention of varicella. MMWR Morb Mortal Wkly Rep 1999;48:1–6.
13. Meyers J. Congenital varicella in term infants: risk reconsidered. J Infect Dis 1974;129:215–217.
14. Remington J, Klein JO. Infectious Diseases of the Fetus and Newborn Infant, 4th ed. Philadelphia: Saunders, 2001.
15. Gershon A. Varicella in mother and infant: problems old and new. In: Krugman S, Gershon A, eds. Infection of the Fetus and Newborn Infant. New York: Liss, 1975:79–95.

9

Human Herpesviruses 6 and 7

Charles T. Leach

INTRODUCTION

The identification of human herpesvirus (HHV) 6 (HHV-6) and 7 (HHV-7) was first reported in 1986 and 1990, respectively. HHV-6 was isolated initially from the blood of several immunodeficient adults, including some with acquired immunodeficiency syndrome (AIDS) *(1)*. The existence of HHV-7 was first revealed in the blood of a healthy, human immunodeficiency virus (HIV)-negative adult *(2)*. Extensive investigations since then have established that these viruses are ubiquitous in the general population and are responsible for the majority of cases of roseola, a common febrile rash illness of infants *(3–5)*. This chapter provides a general overview of HHV-6 and HHV-7 and a summary of present knowledge related to the diagnosis of congenital and perinatal infections.

DESCRIPTION OF ORGANISMS

HHV-6 and HHV-7 are closely related to human cytomegalovirus (CMV). Like all herpesviruses, HHV-6 and HHV-7 possess a nucleocapsid containing deoxyribonucleic acid (DNA), surrounded by a dense tegument and a lipid envelope *(6)*. Although HHV-6 and HHV-7 DNAs possess a high degree of homology, there are distinct antigenic differences *(7)*. Two subtypes of HHV-6 (A and B) have been described *(8)*. Most cases of roseola are caused by subtype B *(9,10)*, and the few congenital HHV-6 infections evaluated thus far have also been caused by subtype B. No disease has been consistently associated with subtype A, although it may be found more frequently in African children *(11)*. HHV-7 subtypes have not been reported.

EPIDEMIOLOGY

Seroprevalence

HHV-6 and HHV-7 infections occur early in life. Almost all newborns possess maternally derived antibodies, but by age 6 months, most have lost maternal antibodies and are susceptible to infection. Acquisition of HHV-6 occurs rapidly, with 50–60% of children becoming HHV-6 seropositive by age 12 months and essentially all children infected by age 2–3 years *(12)*. HHV-7 infection typically occurs slightly later than HHV-6, with more than 90% prevalence reached by age 7–10 years *(12)*.

From: *Infectious Disease: Congenital and Perinatal Infections: A Concise Guide to Diagnosis*
Edited by: C. Hutto © Humana Press Inc., Totowa, NJ

Latency and Viral Shedding

HHV-6 and HHV-7, like all other herpesviruses, become latent following primary infection, with limited expression of viral genes. The primary sites of latency for HHV-6 and HHV-7 are the salivary glands and peripheral blood mononuclear cells (PBMCs). During primary infection, high concentrations of each virus can be found in PBMCs *(13)*. Thereafter, viral DNA persists at very low concentrations in PBMCs. Other sites of viral latency probably include the central nervous system and the female genital tract.

Shedding of HHV-6 and HHV-7 reflects sites of viral latency. Approximately 50% of adults shed HHV-6 in saliva, and about 90% shed HHV-7. Another site of shedding is the female genital tract. HHV-6 was found in the genital tracts of 4% of healthy nonpregnant women *(14)* and 3% of women attending a sexually transmitted disease clinic *(15)*. In early pregnancy, reported rates of genital HHV-6 shedding have ranged between 2 *(14)* and 26% *(16)*, whereas 19% of women shed HHV-6 in late gestation *(17)*. In the only published study of HHV-7, 3% of women in late pregnancy shed the virus in the genital tract *(17)*. Women shedding HHV-6 or HHV-7 in the genital tract have no local clinical manifestations.

There is conflicting data on the presence of HHV-6 in breast milk. Dunne and Jevon *(18)*, from the United States, examined 120 samples of breast milk by polymerase chain reaction (PCR) and found none positive. However, investigators from India, also using PCR, found HHV-6 in breast milk from 100% of healthy women and 89% of HIV-positive women *(19)*.

Transmission

For children beyond the neonatal period, saliva is presumed to be the principal source for transmission of HHV-6 and HHV-7. This is based on the frequent shedding of virus in saliva among infected persons and limited molecular epidemiologic studies *(20)*.

The relatively small number of *in utero* HHV-6 infections is presumably attributable to maternal viremia, yet documentation is lacking. Perinatal infections could occur as a result of exposure to contaminated breast milk, genital secretions, saliva, or other sources. Although one of two studies suggested the presence of HHV-6 within breast milk *(19)*, there is no epidemiologic support for breast milk as an important source for HHV-6 acquisition in early infancy *(21)*. Because HHV-6 and HHV-7 may be shed in the female genital tract, exposure to a contaminated birth canal during vaginal delivery or via ascending infection could account for perinatal HHV-6 and HHV-7 infections. One study evaluated the outcome of pregnant women with and without first trimester genital HHV-6 shedding; none of the newborns in either group was determined to have congenital infection based on PCR analysis of cord blood *(16)*. Studies evaluating the association of late-term viral shedding with neonatal infection are lacking.

Incidence in Mothers

Studies among healthy adults, including pregnant women, indicate that past infections with HHV-6 and HHV-7 are extremely common, presumably as a result of viral exposure early in life *(7,14,22,23)*. Thus, like Epstein-Barr virus, primary (initial) HHV-6/HHV-7 infections during adulthood are expected rarely. However, because latent virus exists in all infected persons, there is some risk for "reactivation." Reactivation of HHV-6 or HHV-7 typically is identified by increasing rates of virus shedding or

Table 1
Detection of HHV-6 DNA or HHV-6 IgM Antibodies in Cord Blood

Population	Reference	Year	Country	No. PCR positive/ no. tested (%)	No. IgM positive/ no. tested (%)
Healthy mothers	*42*	1990	US	5/305 (1.6)	ND
	43	1992	US	ND	2/799 (0.3)[a]
	44	1992	Japan	ND	3/100 (3)
	45	1998	UK	ND	0/235 (0)
	22	1999	Sweden	2/211 (2.0)	ND
	46	1999	Japan	0/58 (0)	ND
	47	1999	Thailand	0/13	ND
	48	2004	US	57/5638	ND
	Total			64/6225 (1.0)	5/1134 (0.4)
HIV-positive mothers	*47*	1999	Thailand	3/41 (7.3)	ND
	19	2000	India	7/36 (19.4)	ND
	Total			10/77 (13.0)	ND

ND, not done.
[a]HHV-6 PCR testing was negative on the two HHV-6 IgM-positive samples.

increases in specific immunoglobulin (Ig) G antibody titers. One study indicated that HHV-6 reactivation may occur in approx 5–10% of pregnant women *(22)*. Symptomatic illness in adults as a consequence of primary or reactivated HHV-6 or HHV-7 reactivation is not well described. Some authors have reported a mononucleosis-like illness in nonpregnant adults *(24)*. No illnesses in pregnant women attributable to primary or reactivated HHV-6/HHV-7 infection have been reported.

Incidence in Neonates

Accumulating data from several different sociogeographic areas indicate that the incidence of congenital or perinatal HHV-6 infections is quite low (Table 1); there is no comparable information for HHV-7. Studies have typically measured HHV-6 DNA in cord blood mononuclear cells by qualitative PCR, or HHV-6 IgM antibodies in cord blood serum, or both. In newborns of healthy mothers, the rate of *in utero* HHV-6 infection is 0–3% (Table 1). Congenital HHV-6 infection occurred at slightly higher rates (7–19%) in infants born to HIV-infected mothers (Table 1). Only one study contains data on congenital HHV-7, with no infections identified *(48)*.

Incidence in Children Outside the Neonatal Period

Like CMV, most HHV-6 and HHV-7 infections are clinically silent. The incidence of roseola, the most common symptomatic illness attributable to these agents, is estimated as 30–35% by age 3 years. Other illnesses possibly associated with HHV-6 are very rare.

CONSEQUENCES OF CONGENITAL OR ACQUIRED HUMAN HERPESVIRUS 6 AND 7 INFECTIONS

Although more than 60 newborns with congenital or perinatal HHV-6 infections have been reported in large series (Table 1), most apparently are healthy and have no unusual features. Several case reports have described fetuses or infants with HHV-6 infection, yet most have no abnormalities. Aubin et al. *(25)* first described *in utero* infection with HHV-6. These investigators examined 52 electively aborted fetuses from HIV-infected women from France and noted one fetus (26 weeks) with HHV-6 DNA distributed throughout fetal tissues. No abnormalities were identified. One study from Japan identified HHV-6 antigens in tissues from 2 of 30 (7%) fetuses spontaneously aborted at 6–12 weeks; fetal abnormalities were not described *(26)*. HHV-6 DNA has also been found in fetal tissues of two of eight cases (25%) of fetal hydrops (17 and 19 weeks of gestation) *(27)*. However, both fetuses also had a chromosomal abnormality (Down syndrome and Turner's syndrome) possibly contributing to the hydrops. Fulminant hepatitis in two neonates (aged 3 and 5 days) has purported to be linked to congenital HHV-6 infection based on HHV-6 viremia in mother and baby *(28)*; further documentation of HHV-6 infection of liver tissue was not performed in these cases. Because HHV-6 viremia may occur in asymptomatic neonates *(29)*, there is some question whether these cases are attributable to HHV-6 infection. Illness resembling roseola has also been reported in one neonate (age 3 weeks) despite the presence of maternal HHV-6 antibodies *(30)*. These studies clearly demonstrate that HHV-6 can be transmitted congenitally as early as 6–12 weeks of gestation, However, there is insufficient evidence indicating a characteristic clinical syndrome; most newborns appear healthy. No reports of congenital or acquired HHV-7 infections have appeared.

CLINICAL EVALUATION

Prenatal

Based on current literature, there are few data suggesting the necessity of evaluating a mother or her fetus for HHV-6 or HHV-7 infection. HHV-6 (and probably HHV-7) may be reactivated during pregnancy, but no studies have clearly established serious consequences. Reports of spontaneous abortion *(26)* and fetal hydrops *(27)* purportedly associated with HHV-6 infection require further corroboration before routine diagnostic studies can be recommended.

Neonatal

Although most neonates with congenital or acquired HHV-6 infection appear normal, disease possibly linked to the virus has occurred in a few patients. One child had fever, rash, and aseptic meningitis *(30)*. Two neonates *(28)* and two infants age younger than 3 months *(31,32)* have been described with liver dysfunction. A newborn with congenital HHV-6 infection has been described with seizures and neurological complications *(32a)*.

VIRAL DIAGNOSTIC ASSAYS AND THEIR INTERPRETATION

General

Because of the rarity of congenital or perinatal HHV-6 and HHV-7 infections as well as the apparent absence of serious consequences in the majority of patients, no standards for diagnostic testing have yet been established. However, numerous tests have been developed for the diagnosis of HHV-6 and HHV-7 infection in other age categories and have been used in studies evaluating newborns for suspected congenital and acquired infections. Specific testing for HHV-6 or HHV-7 infection may include

Table 2
Laboratory Tests Used for Distinguishing Active
From Latent HHV-6 and HHV-7 Infections

Specimen type	Tests indicating active infection
Noncellular	
Serum, plasma	IgM antibodies[a]
	IgG seroconversion or fourfold change
	PCR
	Antigen capture
CSF	PCR
Cellular (e.g., PBMCs, tissues)	Virus isolation
	Quantitative PCR
	RT-PCR
	Immunohistochemistry

[a]False-positive and false-negative results can occur. Ig, immunoglobulin; CSF, cerebrospinal fluid; PCR, polymerase chain reaction; RT-PCR, reverse transcriptase PCR; PBMCs, peripheral blood mononuclear cells.

serology, virus culture, PCR, immunohistochemistry, *in situ* hybridization, and antigen detection.

In considering performance of these viral tests, one must remember the latent nature of these herpesviruses and understand that tests differ in their ability to distinguish nonreplicating, latent virus from replicating, active virus (Table 2). The presence of HHV-6 or HHV-7 DNA in PBMCs or other cellular material indicates viral infection but does not necessarily imply viral disease because these viruses persist latently following primary infection. Assays that detect active viral infection are necessary. In cellular specimens, active infection is typically indicated by the isolation of virus, the presence of specific viral ribonucleic acid, or the expression of viral proteins on cell membranes. In cell-free specimens (e.g., serum, plasma, or cerebrospinal fluid [CSF]), viral replication is indicated by the presence of HHV-6 or HHV-7 DNA or antigens. Serologic methods indirectly measure virus infection and are of limited benefit in diagnosing congenital or perinatal HHV-6/HHV-7 infections.

Serology

The most common antibody tests are enzyme immunoassay (EIA) and indirect immunofluorescence assay (IFA); both assays are available commercially. Reference strains of HHV-6 and HHV-7 are typically grown in a susceptible lymphoblastoid cell line or human mononuclear cells, then harvested and attached to plates (for EIA) or slides (for IFA). Commercial EIA and IFA tests cannot distinguish HHV-6 subtypes. One group of investigators has described a serologic test identifying "low-avidity" IgG antibodies to HHV-6, which is claimed to distinguish primary from past infection in older infants *(33)*; however, this test is not used widely, is not available commercially, and has not been evaluated in neonates.

Serologic profiles are best described for infants with HHV-6-associated roseola, in whom an HHV-6 IgM response typically develops by days 5–7 of illness, peaks at 2–3 weeks, and resolves within 2 months. However, false-positive and false-negative results can occur *(34)*; therefore, IgM testing alone is not reliable. Although not timely, seroconversion of IgG antibodies in serum samples collected 2–3 weeks apart is more reliable than a single IgM test for establishing primary infection. However, because most mothers are already infected with HHV-6 and HHV-7 and newborns acquire passive maternal antibodies, IgG seroconversion is expected to occur rarely in this population. Fourfold increases or decreases in IgG antibodies can also suggest infection. Because of the high seroprevalence of HHV-6 and HHV-7 in the general population, a single positive IgG test is of no diagnostic importance. Because HHV-6 and HHV-7 antibodies may cross-react with each other as well as with CMV, diagnosis of HHV-6 or HHV-7 infection by serologic means alone is insufficient and requires concurrent testing for CMV infection. Acute HHV-6 and HHV-7 infections are more reliably demonstrated by more direct viral assays, described next.

Virus Culture

When incubated under suitable conditions, HHV-6 and HHV-7 may be grown in culture. Because no cell lines reliably sustain growth of virus, it is necessary to incubate specimens in the presence of fresh human mononuclear cells. Virus culture requires prolonged (1–3 weeks) incubation in the presence of fetal calf serum, interleukin 6, and other reagents. Rarely, virus has been identified in other biologic specimens.

The presence of HHV-6 or HHV-7 in culture is suggested by ballooning and eventual lysis of infected cells; infection is confirmed by staining with commercially available monoclonal antibodies. Virus culture presently is available only in specialized research laboratories. A rapid shell vial culture for HHV-6 is available commercially but has not been evaluated extensively *(35)*.

Identification of HHV-6 or HHV-7 in blood by virus culture firmly establishes the presence of active infection. No studies to date, however, have reported isolation of HHV-6 or HHV-7 from infants or fetuses. In fact, cord blood is frequently used for co-cultivation with PBMCs from older patients with suspected HHV-6/7 infection (it is assumed that cord blood does not contain HHV-6 or HHV-7).

Polymerase Chain Reaction

Amplification of HHV-6 and HHV-7 DNA by PCR is becoming widely available, and has been utilized in most studies of congenital HHV-6 infection. However, it is important to reemphasize that active, replicating infection is demonstrated only if viral DNA is detected in noncellular specimens such as CSF, serum, or plasma. Detection in other specimens containing cellular material (e.g., PBMCs, tissues) does not necessarily indicate active infection because these viruses exist in latent form in these tissues following primary infection. Quantitative measurement of virus DNA concentration, such as quantitative PCR *(36)*, may help distinguish active from latent infection and is available commercially. However, concentration thresholds indicating active infection have not been established for newborns or older children and adults; for this reason, interpretation of results is problematic.

Reverse transcriptase PCR (RT-PCR) is an assay that detects specific viral messenger ribonucleic acid transcripts, indicating viral replication. Data suggest that RT-PCR is a sensitive and specific method for identifying active HHV-6 infection and correlates well with virus culture *(37,38)*. RT-PCR is typically performed on PBMCs, may be used on bone marrow samples, and is available from at least one commercial laboratory. There is no information on interpretation of results in newborns. Studies in infants and children suggested that certain combinations of PCR tests are more accurate for diagnosis of primary HHV-6 or HHV-7 infections, such as positive PCR of whole blood with negative IgG antibody in serum *(39)* or positive PCR of whole blood with negative PCR of saliva *(13)*. The accuracy of these combination tests in newborns is unknown.

Other Assays

Other diagnostic tests for HHV-6 and HHV-7 may be useful in selected circumstances.

Immunohistochemistry

Viral antigens, indicating expression of HHV-6/HHV-7 proteins, may be detected in infected tissues and have been utilized in studies of aborted fetuses *(26)* and other subjects *(40)*. Monoclonal antibodies for performance of these tests are available commercially, including antibodies directed specifically against HHV-6 antigens, HHV-7 antigens, or common antigens shared by both viruses.

In Situ *PCR*

Tissues may also be evaluated for the presence of HHV-6 or HHV-7 by using *in situ* PCR. This test can detect DNA in tissues using appropriate genomic DNA probes. Typically, probes are labeled with radioactivity (or another tag) and then hybridized to cells or tissues immobilized on glass slides. The presence of intracellular viral DNA by *in situ* PCR indicates viral infection but does not provide evidence of viral replication because these viruses may exist latently in numerous tissues.

Antigen Capture Assay

An HHV-6 antigen capture assay is available for detection of HHV-6 antigens in serum, but this test has not been evaluated in neonates *(41)*. In this test, anti-HHV-6 monoclonal antibodies directed at HHV-6 proteins are immobilized in plastic wells. When serum or another cell-free specimen containing HHV-6 antigen is added, these antibodies bind the viral antigens and are detected by a colorimetric reaction. The presence of viral antigen in noncellular specimens indicates active viral infection. No assays for HHV-7 antigen detection are available.

REFERENCES

1. Salahuddin SZ, Ablashi DV, Markham PD, et al. Isolation of a new virus, HBLV, in patients with lymphoproliferative disorders. Science 1986;234:596–601.
2. Frenkel N, Schirmer EC, Wyatt LS, et al. Isolation of a new herpesvirus from human CD4$^+$ T cells. Proc Natl Acad Sci U S A 1990;87:748–752.
3. Yamanishi K, Okuno T, Shiraki K, et al. Identification of human herpesvirus-6 as a causal agent for exanthem subitum. Lancet 1988;1:1065–1067.
4. Tanaka K, Kondo T, Torigoe S, Okada S, Mukai T, Yamanishi K. Human herpesvirus 7: another causal agent for roseola (exanthem subitum). J Pediatr 1994;125:1–5.
5. Leach CT. Roseola (human herpesvirus types 6 and 7). In: Behrman RE, Kliegman RM, Jenson HB, eds. Nelson Textbook of Pediatrics, 17th ed. Philadelphia: Saunders, 2004:1069–1072.
6. Biberfeld P, Petren AL, Eklund A, et al. Human herpesvirus-6 (HHV-6, HBLV) in sarcoidosis and lymphoproliferative disorders. J Virol Methods 1988;21:49–59.
7. Wyatt LS, Rodriguez WJ, Balachandran N, Frenkel N. Human herpesvirus 7: antigenic properties and prevalence in children and adults. J Virol 1991;65:6260–6265.
8. Ablashi DV, Balachandran N, Josephs SF, et al. Genomic polymorphism, growth properties, and immunologic variations in human herpesvirus-6 isolates. Virology 1991;184:545–552.

9. Dewhurst S, McIntyre K, Schnabel K, Hall CB. Human herpesvirus 6 (HHV-6) variant B accounts for the majority of symptomatic primary HHV-6 infections in a population of US infants. J Clin Microbiol 1993;31:416–418.
10. Yamamoto T, Mukai T, Kondo K, Yamanishi K. Variation of DNA sequence in immediate-early gene of human herpesvirus 6 and variant identification by PCR. J Clin Microbiol 1994;32:473–476.
11. Kasolo FC, Mpabalwani E, Gompels UA. Infection with AIDS-related herpesviruses in human immunodeficiency virus-negative infants and endemic childhood Kaposi's sarcoma in Africa. J Gen Virol 1997;78:847–855.
12. Huang LM, Lee CY, Liu MY, Lee PI. Primary infections of human herpesvirus-7 and herpesvirus-6: a comparative, longitudinal study up to 6 years of age. Acta Paediatr 1997;86:604–608.
13. Clark DA, Kidd IM, Collingham KE, et al. Diagnosis of primary human herpesvirus 6 and 7 infections in febrile infants by polymerase chain reaction. Arch Dis Child 1997;77:42–45.
14. Leach CT, Frantz C, Gao SJ, et al. Human herpesvirus-8 (HHV-8) associated with small non-cleaved cell lymphoma in a child with AIDS. Am J Hematol 1999;60:215–221.
15. Leach CT, Newton ER, McParlin S, Jenson HB. Human herpesvirus 6 infection of the female genital tract. J Infect Dis 1994;169:1281–1283.
16. Maeda T, Okuno T, Hayashi K, et al. Abortion in human herpesvirus 6 DNA-positive pregnant women. Pediatr Infect Dis J 1997;16:1176–1177.
17. Okuno T, Oishi H, Hayashi K, Nonogaki M, Tanaka K, Yamanishi K. Human herpesviruses 6 and 7 in cervixes of pregnant women. J Clin Microbiol 1995;33:1968–1970.
18. Dunne WM Jr, Jevon M. Examination of human breast milk for evidence of human herpesvirus 6 by polymerase chain reaction [letter]. J Infect Dis 1993;168:250.
19. Joshi PJ, Merchant RH, Pokharankar SL, Damania KS, Gilada IS, Mukhopadhyaya R. Perinatally cotransmitted human herpesvirus 6 is activated in children born with human immunodeficiency virus infection. J Hum Virol 2000;3:317–323.
20. Mukai T, Yamamoto T, Kondo T, et al. Molecular epidemiological studies of human herpesvirus 6 in families. J Med Virol 1994;42:224–227.
21. Kusuhara K, Takabayashi A, Ueda K, et al. Breast milk is not a significant source for early Epstein-Barr virus or human herpesvirus 6 infection in infants: a seroepidemiologic study in 2 endemic areas of human T-cell lymphotropic virus type I in Japan. Microbiol Immunol 1997;41:309–312.
22. Dahl H, Fjaertoft G, Norsted T, Wang FZ, Mousavi-Jazi M, Linde A. Reactivation of human herpesvirus 6 during pregnancy. J Infect Dis 1999;180:2035–2038.
23. Ohashi M, Ihira M, Suzuki K, et al. Transfer of human herpesvirus 6 and 7 antibodies from mothers to their offspring. Pediatr Infect Dis J 2001;20:449–450.
24. Akashi K, Eizuru Y, Sumiyoshi Y, et al. Brief report: severe infectious mononucleosis-like syndrome and primary human herpesvirus 6 infection in an adult. N Engl J Med 1993;329:168–171.
25. Aubin JT, Poirel L, Agut H, et al. Intrauterine transmission of human herpesvirus 6. Lancet 1992;340:482–483.
26. Ando Y, Kakimoto K, Ekuni Y, Ichijo M. HHV-6 infection during pregnancy and spontaneous abortion [letter]. Lancet 1992;340:1289.
27. Ashshi AM, Cooper RJ, Klapper PE, Al-Jiffri O, Moore L. Detection of human herpes virus 6 DNA in fetal hydrops. Lancet 2000;355:1519–1520.
28. Mendel I, de Matteis M, Bertin C, et al. Fulminant hepatitis in neonates with human herpesvirus 6 infection. Pediatr Infect Dis J 1995;14:993–997.
29. Hall CB, Long CE, Schnabel KC, et al. Human herpesvirus-6 infection in children. A prospective study of complications and reactivation. N Engl J Med 1994;331:432–438.
30. Kawaguchi S, Suga S, Kozawa T, Nakashima T, Yoshikawa T, Asano Y. Primary human herpesvirus-6 infection (exanthem subitum) in the newborn. Pediatrics 1992;90:628–630.

31. Asano Y, Yoshikawa T, Suga S, Yazaki T, Kondo K, Yamanishi K. Fatal fulminant hepatitis in an infant with human herpesvirus-6 infection [letter]. Lancet 1990;335:862–863.
32. Tajiri H, Nose O, Baba K, Okada S. Human herpesvirus-6 infection with liver injury in neonatal hepatitis [letter]. Lancet 1990;335:863–863.
32a. Lanari M, Papa I, Venturi V, et al. Congenital infections with human herpesvirus 6 variant B associated with neonatal seizures and poor neurological outcome. J Med Viral 2003;70:628–632.
33. Ward KN, Gray JJ, Fotheringham MW, Sheldon MJ. IgG antibodies to human herpesvirus-6 in young children: changes in avidity of antibody correlate with time after infection. J Med Virol 1993;39:131–138.
34. Suga S, Yoshikawa T, Asano Y, et al. IgM neutralizing antibody responses to human herpesvirus-6 in patients with exanthem subitum or organ transplantation. Microbiol Immunol 1992;36:495–506.
35. Singh N, Carrigan DR. Human herpesvirus-6 in transplantation: an emerging pathogen. Ann Intern Med 1996;124:1065–1071.
36. Cone RW, Hackman RC, Huang ML, et al. Human herpesvirus 6 in lung tissue from patients with pneumonitis after bone marrow transplantation. N Engl J Med 1993;329:156–161.
37. Norton RA, Caserta MT, Hall CB, Schnabel K, Hocknell P, Dewhurst S. Detection of human herpesvirus 6 by reverse transcription-PCR. J Clin Microbiol 1999;37:3672–3675.
38. Van den Bosch G, Locatelli G, Geerts L, et al. Development of reverse transcriptase PCR assays for detection of active human herpesvirus 6 infection. J Clin Microbiol 2001;39:2308–2310.
39. Chiu SS, Cheung CY, Tse CY, Peiris M. Early diagnosis of primary human herpesvirus 6 infection in childhood: serology, polymerase chain reaction, and virus load. J Infect Dis 1998;178:1250–1256.
40. Drobyski WR, Knox KK, Majewski D, Carrigan DR. Brief report: fatal encephalitis due to variant B human herpesvirus-6 infection in a bone marrow-transplant recipient. N Engl J Med 1994;330:1356–1360.
41. Marsh S, Kaplan M, Asano Y, et al. Development and application of HHV-6 antigen capture assay for the detection of HHV-6 infections. J Virol Methods 1996;61:103–112.
42. Farr TJ, Harnett GB, Pietroboni GR, Bucens MR. The distribution of antibodies to HHV-6 compared with other herpesviruses in young children. Epidemiol Infect 1990;105:603–607.
43. Dunne WMJ, Demmler GJ. Serological evidence for congenital transmission of human herpesvirus 6 [letter]. Lancet 1992;340:121–122.
44. Kakimoto K, Ando Y, Moriyama I, Ichijo M. The significance of determination of human herpesvirus-6 (HHV-6) antibody during pregnancy. Nippon Sanka Fujinka Gakkai Zasshi—Acta Obstet Gynaecol Jpn 1992;44:1571–1577.
45. Adams O, Krempe C, Kogler G, Wernet P, Scheid A. Congenital infections with human herpesvirus 6. J Infect Dis 1998;178:544–546.
46. Daibata M, Miyoshi I. Presence of human herpesvirus 6 DNA in cord blood cells. J Infect Dis 1999;179:1046–1047.
47. Kositanont U, Wasi C, Wanprapar N, et al. Primary infection of human herpesvirus 6 in children with vertical infection of human immunodeficiency virus type 1. J Infect Dis 1999;180:50–55.
48. Hall CB, Caserta MT, Schnabel KC, et al. Congenital infections with human herpesvirus 6 (HHV6) and human herpesvirus 7 (HHV7). J Pediatr 2004;145:472–477.

10

Human Herpesvirus 8

Charles Wood and Charles D. Mitchell

INTRODUCTION

Human herpesvirus (HHV) 8 or Kaposi's sarcoma associated herpesvirus (KSHV) is the newest member of the HHV family, discovered almost a decade ago in Kaposi's sarcoma (KS) tissue *(1–3)*. Since it was first identified in KS and is linked to this disease, it is thus termed KSHV. This virus was also the eighth HHV identified; therefore, it is also commonly known as HHV-8. HHV can be divided into three subgroups: the α-, β-, and γ-herpesvirus. The γ-herpesviruses are able to infect human lymphocytes and can be further subdivided into two subgroups, γ-1 or lymphocrytovirus and γ-2 or rhadinovirus. Epstein-Barr virus (EBV) is the prototype γ-1 virus, and the simian herpesvirus saimiri is the prototype γ-2 herpesvirus *(4)*. HHV-8 is classified as a γ-2 rhadinovirus and is the first human virus of this subfamily identified *(5)*. Like other herpesviruses, HHV-8 is a double-stranded deoxyribonucleic acid (DNA) virus. Its genome is linear, is about 165 kbp in length, and contains at least 87 viral genes *(6–8)*.

A feature of some DNA viruses, particularly of herpesviruses and HHV-8, is the ability of these viruses to incorporate or pirate host genes into their genome *(9)*; these genes can then play a role in the replication, survival, and transformation functions of the virus. HHV-8 has been found to encode human homologue genes that regulate cell cycling like cyclin D, growth factors like interleukin 6, or genes that may prevent programmed cell death such as bcl-2. Deciphering the functions of these viral genes will lead to a better understanding of viral pathogenesis and oncogenesis.

HHV-8 is now believed to play a major role in the development of KS. There is a strong association between the presence of the virus and KS. Viral DNA can be detected in more than 95% of KS lesions *(10)*. HHV-8 infection is not a common infection in low-risk populations but occurs commonly among individuals at risk for KS. Furthermore, the detection of viral DNA in the peripheral blood mononuclear cells (PBMCs) of the infected individuals can predict who will subsequently develop KS *(11–13)*. A study of an Amsterdam cohort has shown that individuals infected with human immunodeficiency virus (HIV) who subsequently acquired HHV-8 infection had a higher risk for developing KS than those who were infected by HHV-8 prior to their exposure to HIV-1 *(14)*. Therefore, it is clear that HHV-8 infection plays a major, but not sufficient, role for the development of KS. It is likely that other co-factors, such as immunosuppression, are required for KS development.

From: *Infectious Disease: Congenital and Perinatal Infections: A Concise Guide to Diagnosis*
Edited by: C. Hutto © Humana Press Inc., Totowa, NJ

In addition to KS, HHV-8 is known to be associated with other types of diseases. HHV-8 can be found in all forms of body-cavity-based lymphoma or primary effusion lymphoma, a rare form of B-cell lymphoma that is found most frequently in patients with acquired immunodeficiency syndrome (AIDS) *(15)*. HHV-8 has also been associated with another lymphoproliferative disorder, Castleman's disease *(16)*. HHV-8 can be detected in the bone marrow stromal cells of patients with multiple myeloma, but its link to this malignancy has been controversial and cannot be readily confirmed *(10,17)*.

EPIDEMIOLOGY AND ROUTES OF TRANSMISSION

The prevalence of HHV-8 infection has not yet been firmly established, but it seems to vary among different populations and in different regions of the world. Unlike most other herpesviruses, HHV-8 infection does not seem to be widely distributed in most populations. The frequency of infection appears to be low in the general population in North America, certain Asian countries, and in northern European nations such as the United Kingdom and Germany *(18,19)*. In these countries, the seroprevalence of HHV-8 in different risk groups mirrors the incidence of AIDS KS, with a seroprevalence rate of between 25 and 50% among homosexual men. In other countries such as Italy, Greece, and Israel, especially southern Italy, the infection rate seems to be much higher in the general population and is more variable, ranging between 5 and 35%.

In contrast to North America and Europe, HHV-8 infection is widespread on the African continent. High seroprevalence rates between 40 and 50% have been found in central, west, and South Africa *(20–23)*. Therefore, HHV-8 seroprevalence tracks very closely with KS, with the highest infection rates in geographic areas where classic or endemic forms of KS are more common. KS has a particularly high incidence in central African countries like the Republic of Congo, Uganda, and Zambia; these countries also have the highest HHV-8 infection rates in the world *(21)*.

At the moment, the exact risk factors and routes for HHV-8 transmission are not clear. Epidemiological evidence suggests that the virus is largely transmitted sexually in North America and certain northern European countries. There is a higher rate of infection in homosexual AIDS patients as compared to heterosexual AIDS patients. In the United States, the San Francisco Men's Health study showed that HHV-8 infection in this group of homosexual men was high and was linearly associated with the number of male sexual partners *(24)*. Similarly, a study of a cohort of Danish homosexual men also showed that HHV-8 infection was associated with receptive anal intercourse *(25)*. The likely sources of infection in this population are infected semen and feces.

The virus has not yet been found in fecal matter, but viral DNA can be detected in the semen by the polymerase chain reaction (PCR) technique. It has been reported that HHV-8 can be detected in the PBMCs in between 12 and 25% of homosexual men with KS but has not been consistently detected in semen samples of HIV-infected men without KS or from HIV-negative men *(26–28)*. HHV-8 infections of the urogenital and prostate tissue of healthy men also do not appear to occur frequently. Therefore, the role of HHV-8 transmission via semen is still not clear. Apart from the implication of a linkage between HHV-8 infection and sexual activity suggested by the strong correlation between HHV-8 infection and homosexuality in North America and northern Europe, convincing evidence of heterosexual transmission of HHV-8 has not as yet been found. There are studies suggesting that commercial sex workers are more likely to be infected by HHV-8, and that heterosexual activity appears to be a risk factor for infection *(29,30)*, but other risk factors such as drug use and HIV-1 infection could also play a role in HHV-8 transmission *(31)*. It was suggested that genetic factors might also play a role in infection. A study in French Guinea, where HHV-8 infection is epidemic, suggested that a recessive gene may control susceptibility or resistance to HHV-8 infection *(32)*.

Besides the potential role of sexual contact in HHV-8 transmission, it is likely that nonsexual routes can transmit HHV-8 as well. Among cases of classical KS, even though homosexual transmission may account for some of the cases, an undefined mode of nonsexual transmission must account for most of the other cases of classical KS *(33)*. In developing countries, in contrast to the United States and other Western countries, HHV-8 infection is widespread in both men and women and in children. This suggests that horizontal, nonsexual transmission may be the predominant mode of transmission in these countries.

There could be several routes of nonsexual transmission. One is transmission via blood. However, unlike HIV-1, HHV-8 does not appear to be transmitted readily by blood even though viral DNA can be detected in 10–15% of the PBMCs of healthy HHV-8 seropositive individuals *(13,34)*. However, a history of blood transfusion has been linked to KS in a San Francisco Health study *(24)*, and infectious viruses have been isolated from a blood donor's PBMCs *(35)*. If transfusion-related transmission does occur, it is likely to be uncommon.

HHV-8 transmission, however, has definitely been linked to transplantation. Transplant recipients have been documented to be infected by HHV-8 via allograft transmission. A study involving a cohort of 220 Swiss transplant patients demonstrated that 25 patients seroconverted within a year after transplantation *(36)*. In another case, an organ recipient was shown to be infected after transplant *(37)*. Another study demonstrated that a group of Italian patients who were infected by HHV-8 prior to transplantation developed KS afterward, suggesting that virus reactivation occurred after immunosuppression *(37)*. Therefore, screening of organ donors and recipients for HHV-8 infection, especially in areas with high seroprevalence, should be considered.

A likely route of nonsexual transmission is via saliva. Oral and nasal secretions have been hypothesized to be a source of HHV-8 infection, similar to other herpesviruses. HHV-8 DNA has been detected in saliva *(38)*, tissues *(39)*, and oral KS lesions *(40)*. Even though viruses can be detected in oral secretions, it is unlikely that this is the major route of transmission in North America and northern Europe because of the low seroprevalence rate in the general population. However, this may represent a major route of transmission in endemic regions like Africa, especially in transmissions to children in those areas. This route of transmission may also be responsible for infection among homosexual men *(14)*.

Another potential route of HHV-8 transmission from infected mothers to their infants is via breast milk. A number of human herpesviruses, including cytomegalovirus, EBV, and herpes simplex virus type 1 have been detected in breast milk or shown to be transmitted via breast-feeding. The presence of HHV-8 in breast milk might suggest that this agent may also be transmitted via breast-feeding. A study from Zambia, however, failed to readily detect any HHV-8 DNA in breast milk from HHV-8-seropositive Zambian mothers (both HIV-positive and -negative). In contrast, 21% of the samples studied were positive for EBV DNA *(41)*. This study suggests that breast milk transmission of HHV-8 is an unlikely route of transmission, but further studies will be needed to substantiate this conclusion.

In summary, the exact routes of HHV-8 transmission are unknown. The routes may be different among different populations and in different parts of the world. The sexual mode of transmission may be predominant in the homosexual male population, whereas for other risk groups, nonsexual routes such as horizontal transmission via saliva and organ transplantation may occur.

Infection in Women and Children

Different forms of KS, including African KS and classical KS, occur more commonly in men than in woman and seem to have a bimodal age distribution. Classic KS occurs predominantly in elderly male patients of southern European ancestry. Before the AIDS epidemic, African KS occurred primarily among men. Hormonal differences between genders had previously been implicated as the basis for this observation. In contrast to the known high HHV-8 seroprevalence in the homosexual male population, very little is known about the epidemiology of HHV-8 infection among women. Previous studies have indicated that the rate of HHV-8 infection among HIV-infected women may be much lower than that among HIV-infected homosexual males *(42)*.

A multisite cohort of HIV-infected and high-risk HIV-uninfected women in the United States demonstrated that 15% of the HIV-1-infected and 6.3% of HIV-1-negative women were infected by HHV-8 *(43)*. This was higher than the prevalence rate reported for the heterosexual women population *(44)*. However, much higher rates of infection were reported in KS-endemic regions such as sub-Saharan Africa *(45)*. Of the normal female population, 40% were found to be infected by HHV-8 in Zambia *(22)*, and the infection rate here seems to be as high in the female as the male population.

There are a number of risk factors associated with HHV-8 infection. A history of injection drug use and sexually transmitted diseases such as syphilis are known to be risk factors for infection in women *(29)*. The presence of HIV-1 infection was also found to be consistently associated with HHV-8 infection *(29,43)*. These findings support the notion that HHV-8 can be transmitted sexually in women and through needle sharing during injection drug use. It is likely that the virus is inefficiently transmitted via blood or blood products as HHV-8 infection has only infrequently been linked to transfusion.

Infection by HHV-8 appears to be rare in infants in North America and northern Europe. In endemic countries in sub-Saharan Africa, there seems to be a continuous increase in HHV-8 seroprevalence with age, transmission appears to increase after the age of 2 years, and the infection is likely to be acquired before puberty *(23,46–48)*. Studies suggest that nonsexual transmission may be the predominant mode of transmission in children. In studies from Uganda and Zambia, infants as young as 7 months were documented to have KS *(49,50)*, suggesting that vertical transmission from mother to child is also possible. It has been reported that HHV-8 can be detected in newborn infants in Zambia *(51,52)*, although another study involving a group of Italian women tested during pregnancy and at delivery did not find any evidence of vertical transmission *(53)*. This discrepancy could be caused by different populations in different geographical locations.

Taken together, there is sufficient evidence to show that newborns can acquire HHV-8 infection *in utero*, and that vertical transmission of HHV-8 can occur. The frequency of its occurrence, however, is probably rare. In this regard, the pattern of HHV-8 transmission to infants is very similar to other herpesviruses. The major route of HHV-8 transmission to infants and children may be horizontal, as would occur within families, such as between siblings, and from either parent to the children *(54–56)*.

In conclusion, HHV-8 infection in women and infants varies depending on the geographical location; infection is rare in the Western countries but is quite prevalent in the HIV epidemic countries in Africa. It is not known whether there is an increased risk of HHV-8 infection in pregnant women, but the transmission of HHV-8 from infected mothers to their infants during pregnancies is extremely rare even in the epidemic regions. The majority of the infected children probably acquired the virus horizontally via household contacts.

PRENATAL EVALUATION OF THE MOTHER AND FETUS

Although HHV-8 can be vertically transmitted, as documented in both a report *(52)* and the finding of KS in very young infants, the frequency of vertical transmission is as yet unknown. It probably happens only rarely, with a frequency probably no higher than that of perinatally acquired herpes simplex infection (i.e., 1:2000–1:5000). Unlike perinatally or congenitally acquired herpes simplex infection, however, the natural history of perinatally acquired HHV-8 infection has yet to be determined.

It is uncertain whether there is a greater risk of developing KS, another lymphoproliferative lesion, or any clinical syndrome associated with the acquisition of HHV-8 at an early age. Prior reports from Zambia have documented marked changes in the epidemiology of KS since the beginning of the AIDS pandemic *(57)*. The proportion of women with KS has increased during the last several years. The male-to-female ratio dropped from 10:1 in the early 1980s to 2:1 in the 1990s.

KS has also become one of the most common tumors of early childhood *(49)*. That the majority of pediatric cases are co-infected with HIV-1 suggests that the risk of developing KS may be enhanced following perinatal acquired infection of both agents from the mother. In this scenario, maternal immunosuppression secondary to HIV-1 may facilitate vertical transmission; KS in the infant may be promoted by HIV-1-related immunodeficiency acting in concert with the HIV proteins, such as Tat, which can modulate the immune response. Alternatively, there may be a number of HIV-1-infected infants who acquire HHV-8 as a result of horizontal transmission from other children or adults. The proportion of infants and children who develop KS as a result of perinatal vs horizontal acquisition is unknown.

There are few data regarding the natural history of primary HHV-8 infection. Most primary HHV-8 infections are probably asymptomatic *(58)*, although scattered reports have described the occurrence of symptomatic disease following primary infection among adults and children. Transient angioproliferative lymphadenopathy, fever, asthenia, arthralgia, myalgia, cervical lymphadenopathy, splenomegaly, mildly increased hepatic enzymes, diarrhea, and cytopenia have all been associated with primary HHV-8 infection in adults *(59,60)*. A prospective cohort study of 86 immunocompetent Egyptian children (aged 1–4 years) who presented with a febrile syndrome found that 42% of these children were HHV-8 seropositive *(61)*. Six children had suspected primary

HHV-8 infection. Five of these six had fever plus a prolonged maculopapular rash. Sore throat not associated with painful oral ulcers or reactive cervical lymphadeopathy was also noted. Reactivated HHV-8 infection may also present with symptoms, as evidenced by the case of an immunosuppressed, HHV-8-seropositive adult who developed fever, hepatitis, a maculopapular rash, and pancytopenia secondary to marrow failure in association with detectable HHV-8 DNA in the plasma *(62)*.

CLINICAL EVALUATION OF THE INFANT AFTER BIRTH

All infants considered at risk for acquiring HHV-8 perinatally should have a thorough physical examination to detect any cutaneous lesions. Lymphadenopathy should also be looked for as a number of the Zambian children previously described with early-onset KS presented with the lymphadenopathic form of the disease. All such children who present with persistent lymphadenopathy not secondary to tuberculosis should have a lymph node biopsy to rule out KS. All infants and children who present with cutaneous or lymphadenopathic KS should have a chest x-ray to screen for lung involvement. Patients who present with clinical evidence of either pulmonic or gastrointestinal KS should have a bronchoscopy or endoscopy as warranted to visualize and biopsy any suspicious lesions.

There are as yet no licensed commercial assays available that have been widely adopted for diagnosing HHV-8 infection. Any attempt to document or rule out perinatal transmission will require that specimens drawn for this purpose must be referred to a research laboratory with expertise in performing these assays and the necessary quality control mechanisms in place to verify their results. Initially, PBMCs should be screened at birth by an HHV-8-specific PCR assay, which can detect HHV-8 DNA. Because the virus copy numbers are expected to be extremely low in newly infected infants, the probability of detecting viral DNA even by PCR may be small. Therefore, repeat testing using both the HHV-8 DNA PCR and an HHV-8 immunoglobulin G assay should also be done at 12 months of age to (1) detect active infection, (2) document the clearance of residual maternal HHV-8 antibody if they are not infected, and (3) detect the presence of the infant's antibodies against the virus if they are infected. Any positive assays must be confirmed by repeated testing of additional blood specimens from the same infant. At this point, it appears that antibodies against HHV-8 persist after infection, but it is not clear whether the antibody levels will vary with time. Thus, there is a need to follow infected individuals longitudinally and serially determine their antibody titer to determine whether serological assays can be used to document chronic infection. If the infant is infected, then the family must be counseled regarding the current state of knowledge regarding HHV-8 and its relationship to KS. Although the family should be told of the potential risk of KS (especially if the infant is co-infected with HIV-1), it also should be emphasized that, given our current lack of knowledge, it cannot presently be projected whether the infant will develop KS.

DIAGNOSIS AND ASSAYS FOR HUMAN HERPESVIRUS 8 INFECTION

Diagnosis of HHV-8 infection in asymptomatic individuals relies on the detection of HHV-8 antibodies because viruses cannot be readily detected *(63)*. Viremia can be detected in only 10% of cases of primary infection close to the time of seroconversion *(64)*. A number of studies using a HHV-8-specific PCR have shown that HHV-8 DNA can be found in most KS lesions but not in non-KS tissues from KS patients. In addition, viral DNA can be detected by PCR in the saliva and blood of infected individuals and about 50% of the PBMC samples from KS patients. Detectable viral load appears with increasing tumor burden *(65)*. In asymptomatic HHV-8-infected individuals, the ability to detect HHV-8 DNA in the PBMCs is even lower *(19,66)*.

There are now a number of serological assays that detect antibodies against different viral antigens; however, none has optimal sensitivity and specificity. These assays include immunofluorescence assay (IFA), Western blot, and enzyme-linked immunosorbent assays (ELISA). They use a wide variety of HHV-8 antigens, such as infected whole cells, semipurified or purified virion protein, and various recombinant viral proteins *(67)*.

Among the three prototype assays, whole-cell IFA appears to be most sensitive and has been used most regularly. This assay is performed using HHV-8 chronically infected EBV-negative primary effusion lymphoma cells, such as body-cavity-based lymphoma or BC-3 *(68)*. These cells can either be induced with phorbol esters or butyrate *(69)* to express both nuclear and cytoplasmic lytic antigens or be used without induction to detect antibodies that are specific against latent viral antigens *(70)*. The lytic antigen IFA appears to have the highest sensitivity in detecting HHV-8 infection but also tends to be susceptible to cross-reactivity. This test is also limited by technician subjectivity relative to how the results are interpreted. With this assay, a serum dilution of at least 1:40 is usually used to avoid a nonspecific staining pattern, regardless of virus exposure status.

An alternative, less-subjective serology test for HHV-8 is the ELISA. A test using sucrose-purified virion has been developed *(71)*. This assay has a sensitivity of 90–95% in detecting antibodies in patients with KS, but its ability to detect antibodies in the general population and in epidemic areas like Africa has not been studied extensively. Additional ELISA assays have been developed using recombinant viral antigens, such as capsid protein ORF65.2 and lytic protein K8.1 *(72)*. These assays are comparable to the latent IFA assays in detecting antibodies in KS patients but tend to be more variable in the general blood donor population *(72,73)*. Western blot analyses using either infected whole-cell lysates or recombinant viral proteins have also been used *(44)*. The latency-associated nuclear antigen is the primary antigen detected using the whole-cell lysate *(11)*. These assays in general are much more difficult to perform. They are only about 80–90% sensitive in detecting antibodies in KS patients and are not practical for screening a low-risk population.

In spite of the availability of several serological tests available for detection of HHV-8 antibodies, none have optimal sensitivity or specificity. Although these tests have generally been shown to have good concordance in detecting HHV-8 antibodies in KS or other high-risk individuals, their results have been more variable in the general population. Because of the difficulty in performing the Western blot, the IFA is still the assay of choice, but testing and confirmation by an alternative assay, such as ELISA, is recommended.

REFERENCES

1. Boshoff C, Chang Y. Kaposi's sarcoma-associated herpesvirus: a new DNA tumor virus. Annu Rev Med 2001;52:453–470.
2. Chang Y, Cesarman E, Pessin MS, et al. Identification of herpesvirus-like DNA sequences in AIDS-associated Kaposi's sarcoma. Science 1994;266:1865–1869.
3. Sarid R, Wiezorek JS, Moore PS, Chang Y. Characterization and cell cycle regulation of the major Kaposi's sarcoma-associated herpesvirus (human herpesvirus 8) latent genes and their promoter. J Virol 1999;73:1438–1446.
4. Roizman B, Desrosiers RC, Fleckenstein B, Lopez C, Minson AC, Studdert MJ. The family Herpesviridae: an update. Arch Virol 1992;123:425–449.
5. Moore PS, Gao SJ, Dominguez G, et al. Primary characterization of a herpesvirus agent associated with Kaposi's sarcomae. J Virol 1996;70:549–558.
6. Renne R, Lagunoff M, Zhong W, Ganem D. The size and conformation of Kaposi's sarcoma-associated herpesvirus (human herpesvirus 8) DNA in infected cells and virions. J Virol 1996;70:8151–8154.
7. Russo JJ, Bohenzky RA, Chien MC, et al. Nucleotide sequence of the Kaposi sarcoma-associated herpesvirus (HHV8). Proc Natl Acad Sci U S A 1996;93:14,862–14,867.
8. Zong JC, Metroka C, Reitz MS, Nicholas J, Hayward GS. Strain variability among Kaposi sarcoma-associated herpesvirus (human herpesvirus 8) genomes: evidence that a large cohort of US AIDS patients may have been infected by a single common isolate. J Virol 1997;71:2505–2511.
9. Moore PS, Boshoff C, Weiss RA, Chang Y. Molecular mimicry of human cytokine and cytokine response pathway genes by KSHV. Science 1996;274:1739–1744.
10. Olsen SJ, Moore PS. Kaposi's sarcoma-associated herpesvirus (KSHV/HHV8) and the etiology of KS. In: Bendinelli M, Friedman H, Medveczky PG, eds. Herpesviruses and Immunity. New York: Plenum, 1998:115–147.
11. Gao SJ, Kingsley L, Hoover DR, et al. Seroconversion to antibodies against Kaposi's sarcoma-associated herpesvirus-related latent nuclear antigens before the development of Kaposi's sarcoma. N Engl J Med 1996;335:233–241.
12. Moore PS, Kingsley LA, Holmberg SD, et al. Kaposi's sarcoma-associated herpesvirus infection prior to onset of Kaposi's sarcoma. AIDS 1996;10:175–180.
13. Whitby D, Howard MR, Tenant-Flowers M, et al. Detection of Kaposi sarcoma associated herpesvirus in peripheral blood of HIV-infected individuals and progression to Kaposi's sarcoma. Lancet 1995;346:799–802.
14. Dukers NH, Renwick N, Prins M, et al. Risk factors for human herpesvirus 8 seropositivity and seroconversion in a cohort of homosexual men. Am J Epidemiol 2000;151:213–224.
15. Cesarman E, Chang Y, Moore PS, Said JW, Knowles DM. Kaposi's sarcoma-associated herpesvirus-like DNA sequences in AIDS-related body-cavity-based lymphomas. N Engl J Med 1995;332:1186–1191.
16. Soulier J, Grollet L, Oksenhendler E, et al. Kaposi's sarcoma-associated herpesvirus-like DNA sequences in multicentric Castleman's disease. Blood 1995;86:1276–1280.
17. Rettig MB, Ma HJ, Vescio RA, et al. Kaposi's sarcoma-associated herpesvirus infection of bone marrow dendritic cells from multiple myeloma patients. Science 1997;276:1851–1854.
18. Pellett PE, Wright DJ, Engels EA, et al. Multicenter comparison of serologic assays and estimation of human herpesvirus 8 seroprevalence among US blood donors. Transfusion 2003;43:1260–1268.
19. Schulz TF. KSHV (HHV8) infection. J Infect 2000;41:125–129.
20. Ariyoshi K, Schim van der Loeff M, Cook P, et al. Kaposi's sarcoma in the Gambia, West Africa is less frequent in human immunodeficiency virus type 2 than in human immunodeficiency virus type 1 infection despite a high prevalence of human herpesvirus 8. J Hum Virol 1998;1:193–199.

21. Gao SJ, Kingsley L, Li M, et al. KSHV antibodies among Americans, Italians and Ugandans with and without Kaposi's sarcoma. Nat Med 1996;2:925–928.

22. He J, Bhat G, Kankasa C, et al. Seroprevalence of human herpesvirus 8 among Zambian women of childbearing age without Kaposi's sarcoma (KS) and mother-child pairs with KS. J Infect Dis 1998;178:1787–1790.

23. Olsen SJ, Chang Y, Moore PS, Biggar RJ, Melbye M. Increasing Kaposi's sarcoma-associated herpesvirus seroprevalence with age in a highly Kaposi's sarcoma endemic region, Zambia in 1985. AIDS 1998;12:1921–1925.

24. Martin JN, Ganem DE, Osmond DH, Page-Shafer KA, Macrae D, Kedes DH. Sexual transmission and the natural history of human herpesvirus 8 infection. N Engl J Med 1998;338:948–954.

25. Melbye M, Cook PM, Hjalgrim H, et al. Risk factors for Kaposi's-sarcoma-associated herpesvirus (KSHV/HHV-8) seropositivity in a cohort of homosexual men, 1981–1996. Int J Cancer 1998;77:543–548.

26. Howard MR, Whitby D, Bahadur G, et al. Detection of human herpesvirus 8 DNA in semen from HIV-infected individuals but not healthy semen donors. AIDS 1997;11:F15–F19.

27. Huang YQ, Li JJ, Poiesz BJ, Kaplan MH, Friedman-Kien AE. Detection of the herpesvirus-like DNA sequences in matched specimens of semen and blood from patients with AIDS-related Kaposi's sarcoma by polymerase chain reaction in situ hybridization. Am J Pathol 1997;150:147–153.

28. Pellett PE, Spira TJ, Bagasra O, et al. Multicenter comparison of PCR assays for detection of human herpesvirus 8 DNA in semen. J Clin Microbiol 1999;37:1298–1301.

29. Cannon MJ, Dollard SC, Smith DK, et al. Blood-borne and sexual transmission of human herpesvirus 8 in women with or at risk for human immunodeficiency virus infection. N Engl J Med 2001;344:637–643.

30. Sosa C, Benetucci J, Hanna C, et al. Human herpesvirus 8 can be transmitted through blood in drug addicts. Medicina (B Aires) 2001;61:291–294.

31. Sosa C, Klaskala W, Chandran B, et al. Human herpesvirus 8 as a potential sexually transmitted agent in Honduras. J Infect Dis 1998;178:547–551.

32. Plancoulaine S, Gessain A, van Beveren M, Tortevoye P, Abel L. Evidence for a recessive major gene predisposing to human herpesvirus 8 (HHV-8) infection in a population in which HHV-8 is endemic. J Infect Dis 2003;187:1944–1950.

33. Grulich AE, Olsen SJ, Luo K, et al. Kaposi's sarcoma-associated herpesvirus: a sexually transmissible infection? J Acquir Immune Defic Syndr Hum Retrovirol 1999;20:387–393.

34. Lefrere JJ, Mcyohas MC, Mariotti M, Meynard JL, Thauvin M, Frottier J. Detection of human herpesvirus 8 DNA sequences before the appearance of Kaposi's sarcoma in human immunodeficiency virus (HIV)-positive subjects with a known date of HIV seroconversion. J Infect Dis 1996;174:283–287.

35. Blackbourn DJ, Ambroziak J, Lennette E, Adams M, Ramachandran B, Levy JA. Infectious human herpesvirus 8 in a healthy North American blood donor. Lancet 1997;349:609–611.

36. Regamey N, Cathomas G, Schwager M, Wernli M, Harr T, Erb P. High human herpesvirus 8 seroprevalence in the homosexual population in Switzerland. J Clin Microbiol 1998;36:1784–1786.

37. Parravicini C, Olsen SJ, Capra M, et al. Risk of Kaposi's sarcoma-associated herpes virus transmission from donor allografts among Italian posttransplant Kaposi's sarcoma patients. Blood 1996;90:2826–2829.

38. Blackbourn DJ, Lennette ET, Ambroziak J, Mourich DV, Levy JA. Human herpesvirus 8 detection in nasal secretions and saliva. J Infect Dis 1998;177:213–216.

39. Di Alberti L, Ngui SL, Porter SR, et al. Presence of human herpesvirus 8 variants in the oral tissues of human immunodeficiency virus-infected persons. J Infect Dis 1997;175:703–707.

40. Flaitz CM, Jin YT, Hicks MJ, Nichols CM, Wang YW, Su IJ. Kaposi's sarcoma-associated herpesvirus-like DNA sequences (KSHV/HHV-8) in oral AIDS-Kaposi's sarcoma: a PCR and clinicopathologic study. Oral Surg Oral Med Oral Pathol Oral Radiol Endod 1997;83:259–264.
41. Brayfield BP, Kankasa C, West JT, et al. Distribution of kaposi sarcoma-associated herpesvirus/human herpesvirus 8 in maternal saliva and breast milk in Zambia: implications for transmission. J Infect Dis 2004;189:2260–2270.
42. Kedes DH, Ganem D, Ameli N, Bacchetti P, Greenblatt R. The prevalence of serum antibody to human herpesvirus 8 (Kaposi sarcoma-associated herpesvirus) among HIV-seropositive and high-risk HIV-seronegative women. JAMA 1997;277:478–481.
43. Greenblatt RM, Jacobson LP, Levine AM, et al. Human herpesvirus 8 infection and Kaposi's sarcoma among human immunodeficiency virus-infected and uninfected women. J Infect Dis 2001;183:1130–1134.
44. Simpson GR, Schulz TF, Whitby D, et al. Prevalence of Kaposi's sarcoma associated herpesvirus infection measured by antibodies to recombinant capsid protein and latent immunofluorescence antigen. Lancet 1996;348:1133–1138.
45. Serraino D, Franceschi S, Dal Maso L, La Vecchia C. HIV transmission and Kaposi's sarcoma among European women. AIDS 1995;9:971–973.
46. Cattani P, Cerimele F, Porta D, et al. Age-specific seroprevalence of human herpesvirus 8 in Mediterranean regions. Clin Microbiol Infect 2003;9:274–279.
47. Gessain A, Mauclere P, van Beveren M, et al. Human herpesvirus 8 primary infection occurs during childhood in Cameroon, Central Africa. Int J Cancer 1999;81:189–192.
48. Mayama S, Cuevas LE, Sheldon J, et al. Prevalence and transmission of Kaposi's sarcoma-associated herpesvirus (human herpesvirus 8) in Ugandan children and adolescents. Int J Cancer 1998;77:817–820.
49. Athale UH., Patil PS, Chintu C, Elem B. Influence of HIV epidemic on the incidence of Kaposi's sarcoma in Zambian children. J Acquir Immune Defic Syndr Hum Retrovirol 1995;8:96–100.
50. Ziegler JL, Katongole-Mbidde E. Kaposi's sarcoma in childhood: an analysis of 100 cases from Uganda and relationship to HIV infection. Int J Cancer 1996;65:200–203.
51. Brayfield BP, Phiri S, Kankasa C, et al. Postnatal human herpesvirus 8 and human immunodeficiency virus type 1 infection in mothers and infants from Zambia. J Infect Dis 2003;187:559–568.
52. Mantina H, Kankasa C, Klaskala W, et al. Vertical transmission of Kaposi's sarcoma-associated herpesvirus. Int J Cancer 2001;94:749–752.
53. Sarmati L, Carlo T, Rossella S, et al. Human herpesvirus-8 infection in pregnancy and labor: lack of evidence of vertical transmission. J Med Virol 2004;72:462–466.
54. Bourboulia D, Whitby D, Boshoff C, et al. Serologic evidence for mother-to-child transmission of Kaposi sarcoma-associated herpesvirus infection. JAMA 1998;280:31–32.
55. Lyall EG, Patton GS, Sheldon J, et al. Evidence for horizontal and not vertical transmission of human herpesvirus 8 in children born to human immunodeficiency virus-infected mothers. Pediatr Infect Dis J 1999;18:795–799.
56. Mbulaiteye SM, Pfeiffer RM, Whitby D, Brubaker GR, Shao J, Biggar RJ. Human herpesvirus 8 infection within families in rural Tanzania. J Infect Dis 2003;187:1780–1785.
57. Chintu C, Athale UH, Patil PS. Childhood cancers in Zambia before and after the HIV epidemic. Arch Dis Child 1995;73:100–104;discussion 104–105.
58. Moore PS, Chang Y. Molecular virology of Kaposi's sarcoma-associated herpesvirus. Philos Trans R Soc Lond B Biol Sci 2001;356:499–516.
59. Marcelin AG, Dupin N, Simon F, Descamps D, Agut H, Calvez V. Primary infection with human herpesvirus 8 in an HIV-1-infected patient. AIDS 2000;14:1471–1473.
60. Oksenhendler E, Cazals-Hatem D, Schulz TF, et al. Transient angiolymphoid hyperplasia and Kaposi's sarcoma after primary infection with human herpesvirus 8 in a patient with human immunodeficiency virus infection. N Engl J Med 1998;338:1585–1590.

61. Andreoni M., Sarmati L, Nicastri E, et al. Primary human herpesvirus 8 infection in immunocompetent children. JAMA 2002;287:1295–1300.
62. Luppi M, Barozzi P, Schulz TF, et al. Nonmalignant disease associated with human herpesvirus 8 reactivation in patients who have undergone autologous peripheral blood stem cell transplantation. Blood 2000;96:2355–2357.
63. Harrington WJ Jr, Bagasra O, Sosa CE, et al. Human herpesvirus type 8 DNA sequences in cell-free plasma and mononuclear cells of Kaposi's sarcoma patients. J Infect Dis 1996;174:1101–1105.
64. Goudsmit J, Renwick N, Dukers NH, et al. Human herpesvirus 8 infections in the Amsterdam Cohort Studies (1984–1997): analysis of seroconversions to ORF65 and ORF73. Proc Natl Acad Sci U S A 2000;97:4838–4843.
65. Whitby D, Luppi M, Barozzi P, Boshoff C, Weiss RA, Torelli G. Human herpesvirus 8 seroprevalence in blood donors and lymphoma patients from different regions of Italy. J Natl Cancer Inst 1998;90:395–397.
66. Bigoni B, Dolcetti R, de Lellis L, et al. Human herpesvirus 8 is present in the lymphoid system of healthy persons and can reactivate in the course of AIDS. J Infect Dis 1996;173:542–549.
67. Rabkin CS, Schulz TF, Whitby D, et al. Interassay correlation of human herpesvirus 8 serologic tests. HHV-8 Interlaboratory Collaborative Group. J Infect Dis 1998;178:304–309.
68. Cesarman E, Moore PS, Rao PH, Inghirami G, Knowles DM, Chang Y. In vitro establishment and characterization of two acquired immunodeficiency syndrome-related lymphoma cell lines (BC-1 and BC-2) containing Kaposi's sarcoma-associated herpesvirus-like (KSHV) DNA sequences. Blood 1995;86:2708–2714.
69. Lennette ET, Blackbourn DJ, Levy JA. Antibodies to human herpesvirus type 8 in the general population and in Kaposi's sarcoma patients. Lancet 1996;348:858–861.
70. Kedes DH, Lagunoff M, Renne R, Ganem D. Identification of the gene encoding the major latency-associated nuclear antigen of the Kaposi's sarcoma-associated herpesvirus. J Clin Invest 1997;100:2606–2610.
71. Chatlynne LG, Lapps W, Handy M, et al. Detection and titration of human herpesvirus-8-specific antibodies in sera from blood donors, acquired immunodeficiency syndrome patients, and Kaposi's sarcoma patients using a whole virus enzyme-linked immunosorbent assay. Blood 1998;92:53–58.
72. Chandran B, Bloomer C, Chan SR, Zhu L, Goldstein E, Horvat R. Human herpesvirus-8 ORF K8.1 gene encodes immunogenic glycoproteins generated by spliced transcripts. Virology 1998;249:140–149.
73. Raab MS, Albrecht JC, Birkmann A, et al. The immunogenic glycoprotein gp35–37 of human herpesvirus 8 is encoded by open reading frame K8.1. J Virol 1998;72:6725–6731.

11
Rubella

Cecelia Hutto

INTRODUCTION

Rubella, also called German measles or the 3-day measles, is a mild, self-limited infection in most individuals who acquire the infection after birth. A primary rubella infection during pregnancy, however, can cause significant problems for the fetus, including fetal death, miscarriage, or congenital anomalies. The teratogenic potential for rubella was first reported by Sir Norman Gregg, an ophthalmologist, in 1941 when he noted cataracts and congenital heart disease in a large number of newborns whose mothers had rubella during their pregnancy *(1)*. An association between maternal rubella and birth defects was confirmed during the worldwide rubella pandemic that occurred between 1962 and 1964, when there were an estimated 12.5 million cases of rubella, 11,000 fetal deaths, and 20,000 newborns with congenital birth defects *(2)*. The routine use of the rubella vaccine beginning in 1969 in the United States resulted in a marked decline in the incidence of rubella and congenital rubella in this country. However, sporadic cases continue to occur, particularly among individuals immigrating from countries in which rubella continues to be endemic.

EPIDEMIOLOGY AND TRANSMISSION

The virus that causes rubella is a ribonucleic acid virus and a member of the Togaviridae family, which also includes the arboviruses. The rubella virus, however, is not related serologically to arboviruses or any other known viruses. Rubella is spread either by the direct contact with nasopharyngeal secretions of an infected individual or through droplets. Congenital infections in infants result from transplacental spread of virus associated with maternal viremia during a primary infection.

Rubella occurs throughout the world, but the epidemiology varies globally. In temperate climates, the peak incidence for infection is the late winter and spring. Rubella remains prevalent in many areas of the world in which the rubella vaccine is not used. In the United States and other countries where the vaccine has been given routinely since the early 1970s, the epidemiology of rubella has changed dramatically. Epidemics of rubella, which occurred in 6- to 9-year cycles prior to vaccine use, have been disrupted, and endemic rubella has been almost eradicated in the United States *(3)*. A 99% reduction in reported cases of rubella and the congenital rubella syndrome (CRS) occurred in the United States between 1965, when the last epidemic occurred, and

From: *Infectious Disease: Congenital and Perinatal Infections: A Concise Guide to Diagnosis*
Edited by: C. Hutto © Humana Press Inc., Totowa, NJ

1998 *(4)*. With the exception of 1998, there were fewer than 300 reported cases of rubella each year in the United States between 1992 and 1999 *(5)*.

The demographic characteristics of individuals with rubella reported to the Centers for Disease Control and Prevention also changed significantly during the decade of the 1990s. During this decade, rubella occurred more commonly in older individuals than children. Children younger than 15 years of age accounted for only 11% of the cases in 1996 compared with 69% in 1990 *(5)*. The incidence of rubella among individuals 15–44 years was twice as high in the latter half of the decade as compared to 1990.

Changes were also seen in the distribution of cases by ethnicity. Most of the reported cases occurred in individuals of Hispanic ethnicity, many of whom were born outside the United States. A study of 49 infants with CRS who were born in California between 1990 and 1999 identified maternal risk factors for rubella *(4)*. The mothers of infants with CRS were young, with a mean age of 23 years (range 15–33 years), 73% were Hispanic, and 60% of the mothers were born outside the United States. Most received prenatal care, but a fourth received no prenatal care or received care late in pregnancy only. Outbreaks of rubella have also occurred among individuals in closed religious communities over the past decade *(6)*. Rubella and congenital rubella, however, have affected the Hispanic population of the United States disproportionately over the past decade *(5)*. These changes underscore the role of international travel and immigration in the changing epidemiology of rubella and other infections and emphasize the continuing importance, for clinicians responsible for the care of pregnant women and infants, of being cognizant of the clinical presentation of rubella and its effects on the fetus.

RISK OF MATERNAL INFECTION

In the United States at this time, the risk of rubella infection in a woman during pregnancy who is born in this country is low. However, there continue to be populations of women of childbearing age who are susceptible to rubella infection. Premarital screening programs in some states have found 6–11% of postpubertal females are seronegative *(7,8)*. A similar rate was reported in a study that identified risk factors for rubella susceptibility among Mexican-born and US-born workers at a chicken processing plant in the southern United States in which an outbreak occurred *(9)*. The rate for Mexican-born women in this study was three times that of US-born women, but the rate of susceptibility among US-born females was 9%.

RISK OF CONGENITAL INFECTION

Intrauterine transmission of rubella occurs during viremia in the mother. Because antibody protects against significant viremia, neonates born to women without preexisting immunity are at risk for congenital infection if the mother has an infection during her pregnancy. Reinfection of women during pregnancy may occur, but the risk of fetal infection with reinfection is felt to be very low *(10)*.

Although transmission of infection to the fetus has been documented after maternal exposure during any trimester of pregnancy, both the risk of infection and the risk of associated birth defects are related to the trimester of maternal exposure, with infection during the first trimester having the greatest risk. Congenital infection occurred in 81% of infants born to mothers having serologically confirmed rubella during the first trimester in one study *(11)*. The rate of infection in infants whose mothers had exposure before 11 weeks of gestation was 90%. With maternal infection during the second and third trimester, the rate of infection in neonates was 39 and 53%, respectively. In another study, the rate of congenital infection based on demonstration of an immunoglobulin (Ig) M response in the infant was 28% if maternal infection occurred during the second trimester and 29% with maternal infection during the third trimester *(12)*.

For infants with congenital infection, the risk of congenital anomalies is also closely associated with the gestational age of the fetus at the time of maternal infection. The risk for defects in neonates infected during the first trimester of pregnancy is very high. As many as 85% of neonates of mothers with infection during the first 4 weeks of gestation have congenital anomalies, but the risk falls to 20–30% during the second month of gestation and 5% during the third month *(13)*. Infection after the 16th week of gestation rarely results in congenital defects in the infant that are detectable at birth *(3)*. A number of abnormalities may not be present or not detected at birth but can present months to years later *(10)*. These include deafness, ocular abnormalities, endocrinopathies, and central nervous system disease.

EVALUATION OF PREGNANT WOMAN

Most acquired rubella infections are asymptomatic or cause only mild disease. Low-grade fever, an erythematous nonconfluent macular papular rash that begins on the face and spreads to the trunk, and generalized lymphadenopathy are the typical signs of infection. Cough, coryza, and conjunctivitis may also be present; in adults, arthritis or arthralgias may occur at the time of the onset of the rash or soon after its appearance. The arthritis is often slow to resolve, but it usually does not cause chronic symptoms. Women are affected more frequently than men with arthritis; as many as one-third of women may have joint symptoms *(14,15)*.

In the United States, rubella serology is obtained prenatally to document the woman's susceptibility to rubella. If rubella immunity is documented, the woman is protected from primary infection, and the fetus is not at risk for congenital anomalies. Rubella immunity is defined according to the type of serologic assay used. For example, assays measuring antibodies using the hemagglutinin inhibition require a titer above 1:8 for immunity, whereas the optical density required by the enzyme immunoassay (EIA) depends on the limit set by the assay's manufacturer *(16)*. Any pregnant woman who is not seroimmune and has exposure to rubella during her pregnancy should be followed carefully for the next few weeks after exposure. (The incubation period for rubella is 2–3 weeks.) If she has fever, a rash, lymphadenopathy, arthralgias, or arthritis, an evaluation for infection is indicated.

Diagnosis of an acute rubella infection in a woman during pregnancy may be made by culture of the nose or throat. In acquired rubella, virus shedding is most consistent and intense in the nasopharynx, but the period of shedding is limited to the period from about 1 week prior to the rash to about 14 days after the rash *(10)*. A more common and practical approach for diagnosis is the use of rubella-specific IgM antibody. IgM antibodies can be detected at low levels at the time of onset of the rash and are generally present within 5–10 days after the onset of the rash *(10)*. After reaching their peak in titer at about 3 weeks after the rash begins, they then decline rapidly (Fig. 1). Knowledge of the kinetics of the IgM response to infection will allow serum to be obtained at

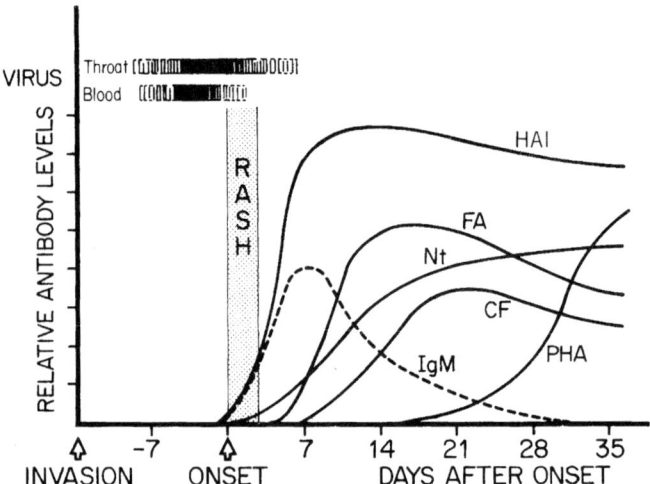

Fig. 1. Schematic of the immune response in acute rubella infection. CF, complement fixation; EIA, enzyme immunoassay; FIA/FIAX and IFA, immunofluorescence; HI, hemagglutination inhibition; IgM, immunoglobulin M; LA, latex agglutination; Nt, neutralization; PHA, passive agglutination; RIA, radioimmunoassay. (From refs. *10* and *17*, with permission.)

a time when the antibodies are most likely to be present. If IgM antibodies are not present in the initial serum, consideration should be given to obtaining another sample from the woman for testing because the initial test may have been done prior to the development of IgM. The presence of IgM antibody in high titers is diagnostic of a recent infection with rubella.

Because false-positive and false-negative IgM antibodies may occur, serological evidence of infection should be confirmed with rubella IgG antibody measurement. Serum collected at the time of exposure or as soon as possible after the onset of rash and 2–4 weeks later is tested for IgG antibody to determine if seroconversion has occurred. If seroconversion has occurred, the IgM is positive in high titers, or the culture is positive, the risk of fetal infection and malformation is considerable if the mother was exposed during the first trimester. Because of the risk associated with congenital rubella and the not-infrequent problems with serological assays, the assays should be repeated to confirm the accuracy of the diagnosis. Because rubella may be asymptomatic or very mild in some individuals, evaluating a pregnant woman for evidence of a recent infection should also be considered in any woman with known exposure to rubella even if she has had no symptoms.

EVALUATION OF THE NEWBORN

Intrauterine infection with rubella can affect any organ system, and infants often have multiple organ systems involved. The spectrum of clinical abnormalities reported with congenital rubella is extremely diverse. The most common abnormalities, however, are ophthalmological, cardiac, auditory, and neurological. Common ophthalmological abnormalities include cataracts, retinopathy, and congenital glaucoma. Patent ductus arteriosus, the most common cardiac anomaly, occurs in about one-third of infants with symptomatic infection. Pulmonary artery stenosis and pulmonary valvular stenosis are also common. Sensorineural hearing loss occurs more frequently than any other anomaly, may be the only manifestation of infection, and may not be detected at birth *(4)*. Meningoencephalitis and microcephaly are two of the most common central nervous system abnormalities that may be present at birth in some infants. Infants often have growth retardation at birth, and other frequently associated findings are hepatomegaly, splenomegaly, thrombocytopenia, and the "blueberry muffin" skin rash. These symptoms are often self-limited and resolve with time *(15)*.

For an infant born to a mother with known exposure to rubella, the diagnosis of rubella is usually not difficult if the infant has any of these anomalies at birth. Virologic or serologic confirmation, however, is important because the clinical disease associated with rubella can mimic disease caused by other microbial pathogens that can be transmitted to an infant *in utero*, including cytomegalovirus, toxoplasmosis, and syphilis. In the absence of known maternal exposure, rubella should be considered in infants with intrauterine growth retardation who have other clinical anomalies consistent with rubella. Consideration of rubella is particularly important in infants if their mother's rubella serology is not known, if their mother did not receive prenatal care, or if their mother immigrated from a country where rubella vaccine is not routinely given.

The diagnosis of congenital rubella can be confirmed with virus isolation, which is the most reliable method of making the diagnosis. Unlike individuals who acquire rubella postnatally, infants with congenital rubella excrete the virus for months. Cultures are most sensitive for isolation of virus when done soon after birth because the quantity of virus present decreases over time. The nasopharynx and throat are probably the best sites for isolation of virus, but it may also be cultured from the urine, blood, feces, and cerebrospinal fluid *(10)*.

For most clinicians, a more practical approach to diagnosis is the use of serology because diagnosis of infection may be made with rubella-specific IgM antibody. Either cord blood or neonatal serum may be used. A limitation of IgM antibody for diagnosis includes the occurrence of false-positive assays because of the presence of rheumatoid factor. False-negative assays may also occur because the infant does not make detectable levels of antibody, IgM antibodies are no longer present when the diagnosis is considered, or there is variation in the performance of serologic assays. To enhance the sensitivity of the IgM assay for diagnosis, it has been recommended that the test be done within the first 2 months of life *(4)*.

IgG antibodies can also be used to diagnose congenital infection by observing the pattern of antibody in the serum over time. Titers should be obtained at birth, 3 months, and at about 6 months and then run concurrently *(10)*. If IgG antibodies persist at 6–12 months with a titer that is similar to or greater than that which occurred at birth, it is likely the infant had an intrauterine infection. A potential confounding factor when IgG antibodies are used for diagnosis is that infants can become infected with rubella after birth, and IgG antibodies would be present in response to a postnatal infection. Diagnosis of intrauterine infection using IgG antibodies requires consideration of the possibility that rubella exposure and infection occurred after birth.

SEROLOGIC ASSAYS FOR RUBELLA

As shown in Fig. 1, there are a number of serologic assays available for measuring rubella IgG antibodies. The hemagglutinin inhibition assay was the standard for many years because of its reliability. Other assays that are now more available commercially and used more commonly are the EIA, immunofluorescent assay, and the latex agglutination assay. Because rubella titers vary according to the test used, the same assay should be used for testing acute and convalescent sera for rubella seroconversion. Several serologic assays are also available for IgM measurements and include the EIA, immunofluorescent assay, and hemagglutinin inhibition assay. Experts at a workshop in 2000 about congenital rubella in the United States proposed the EIA IgM capture assay as the preferred initial assay for use *(4)*.

SUMMARY

In the United States and areas of the world where rubella vaccine is routinely used, congenital rubella is no longer commonly seen. Cases do continue to be reported, however, and occur mostly in infants born to mothers who immigrated from countries where rubella continues to occur because the vaccine is not yet widely or routinely given. Women without prenatal care, particularly if they immigrated from these countries, or pregnant women in whom rubella serology is negative at the time of prenatal care should be evaluated for rubella if they are exposed to rubella or a person with symptoms of rubella. Cultures are sensitive and reliable for diagnosis of rubella in infants suspected of having congenital rubella. Diagnosis may also be made with a rubella-specific IgM antibody assay, but limitations of the assay should be considered.

REFERENCES

1. Gregg NM. Congenital cataract following German measles in the mother. Trans Ophthalmol Soc Aust 1941;3:35–46.
2. Rubella Surveillance. National Communicable Disease Center, US Department of Health, Education, and Welfare, no. 1, June 1969.
3. Plotkin SA. Rubella eradication. Vaccine 2001;19:3311–3319.
4. Reef SE, Plotkin S, Cordero JF, et al. Preparing for elimination of congenital rubella syndrome (CRS): summary of a workshop on CRS elimination in the US. Clin Infect Dis 2000:31:85–95.
5. Reef SE, Frey TK, Theall K, et al. The changing epidemiology of rubella in the 1990s. On the verge of elimination and new challenges for control and prevention. JAMA 2002;287:464–472.
6. Mellinger AK, Cragan JD, Atkinson WL, et al. High incidence of congenital rubella syndrome after a rubella outbreak. Pediatr Infect Dis J 1995;4:573–578.
7. Stehr-Green PA, Cochi SL, Preblud SR, Orestein WA. Evidence against increasing rubella seronegativity among adolescent girls. Am J Public Health 1990;80:88.
8. Schum TR, Nelson DB, Duma MA, Senmak GV. Increasing rubella seronegativity despite a compulsory school law. Am J Public Health 1989;79:66–69.
9. Danovaro-Holliday MC, Gordon ER, Woernle C , et al. Identifying risk factors for rubella susceptibility in a population at risk in the United States. Am J Public Health 2003;93:289–291.
10. Cooper LZ, Alford CA. Rubella. In: Remington JS, Klein JO, eds. Infectious Diseases of the Fetus and Newborn, 5th ed. Philadelphia: Saunders, 2001:347–388.
11. Miller E, Cradock-Watson JD, Pollock TM. Consequences of confirmed maternal rubella at successive stages of pregnancy. Lancet 1982;2:782–785.
12. Cradock-Watson JE, Ridehalgh MK, Anderson MJ, et al. Fetal infection resulting from maternal rubella after the first trimester of pregnancy. J Hyg Camb 1980;85:381–391.

13. American Academy of Pediatrics. Rubella. In: Pickering LK, ed. Red Book, 2003 Report of the Committee on Infectious Diseases, 26th ed. Elk Grove Village, IL: American Academy of Pediatrics, 2003:536–541.
14. Johnson RE, Hall AP. Rubella arthritis. N Engl J Med. 1958;258:743–745.
15. Krugman S, ed. Rubella symposium. Am J Dis Child 1965;110:345.
16. Plot S. Rubella vaccine. In: Plotkin SA, Orenstein WA, eds. Vaccines, 3rd ed. Philadelphia: Saunders, 1999:409–439.
17. Hermann KL. Rubella virus. In: Lennette EH, Schmidt NJ, eds. Diagnostic Procedures for Viral, Rickettsial and Chlamydial Infections. Wasington, DC: American Public Health Association, 1979:725.

Mobeen H. Rathore

INTRODUCTION

Parvoviruses belong to the family Parvoviridae. They are single-stranded, relatively uniform, isometric, nonenveloped deoxyribonucleic acid (DNA) viruses that infect many animals, including humans. The parvoviruses are extremely resistant to inactivation and can survive in a wide pH range (3.0–9.0) and at 60°C for up to 12 hours. Parvovirus B19 is the only genus of parvovirus proven to cause human infection. First discovered in 1975, parvovirus was not linked to human disease until 1981 (1,2). In 1983, parvovirus B19 was associated with erythema infectiosum; in 1984, this virus was associated with poor outcome of pregnancy and in 1985 with arthropathy (3–5). Parvoviruses are 20–25 nm in diameter, and the B19 genome has been completely sequenced (6,7). There is some antigenic variability between strains; however, the significance of this variability is not known (8). Cultivation of the virus requires red blood cell precursors, but none of the cultivation techniques have practical use for clinical diagnosis. Parvovirus B19 causes a number of diseases in humans. Most parvovirus B19 infections, however, are likely to be asymptomatic or not recognized.

PATHOGENESIS

During the first week after infection, parvovirus B19 causes a viremia that may be associated with fever, malaise, and other constitutional symptoms. During this period of viremia, the bone marrow is also infected, and the virus replicates in and kills the erythroid progenitor cells, resulting in their depletion. The reticulocyte count drops precipitously and is followed by anemia. In most otherwise healthy individuals, these changes are inconsequential with complete recovery of the bone marrow. However, in individuals with red blood cells that have a shorter than normal life span and who have underlying chronic anemia, parvovirus infection can result in serious anemia. This could be a potential problem in pregnant women who are already severely anemic. Parvovirus B19 can also occasionally infect other cell lines, causing leukopenia and thrombocytopenia (9,10). The immune response to parvovirus is primarily through antibody production and immunity is lifelong.

Parvovirus B19 infection in the animal model suggests that the virus can easily overcome the placental barrier. Parvovirus B19 is pathogenic throughout pregnancy, and

From: *Infectious Disease: Congenital and Perinatal Infections: A Concise Guide to Diagnosis*
Edited by: C. Hutto © Humana Press Inc., Totowa, NJ

because it destroys the dividing cells rather than just inhibiting mitotic activity, it is more embryocidal and less teratogenic *(11)*.

TRANSMISSION

Parvovirus B19 infections usually occur in winter and spring but can occur through-out the year *(12)*. Although direct proof of the routes of transmission and spread are lacking, it is most likely that parvovirus B19 is transmitted from person to person by direct contact with the respiratory secretions of infected individuals. Indirect proof of spread by respiratory secretions is provided by studies in which parvovirus B19 was isolated from respiratory secretions of infected individuals and by studies of human volunteers infected by intranasal inoculation of the virus *(13–15)*.

Spread of infection by direct contact rather than airborne spread is supported by the epidemiology of parvovirus B19. Infection spreads slowly, and the virus causes infec-tions in contacts over long periods of time rather than by rapid spread over short peri-ods of time, a pattern that is typical of infections spread by aerosol droplets. Vertical transmission is the only proven natural method for transmission of parvovirus B19. Contaminated blood products and needles can also transmit the infection. Parvovirus B19 in secretions of infected persons can cause environmental contamination, and chemicals commonly used to clean environmental surfaces may not always be effec-tive in eliminating the virus from surfaces and fomites. As a result, nosocomial trans-mission of parvovirus B19 without direct contact with an infected individual can occur *(16,17)*. Because environmental decontamination and eradication of parvovirus B19 from surfaces is difficult, this virus can be transmitted in many settings in which sur-face contamination by respiratory secretions occurs. In day care centers, homes, and schools where young children live and play, contamination of the environment with saliva occurs, and there is a high risk of transmission of infection to others sharing the space, including susceptible pregnant women.

RISK OF MATERNAL INFECTION DURING PREGNANCY

There are no data that provide direct evidence of the incidence of acute parvovirus B19 infection during pregnancy. Seroprevalence studies in the general population sug-gest that 28–86% of women of reproductive age do not have antibodies to parvovirus B19 and may be at risk for acute parvovirus B19 infection *(18–20)*. Seroprevalence increases with age; therefore, younger women are at a higher risk for acute infection compared with older women (Table 1).

There are few data about the incidence of acute parvovirus B19 infection in pregnant women. One study suggested an annual seroconversion rate of 1.4% in the absence of an outbreak *(19)*. This would give an infection rate of 1.1% for susceptible women over the 40-week period of pregnancy. In another study of 1610 pregnant women, 35% had serologic evidence of prior parvovirus B19 infection at the time of study entry. Of the women, 2% had serologic evidence of acute infection at entry, and another 2% of the women seroconverted prior to delivery. This study had a total infection rate of 4% (60 women) during pregnancy *(21)*. Another study noted a seroconversion rate of 13% during an epidemic of parvovirus B19 infection compared with 1.5% in nonepidemic periods *(22)*.

Table 1
Age-Related Prevalence of Parvovirus B19 Infection[a]

Age	Prevalence
<1 year	Unknown[b]
1–5 years	2–15%
5–19 years	15–60%
>20 years	45–75%

[a]By anti-B19 IgG.
[b]Because of transplacentally acquired antibodies. (Adapted from refs. *38* and *39*.)

FETAL AND NEONATAL RISK WITH MATERNAL INFECTION

Transplacental parvovirus B19 infection is well documented; however, the incidence of intrauterine parvovirus B19 infection, although considered low, is not known. One study estimated a perinatal infection rate of 33% *(23)*. In another study, 56 infants born to 55 women who were infected during pregnancy showed no *in utero* ultrasonographic evidence of hydrops fetalis. Six (11%) of these infants had serological evidence of congenital parvovirus B19 infection at birth. All newborns were healthy at birth and were without evidence of congenital abnormalities. Forty-eight of these infants were followed up to 12 months of age and remained clinically well, and all of them had serology for parvovirus B19 performed around 12 months of age. Based on confirmed infection at 12 months of age, it was determined that in mothers infected after 20 weeks of gestation, the risk of infection was more than double that for those infected before 20 weeks of gestation (35 vs 16%) *(21)*.

Most neonates born to women infected with parvovirus B19 during pregnancy will appear normal, and less than one-third of the women who are infected during pregnancy become symptomatic. Therefore, most infections will often not be recognized in either the pregnant woman or the newborn. However, parvovirus B19 infection during pregnancy can have an adverse outcome. In one study, 5 of the 60 women infected during pregnancy had spontaneous abortions, but evidence of parvovirus B19 infection was present in only one abortus. This study had a fetal death rate directly attributable to parvovirus B19 of fewer than 1 in 1000 pregnancies *(21)*.

Parvovirus B19 intrauterine infection is a known cause of fetal demise *(24)*; however, the frequency of B19 as a cause of fetal death is unknown. Although parvovirus B19 may contribute to only a limited number of fetal deaths, the estimates of 1–3% may be low *(25)*. In a study that enrolled pregnant women with serologically confirmed parvovirus B19 infection, the overall fetal death rate was 33% *(26)*. However, in a much smaller cohort of women infected during an outbreak of parvovirus B19 infection, the fetal death rate was only 3% *(27)*. Other studies have shown that the risk of fetal death is higher if infection occurs before 22 weeks of gestation *(28,29)*.

Nonimmune fetal hydrops is a well-described result of maternal parvovirus B19 infection, although its frequency is not clear. Reported frequencies varying from less than 1 to 27% have been reported in various studies *(30,31)*. More recent data suggested a much lower incidence of nonimmune hydrops associated with parvovirus B19 infection in the fetus.

Most live neonates with parvovirus B19 infection are either asymptomatic or have nonimmune hydrops. Reports of an association of parvovirus B19 infection with birth defects are growing. There is a possible association of parvovirus B19 infection with ophthalmological, cardiac, and neurological birth defects, but there is no epidemiological information to confirm this association *(4)*. The frequency of developmental delay in children with congenital parvovirus B19 infection followed up to 10 years of age is not different from that in the general population *(28)*.

COUNSELING OF PREGNANT WOMEN

Pregnant women with parvovirus infection should be counseled about the limitations of current data concerning the risk to the fetus and the long-term outcome for the infant. Routine antenatal screening for parvovirus B19 is not recommended because it is not possible to prevent the risk of infection. It should be stressed that the current state of knowledge indicates that the risk for an adverse pregnancy outcome, although not zero, is low. Women should be further counseled that they should report exposure to parvovirus B19-infected persons to their physician, and that the probability of a good outcome of pregnancy is high even if infection occurs during pregnancy.

Although a large number of women of childbearing age are potentially susceptible to parvovirus B19, the risk of intrauterine infection is low. Because of this, exclusion of pregnant women from work cannot be supported and is not recommended. In addition, the majority of infected individuals are asymptomatic, and those having symptoms are contagious prior to developing symptoms.

A discussion of risk factors is warranted with all pregnant women, especially those who are around children. Preconceptional counseling of these women should include discussion about the fetal risk of parvovirus B19 infection during pregnancy. Some women may choose to get tested for parvovirus B19 prior to getting pregnant, and serology would be the recommended test in these women. The presence of immunoglobulin (Ig) G antibody to parvovirus indicates that a woman is not at risk for parvovirus B19 infection. Currently, exclusion of pregnant women from the workplace (and other high-risk groups) during an outbreak of parvovirus B19 is not recommended. Women at greatest risk are those who work in the health care industry (especially with children), teachers, day care center workers, and mothers with an infected child in the household *(12,32)*.

Clinicians are frequently faced with the situation of a pregnant woman with work-related exposure to parvovirus B19 infection. In this circumstance, testing using serology is recommended. Interpretation of the mother's serology and risk for the fetus are described in Table 2. Exposure during a workplace outbreak may warrant diagnostic testing for the mother (Fig. 1).

Prenatal Evaluation of the Mother and Fetus

The prenatal evaluation and diagnosis of parvovirus B19 infection in the mother is not difficult, but determination of infection in the fetus may be complicated. Universal screening for parvovirus B19 is not recommended because of the low risk of maternal infection and low risk of adverse outcome to the fetus *(33)*. Screening is recommended for pregnant women exposed to individuals with erythema infectiosum, in an aplastic crisis, and in an outbreak (because of a high attack rate in some situations) *(26–*

Table 2
Maternal Parvovirus B19 Serology
and Associated Fetal Risk

IgG	IgM	Maternal infection	Fetal risk
+	–	Past infection	No risk
+	+	Recent acute infection	At risk
–	+	Active infection	At risk
–	–	No infection	No risk

+, positive; –, negative.

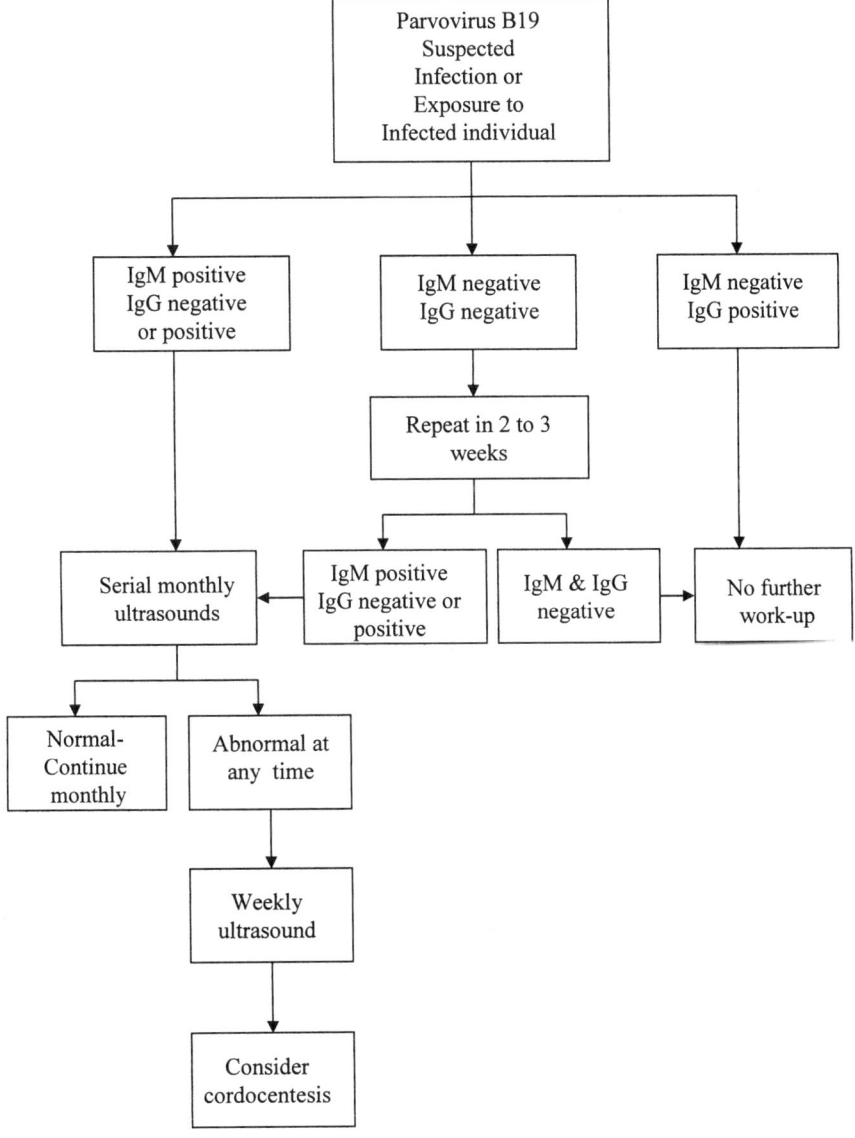

Fig. 1. Algorithm for maternal evaluation for parvovirus B19 infection during pregnancy.

28,30,31,33,34). A pregnant woman presenting with rash and arthropathy should be evaluated for parvovirus B19 infection. If maternal infection is suspected, this should be confirmed by laboratory tests. An algorithm for evaluation of mother and fetus is shown in Fig. 1.

The diagnosis of parvovirus B19 infection in pregnant women is not different from any other individual with suspected parvovirus B19 infection. Clinical presentation and disease caused by parvovirus B19 infection in pregnant women may not be very different from otherwise healthy individuals. The infection presents as a self-limited, mild, viral-like illness in 50% of individuals; 25% remain asymptomatic, and the remaining 25% may present with a rash (classically slapped-cheek appearance in children) or joint symptoms *(35)*. Asymptomatic pregnant women may be diagnosed with parvovirus B19 infection because of serologic testing during a community outbreak of the infection or exposure of a pregnant woman to an individual with the infection. Women who are immunosuppressed or those with an unstable red cell population and short red cell life span (e.g., hemoglobinopathies) can have a severe and prolonged illness. There are no data to suggest that pregnancy has an effect on parvovirus B19 infection, making disease caused by this infection worse.

Both IgG and IgM antibodies to parvovirus B19 should be tested. Parvovirus B19 IgM is detectable 1–3 weeks after infection, and high titers are present during the second week after infection and can persist for up to 3 months *(14)*. The parvovirus B19 IgM is usually present when the patient is symptomatic with a rash. Parvovirus B19-specific IgG is detectable within 1–2 weeks and at the time of the appearance of rash and arthropathy and can persist for prolonged periods of time *(14)*. The presence of IgM only or IgM and IgG anti-B19-specific antibodies is diagnostic of an acute infection (Table 2). Because of the appearance of both IgG and IgM anti-parvovirus B19 antibodies in such close temporal proximity, it is not unusual for both IgG and IgM antibodies to be present simultaneously in acute infection. The presence of IgG antibodies only is evidence of past infection, and the patient is considered immune. The absence of both IgG and IgM anti-parvovirus B19 antibodies is an indication that the patient is susceptible to parvovirus B19 infection.

Because intrauterine parvovirus B19 infection cannot always be diagnosed with serology, detection of viral DNA may be needed to make a diagnosis. Parvovirus B19 polymerase chain reaction (PCR) can detect DNA in amniotic fluid and maternal and fetal blood in infected patients. Prenatal diagnosis of fetal parvovirus B19 infection can be confirmed using amniotic fluid, fetal blood, and other fetal tissue specimens. Because the incidence of intrauterine infection and disease (including hydrops) is low, the benefits of performing such tests cannot be justified because of the associated risks of the procedures for obtaining these specimens. The role of maternal α-fetoprotein levels in diagnosis of fetal parvovirus B19 disease is uncertain. Maternal α-fetoprotein levels may be elevated in some cases, and some authorities recommend serial levels in mothers who are infected during pregnancy. Because maternal α-fetoprotein levels have not been evaluated as an indication of fetal parvovirus B19 disease, their sensitivity and specificity are not known. It cannot be recommended as a routine test for evaluation of fetal parvovirus B19 disease.

Diagnosis of intrauterine parvovirus B19 disease requires careful follow-up of the fetus once exposure and infection with parvovirus during pregnancy is confirmed or highly suspected. The diagnosis of parvovirus B19 disease in the fetus is primarily based on the diagnosis of hydrops. A baseline fetal ultrasound is recommended. The use of serial ultrasound examinations throughout pregnancy, however, is not universally recommended *(34)*. Because a fetal infection will most likely be manifested within 3 months of maternal infection, serial ultrasounds should at least be considered during this time period. Serial ultrasonography can detect signs of hydrops, such as scalp edema and ascites, as well as pericardial and pleural effusions. The placenta may also appear large in these cases.

If hydrops is diagnosed after a maternal parvovirus B19 infection, the fetus should be followed. A conservative approach with weekly ultrasonographic evaluation is recommended. If the hydrops does not resolve, cordocentesis should be considered to assess the fetal hematocrit. Cordocentesis is not without risk to the fetus, and the risks should be considered when performing this procedure. The ability to perform an intrauterine transfusion should be available if one is needed.

Clinical Evaluation of the Infant

As with older children and adults, most parvovirus B19 infections in newborn infants are asymptomatic *(19)*. Therefore, the diagnosis of perinatally acquired parvovirus B19 infection depends largely on a high index of suspicion, a history of maternal exposure to or infection with parvovirus B19, and serological evaluation of the mother and the newborn. However, serological evaluation of an asymptomatic newborn is fraught with difficulties because of an unpredictable immunological response in the baby.

First, the baby may have transplacentally acquired maternal anti-B19 IgG antibodies, which may take up to 1 year to become undetectable. The use of anti-B19 IgM antibodies for diagnosis of newborn infection is insensitive. A number of studies have shown a very small percentage of newborn infants infected with parvovirus B19 have detectable anti-B19 IgM antibodies at birth. In addition, in some infants with detectable anti-B19 IgM antibodies at birth, neither anti-B19 IgM nor IgG antibodies were found later in infancy. The use of anti-B19 IgA antibodies for diagnosis of infection is even less well studied and remains largely a research tool *(36)*.

There is no single test that is diagnostic for congenital parvovirus B19 infection if the neonate is asymptomatic. Although parvovirus B19 infection may be diagnosed by use of electron microscopy to visualize virus in tissue specimens, the need for tissue specimen limits the utility of this test. The use of PCR or DNA hybridization to detect parvovirus B19 viral DNA provides much more promising tests for clinical diagnosis. Parvovirus B19 PCR has been used to detect the virus in urine and saliva *(19)*.

All newborns with nonimmune hydrops should be evaluated for a possible parvovirus B19 infection. Some authorities have suggested that all abortuses should also be evaluated for parvovirus B19 infection.

The clinical presentations of symptomatic parvovirus B19 infection, including neonates, are shown in Table 3. The current state of knowledge about parvovirus B19 infection in the newborn and the available diagnostic tests dictate a follow-up of an

Table 3
Clinical Presentations of Symptomatic Parvovirus B19 Infection

Erythema infectiosum (fifth disease)
Arthropathy
Hematological complications (including congenital anemia[a])
Chronic infection in immunocompromised
Hydrops fetalis[a]
Fetal death[a]
Congenital abnormalities (neurological, cardiac, ophthalmological)[a]
Myocarditis[a]
Neurological diseases[a]
Vasculitis

[a]Specific for newborns. (From refs. *40–46.*)

Table 4
Diagnostic Tests for Parvovirus B19 Infection

Antibody assays (IgM and IgG)
    Capture radioimmunoassay
    Enzyme immunoassays
    Immunofluorescent assays
    Immunoblot assays
    Western blot
Counter immunoelectropheresis
Viral antigen detection
    Counter immunoelectropheresis
    Enzyme immunoassays
    Immunohistochemistry
Viral DNA detection
    Hybridization assay
    Polymerase chain reaction
Electron microscopy

asymptomatic child for at least 1 year. At about 1 year of age, serological tests should be repeated to diagnose or exclude parvovirus B19 infection.

ASSAYS FOR DIAGNOSIS

Diagnostic tests for parvovirus B19 are shown in Table 4. Serology is the mainstay for diagnosis of parvovirus B19 infection. Serology is most readily available to clinicians and most frequently used for the diagnosis of parvovirus B19 infection. Various techniques can be used to determine both IgG and IgM anti-parvovirus B19 antibodies. Because these tests are not standardized, there is significant inter- and intralaboratory variation. The sensitivity and specificity of the test often depend on the expertise and experience of the technician and the laboratory. In some individuals with serologically confirmed acute parvovirus B19 infection, the parvovirus B19 DNA may not be detected by the routinely used techniques. In one study, only 45% of the serologically confirmed acute parvovirus B19 infections had parvovirus B19 DNA detected using

PCR *(37)*. Therefore, serology is preferable to PCR for the diagnosis of acute parvovirus B19 infection. Of the various parvovirus B19 antibody detection tests available, the capture immunoassay is more sensitive and specific than the enzyme immunoassay *(37)*. However, the enzyme immunoassay is the only test approved by the Food and Drug Administration and is most commonly used in the United States by commercial laboratories.

Detection of viral antigen is available mostly in research laboratories and is not frequently used in clinical practice. This assay may have a role in the detection of parvovirus B19 infection in abortuses and placentas under evaluation for congenital infection.

Viral DNA detection tests are not approved by the Food and Drug Administration but are available in research and some commercial laboratories. These tests may have a value in the fetal and neonatal diagnosis of parvovirus B19 infection. They are of limited use in diagnosis of clinical infection in the mother. These tests are very specific, but their sensitivity is variable. The presence of viral DNA is diagnostic of parvovirus B19 infection.

Electron microscopy, although beneficial, is of limited use because of the need for a tissue specimen. Its sensitivity and specificity is very operator dependent, and this diagnostic modality is not readily available to most clinicians.

REFERENCES

1. Cossart YE, Field AM, Cant B, et al. Parvovirus-like particles in human sera. Lancet 1975;1:72–73.
2. Pattison JR, Jones SE, Hodgson J, et al. Parvovirus infections and hypoplastic crisis in sickle-cell anemia. Lancet 1981;1:664–665.
3. Anderson MJ, Jones SE, Fisher-Hoch SP, et al. Human parvovirus the cause of erythema infectiosum (fifth disease)? Lancet 1983;1:1378.
4. Brown T, Anand A, Ritchie RD. Intrauterine parvovirus infection associated with hydrops fetalis. Lancet 1984;2:1033–1034.
5. Reid DM, Reid TMS, Brown T, et al. Human parvovirus-associated arthritis: a clinical and laboratory description. Lancet 1985;1:422–425.
6. Deiss V, Tratschin JD, Weitz M, et al. Cloning of the human parvovirus B19 genome and structural analysis of its palindromic termini. Virology 1990;175:247–254.
7. Blundell MC, Beard C, Astell CR, et al. In vitro identification of a B19 parvovirus promoter. Virology 1987;157:534–538.
8. Brown CS, Jensen T, Melten RH, et al. Localization of an immunodominant domain on baculovirus-produced parvovirus B19 capsids: correlation to a major surface region on the native virus particle. J Virol 1992;66:6989–6996.
9. Anderson MJ, Higgins PG, Davis LR, et al. Experimental parvoviral infection in humans. J Infect Dis 1985;152:257–265.
10. Potter CG, Potter AC, Hatton CS, et al. Variation of erytheroid and myeloid precursors in the marrow and peripheral blood of volunteer subjects infected with human parvovirus (B19). J Clin Invest 1987;79:1486–1492.
11. Margolis G, Kilham L. Problems of human concerns arising from animal models of intrauterine and neonatal infections due to viruses: a review. II Pathological studies. Prog Med Virol 1975;20:144–179.
12. Anderson MJ, Cohen BJ. Human parvovirus B19 infections in the United Kingdom 1984–1986 [letter]. Lancet 1987;1:738–739.
13. Plumme FA, Hammond GW, Forward K, et al. An erythema infectiousum-like illness caused by human parvovirus infection. N Engl J Med 1985;313:74–79.

14. Anderson MJ, Higgins PG, Davis LR, et al. Experimental parvoviral infection in humans. J Infect Dis 1985;152:257–265.

15. Potter CG, Potter AC, Hatton CSR, et al. Variation of erythroid and myeloid precursors in the marrow of volunteer subjects infected with human parvovirus B19. J Clin Invest 1987;79:1486–1492.

16. Bell LM, Naides SJ, Stoffman P, et al. Human parvovirus B19 infection among hospital staff members after contact with infected patients. N Engl J Med 1989;321:485–491.

17. Dowell SF, Torok TJ, Thorp JA, et al. parvovirus B19 infection in hospital workers: community or hospital acquisition? J Infect Dis 1995;172:1076–1079.

18. Cohen BJ, Buckley MM. The prevalence of antibody to human parvovirus B19 in England and Wales. J. Med Microbiol 1988;25:151–153.

19. Koch WC, Adler SP. Human parvovirus B19 infections in women of child bearing age and within families. Pediatr Infect Dis J 1989;8:83–87.

20. Anderson LJ. Role of parvovirus B19 in human disease. Pediatr Infect Dis J 1987;6:711–718.

21. Gratacos E, Torres PJ, Vidal J, et al. The incidence of human parvovirus B19 infection during pregnancy and its impact on perinatal outcome. J Infect Dis 1995;171:1360–1363.

22. Valeur-Jensen A, Pedersen CB, Westergaard T, et al. Risk factors for parvovirus B19 infection in pregnancy. JAMA 1999;281:1099–1105.

23. Public Health Laboratory Service Working Party on Fifth Disease. Prospective Study of human parvovirus (B19) infection in pregnancy. BMJ 1990;300:1166–1170.

24. Teuscher T, Baillod B, Holzer BR. Prevalence of human parvovirus B19 in sickle cell disease and healthy controls. Trop Geogr Med 1991;43:108–110.

25. Kinney JS, Anderson LJ, Farrar J, et al. Risk of adverse outcomes of pregnancy after parvovirus B19 infection. J Infect Dis 1988;157:663–667.

26. Mark Y, Rogers BB, Oyer CE. Diagnosis and incidence of fetal parvovirus infection in an autopsy series: II: DNA amplification. Pediatr Pathol 1993;13:381–386.

27. Rodis JF, Quinn DL, Gravy GW Jr, et al. Management and outcomes of pregnancies complicated by human B19 parvovirus infection: a prospective study. Am J Obstet Gynecol 1990;163:1168–1171.

28. Miller E, Fairley CK, Cohen BJ, et al. Immediate and long-term outcome of human parvovirus B19 infection in pregnancy. Br J Obstet Gynaecol 1998;105:174–178.

29. Yaegashi N, Niimua T, Chisakra H, et al. The incidence of, and factors leading to, parvovirus B19-related hydrops fetalis following maternal infection; report of 10 cases and meta-analysis. J Infect 1998;37:28–35.

30. Morey AL, Keeling JW, Porter HJ, et al. Clinical and histopathological features of parvovirus B19 infection in the human fetus. Br J Obstet Gynaecol 1992;99:566–574.

31. Rogers BB, Mark Y, Oyer CE. Diagnosis and incidence of fetal parvovirus infection in an autopsy series: I: Histology. Pediatr Pathol 1993;13:371–379.

32. Gillespie SM, Cartter ML, Asch S, et al. Occupational risk of human parvovirus B19 infection for school and daycare personnel during an outbreak of erythema infectiosum. JAMA 1990;263:2061–2065.

33. Rodis JF, Hovick TJ, Quinn DL, et al. Human parvovirus B19 infection in pregnancy. Obstet Gynecol 1988;2:733–738.

34. Harger JH, Adler SP, Koch WP, et al. Prospective evaluation of 618 pregnant women exposed to parvovirus B19 infection, risks and symptoms. Obstet Gynaecol 1998;91:413–420.

35. Woolf AD, Capion GV, Chishick A, et al. Clinical manifestations of human parvovirus B19 in adults. Arch Intern Med 1989;149;1153–1156.

36. Koch WC, Harger JH, Barnstein B, et al. Serologic and virologic evidence for frequent intrauterine transmission of human parvovirus B19 with a primary maternal infection during pregnancy. Pediatr Infect Dis 1998;17:489–494.

37. Jordan JA. Diagnosing human parvovirus B19 infection: guidelines for test selection. Mol Diagn 2001;6:307–312.

38. Török TJ. Human parvovirus B19. In: Remington J, Klein J, eds. 2001. Infectious Diseases of the Fetus and Newborn Infant. 5th Ed. Philadelphia, PA: WB Saunders.

39. Centers for Disease Control. Risks associated with human parvovirus B19 infection. MMWR 1989;38:81–88, 97–97.

40. Ager EA, Chin TDY, Poland JD. Epidemic erythema infectiosum. N Engl J Med 1966;275:1326–1331.

41. Chorba T, Coccia R, Holman RC, et al. The role of parvovirus E19 in aplastic crisis and erythema infectiosum (fifth disease). J Infect Vis 1986;154:383–393.

42. Cramp HE, Armstrong EDJ. Erythema infectiosum: an outbreak of "slapped cheek" disease in north Devon. Br Med J 1976;1:885–886.

43. Lauer EA, MacCormack IN, Wifert C. Erythema infectiosum: an elementary school outbreak. Am J Dis Child 1976;130:252–254.

44. Lefrere JJ, Courouce AM, Eertrand Y, et al. Human parvovirus and aplastic crisis in chronic hemolytic anemias: a study of 24 observations. Am J Hematol 1986;23:271–275.

45. Anderson MJ, Lewis E, Kidd IM, et al. An outbreak of erythema infectiosum associated with humam parvovirus infection. J Hyg (Camb) 1994;93:85–93.

46. Brown KE, Green SW, Antunez de Mayolo J, et al. Congenital anaemia after transplacental B19 parvovirus infection. Lancet 1994;343:895–896.

13

Enteroviruses

Mark J. Abzug

INTRODUCTION

Enteroviruses (EVs) comprise a genus in the Picornaviridae family, so named because they are small, single-stranded ribonucleic acid (RNA)-containing viruses. The EVs are divided into the subgroups of polioviruses, coxsackie A viruses, coxsackie B viruses, and echoviruses based on replication properties in tissue culture and animal models. Newer EVs are simply designated by number (e.g., EV 71), rather than by subgroup designation. The human EVs have been recently reclassified based on nucleotide and amino acid sequences into five species, polioviruses and human EVs A–D. EV serotypes are distinguished by antigenic differences.

EVs are extremely common causes of human infection. Polioviruses, the cause of paralytic poliomyelitis, continue to be prevalent in some areas of the developing world. The more than 60 serotypes of nonpoliovirus EVs cause a large number and wide variety of diseases, ranging from mild illnesses such as respiratory infections, nonspecific febrile illnesses, herpangina, and uncomplicated hand-foot-and-mouth disease to more severe illnesses such as meningitis, encephalitis, paralytic disease, myocarditis, and chronic or disseminated infection in immunocompromised hosts (e.g., hypogammaglobulinemic patients or bone marrow transplant recipients). In general, the incidence and severity of EV infections are inversely related to age. In temperate climates, EV infections have a distinct seasonality, with infections occurring predominantly in the summer and fall months (1).

EFFECTS ON THE FETUS AND NEONATE

Although maternal poliomyelitis in the first two trimesters can be associated with spontaneous abortion or stillbirth and can predispose to intrauterine growth retardation and premature delivery, poliovirus infection of the fetus was an infrequent occurrence in the prevaccine era (2–7). Maternal poliovirus infection was not linked to an increased incidence of congenital anomalies (8). Neonatal poliomyelitis was a complication of maternal infection, however. Cases presented from birth to 28 days of age, with most cases occurring between days 5 and 21. The incubation period of neonatal poliomyelitis was often shorter (<11 days) than that observed with poliomyelitis acquired at a later age. Symptoms included anorexia and lethargy, and paralytic disease was frequent. Fever was variable, and diarrhea occasionally was present. Reports of neonatal

From: *Infectious Disease: Congenital and Perinatal Infections: A Concise Guide to Diagnosis*
Edited by: C. Hutto © Humana Press Inc., Totowa, NJ

poliovirus emphasized the seriousness of the condition, with half of reported cases dying and one-quarter showing residual paralysis *(3)*.

Among the most significant infections that the nonpoliovirus EVs cause are infections affecting the fetus or newborn infant. *In utero* infection can cause spontaneous abortion or stillbirth, with evidence of infection of amniotic fluid, placenta, and many fetal organs or fluids, including brain, heart, liver, adrenal glands, kidney, spleen, blood, and cerebrospinal fluid *(9–15)*. Several stillbirths with evidence of fetal myocarditis or pancarditis and demonstration of coxsackie B virus antigens in myocardia have been described *(16,17)*.

Seroepidemiologic studies have suggested that maternal infections with certain EV serotypes can result in congenital anomalies. Maternal coxsackie B3 and B4 infections were associated with increased rates of cardiovascular anomalies, coxsackie B2 and B4 infections with urogenital abnormalities, and coxsackie A9 infections with gastrointestinal anomalies in one study *(18)*. Another report described increases in titers to coxsackie B5 virus in mothers of infants with congenital anomalies, but no specific organ system was singled out *(19)*. Coxsackie B6 virus was implicated in several neonates with abnormalities of the central nervous system (hydranencephaly, meningocele, hydrocephalus, aqueductal stenosis) by detection of neutralizing antibody in cerebrospinal fluid; viral cultures were negative, however *(20)*. A more recent study linked EVs to central nervous system and cardiac defects by identifying EV RNA in amniotic fluid by polymerase chain reaction (PCR) *(21)*. It should be noted that, with the exception of a report linking cardiac and other defects to a community EV outbreak, most reports have not identified an increase in congenital anomalies as a result of large community EV epidemics *(22–27)*. In addition, a temporal pattern of birth defects matching the seasonality of EV infections has not been observed.

Several epidemiologic studies have suggested that congenital or neonatal EV (poliovirus or nonpoliovirus) infection may predispose to schizophrenia and type I diabetes mellitus *(28–30)*. Increased levels of IgM antibody to coxsackieviruses have been measured during pregnancy in mothers whose children subsequently developed diabetes. EV RNA has been detected by PCR in sera obtained in the first trimester from a small number of these women *(31)*. Exposure to EVs both *in utero* and in the neonatal period has been linked to later development of diabetes *(32)*.

Neonatal infections by the nonpoliovirus EVs can be asymptomatic, cause benign illness, or produce life-threatening, severe disease *(33,34)*. The majority are asymptomatic *(35)*. Most affected neonates are full term, with uncomplicated pregnancies, deliveries, and neonatal courses prior to the onset of EV disease *(33,36,37)*. History often reveals a maternal viral illness preceding or immediately following delivery, with symptoms including fever, respiratory symptoms, or abdominal pain that may suggest chorioamnionitis or abruptio placentae. Viral symptoms are also frequently present in other family members *(33,34,36–38)*. Newborns can present with symptoms throughout the neonatal period; some cases present as early as day 1 of life. Symptoms and signs include fever in the majority, hypothermia, irritability, lethargy, anorexia, respiratory findings (tachypnea, cough, grunting, retracting, wheezing, rhinorrhea, apnea), decreased perfusion, jaundice, abdominal distension, emesis, and occasionally diarrhea *(33,36,37)*. Although diarrhea can be prominent and may occasionally be bloody or severe *(39)*, in most series it is not a dominant clinical feature. Macular or maculo-papular rashes are frequently present and may be diagnostically helpful.

The majority of affected neonates have mild illness with resolution of fever in an average of 3 days and other symptoms in approx 7 days, with no sequelae *(33,36,37)*. A subset of infected newborns have more severe disease, characterized by any combination of sepsis, meningoencephalitis, myocarditis, pneumonia, hepatitis, and coagulopathy. Encephalitis may be manifested by extreme lethargy progressing to depressed consciousness, seizures, or focal neurologic abnormalities. Bulging fontanelle or nuchal rigidity may occasionally be present *(36,40–42)*. Cardiomegaly, congestive heart failure, arrhythmias, or myocardial infarction suggest myocarditis, which may be accompanied by pericarditis *(43–45)*. Pneumonia can be rapidly progressive *(15,46,47)*. Hepatitis, characterized by jaundice, hepatomegaly, and elevated transaminases and bilirubin, is frequently associated with thrombocytopenia and coagulopathy. Acute hepatic necrosis, liver failure, and bleeding complications may ensue *(36,38,48)*. Intracranial hemorrhage can be a particularly severe, life-threatening complication *(49)*. Other complications of neonatal EV infections include necrotizing enterocolitis, myositis, hemophagocytic syndrome, and hyponatremia with inappropriate antidiuretic hormone secretion *(36,37,39,50)*.

Mortality rates ranging between 0 and 83% have been reported in retrospective reports and literature reviews of neonatal EV infections *(33,34,36,37)*. Myocarditis and hepatitis and coagulopathy are associated with the highest mortality *(34,36,48)*. The mortality rate associated with hepatitis or coagulopathy was 31% in one report, with particularly high mortality noted when hepatitis and myocarditis occurred together *(48)*. Fortunately, the prognosis for survivors is generally favorable, even following severe disease. Although residual myocardial dysfuntion and chronic, calcific myocarditis with chronic heat failure and dysrhythmias have been reported after neonatal myocarditis, most survivors do not have long-term cardiac sequelae *(43,44,51)*. Hepatic dysfunction following hepatitis may persist into infancy and residual hepatic calcification may develop, but most survivors eventually demonstrate normalization of liver function and satisfactory growth *(48)*. The neurological prognosis for neonates with central nervous system involvement is more difficult to predict. Some reports have identified long-term sequelae such as delayed speech and language development, intellectual deficits, motor abnormalities (spasticity, hypotonicity, and weakness), seizure disorders, ocular defects, and microcephaly, whereas other series found no evidence of long-term neurological deficits *(36,52–58)*. Severe encephalitis may be associated with increased risk of necrosis and neurological compromise, including decreased intelligence, motor abnormalities, and hydrocephalus *(42,52,53)*.

TIMING AND ROUTES OF TRANSMISSION

Polioviruses have infrequently been recovered from placental or fetal tissue, suggesting that *in utero* infection early in pregnancy is uncommon *(3,8)*. Neonatal poliomyelitis most often occurred via acquisition from an infected mother; maternal illness between 1 week prior to delivery and 4 weeks after delivery posed the highest risk of neonatal disease *(7)*. A minority of affected newborns had onset of illness at birth or within the first 5 days of life, suggesting intrauterine infection *(3,59)*. Infection in the remainder was likely via contact with maternal blood or secretions during or after delivery. Exposure to nonmaternal contacts was also occasionally implicated *(8)*.

The clearest evidence for *in utero* infection by nonpolio EVs comes from cases of spontaneous abortion or stillbirth with demonstration of EV infection in fetal tissues *(9,10,16,17,60)*. Most abortions have been reported between the third and fifth months of pregnancy, although spontaneous abortion in the first trimester has also been described *(9,10,60)*. Stillbirths have been reported between the fifth and ninth months of gestation *(11,12,16,17)*. It should be noted that some stillbirths have occurred following EV infection of the placenta in the absence of evidence of direct fetal infection *(14)*.

Further evidence of *in utero* infection is provided by the small number of reported cases of neonatal EV disease with onset in the first few hours after birth. *In utero* infection has been substantiated in these cases by viral culture of amniotic fluid and umbilical cord blood, antigen detection in myocardia hours after birth, culture of neonatal organs a few hours after delivery, and detection of serum-neutralizing immunoglobulin (Ig) M antibody on the first day of life *(17,46,61–64)*. Identification of EVs in placentas, often in association with placentitis, villitis, villous necrosis, vasculitis, thrombosis, or other placental pathology, suggests that some fetal infections occur via a transplacental route *(10,12,14,65)*. Shedding of EVs from the stool and cervixes of pregnant women, demonstration of susceptibility of amnion cells to EV infection in vitro, and growth of EVs from amniotic fluid in vivo point to the potential for ascending infection also *(11,12,36,61,66–69)*. Based on the occurrence of viremia or symptoms in the first 1–2 days of life, it has been estimated that approx 22% of fatal neonatal coxsackie B virus infections and 11% of neonatal echovirus infections were acquired *in utero* *(15,34,36,40)*.

Most EV-infected neonates are thought to be infected either intrapartum by exposure to maternal blood or genital secretions or after delivery by exposure to oropharyngeal secretions or stool of mothers or other contacts *(6,34,37)*. EVs have been grown from cervical swabs obtained from symptomatic pregnant women and from mothers of infected, ill neonates *(62,66–68)*. Shedding of virus from maternal throat and rectum during pregnancy has also been documented, with or without symptoms *(69)*. These observations lend support to the potential for viral transmission from mother during or after delivery. High rates of viral illness in the peripartum period among siblings and fathers of EV-infected newborns also suggest potential viral transmission from these family members *(33)*.

Many episodes of both sporadic transmission and epidemic spread of EVs in hospital nurseries have been reported *(34,36,39,62,64,70–75)*. Full-term and premature infants have been affected, and asymptomatic and symptomatic infections have resulted. Several outbreaks could be traced to vertically infected neonates, with spread by hospital staff. In other epidemics, adults likely introduced EVs into nurseries *(34)*.

RISK OF MATERNAL INFECTION DURING PREGNANCY

In the prevaccine era, paralytic poliomyelitis occurred in pregnant women at a rate greater than age-adjusted expected rates *(2,3,5,6,76)*. This increased risk was not trimester specific. In addition, pregnant women with poliomyelitis had a higher mortality rate than nonpregnant women in some series, with the risk greatest in the last trimester and puerperium in some reports *(3,6)*. Among survivors, sequelae such as paralysis were not more common following infection during gestation *(3)*.

Nonpoliovirus EV infections, both asymptomatic and symptomatic, occur frequently during pregnancy. In one seroepidemiologic survey conducted over a 10-year period, 42% of pregnant women were infected with EVs *(18)*. In another study, coxsackie B virus infections were identified serologically in 9% of women during pregnancy *(77)*. Twenty-five percent of pregnant women had serologic evidence of an EV infection during the 3-month period surrounding delivery in a study conducted in peak EV season. Of pregnant women, 3–4% shed EVs from the throat or rectum near delivery during EV season, frequently with minimal or no symptoms *(69)*. In several reports of stillbirths following EV infection, maternal illnesses suggestive of chorioamnionitis, influenzalike disease, or meningitis are described *(11–14)*.

RISK OF FETAL AND NEONATAL INFECTION

Although direct fetal infection by polioviruses in early gestation is uncommon, almost half of pregnancies complicated by maternal poliomyelitis in the first trimester ended with fetal loss *(8)*. Fetal loss was greatest with severe maternal illness, although spontaneous abortion also occurred with mild, nonparalytic maternal disease *(6)*. Pathologic evidence of direct fetal infection was lacking in most cases. Neonatal infection was also relatively uncommon compared with the incidence of poliomyelitis in later childhood. However, among mothers with poliomyelitis near the time of delivery, almost 40% of their neonates developed clinical poliomyelitis *(7)*. In the absence of maternal disease at or within the first week after delivery, neonatal poliomyelitis was infrequent *(7)*. Neonatal poliomyelitis is now extremely rare in countries with widespread vaccination but continues to occur in regions with underimmunized populations.

Information on *in utero* infection by nonpoliovirus EVs is derived primarily from case reports of spontaneous abortion and stillbirths. Maternal infection may lead to fetal demise with or without direct evidence of fetal infection *(78)*; stillbirths in which EV infection was documented in placental tissue but not fetal tissue have been described *(14)*. Large population-based studies that can provide estimates of the risk of fetal infection and adverse outcome following maternal infection during gestation have not been performed *(66)*. In several reports describing large echovirus 9 and coxsackie B virus epidemics, maternal infections were not associated with increases in spontaneous abortions, stillbirths, or congenital anomalies *(23–27,79)*.

Neonatal nonpoliovirus EV infections are common. In one study, 13% of infants younger than 1 month were infected by an EV during the summer and fall months; 21% of infected newborns were symptomatic. Infection was associated with non-breast-feeding and lower socioeconomic status *(35,80)*. EVs were responsible for 65% of hospital admissions of those younger than 3 months with suspected sepsis in the summer and fall in the same community *(81)*. In another report, asymptomatic or symptomatic neonatal EV infections were detected by culture in 5% of infants and by serology in 7% during EV season *(69)*. In a series of neonates evaluated for possible sepsis over a 13-month period, 4% were found to have EV infection by culture or antigen detection *(82)*. Review of cases of neonatal meningitis at one institution found EVs to be the most frequently identified cause between days 8 and 29 of life, comprising at least one-third of cases *(83)*. Overall, estimates suggest that the incidence of neonatal EV disease is greater than or equal to that of group B streptococcus, herpes simplex virus, and cytomegalovirus *(34–36)*.

Maternally derived neutralizing antibody does not necessarily protect against neonatal infection, although it does provide some protection against neonatal EV disease. Conversely, absence of or low neutralizing titer to an infecting EV serotype is a significant risk factor for development of symptomatic infection *(38,72,73,84)*. Route of delivery has not been demonstrated to affect the incidence or severity of neonatal EV disease; cases following cesarean section are described *(3,34,38,72)*. Factors that are associated with severe neonatal disease include maternal illness prior to or at delivery, prematurity, early age of onset of illness (especially the first few days of life), multiorgan disease, severe hepatitis/hepatic necrosis, positive serum viral culture, specific infecting serotypes (e.g., group B coxsackieviruses and echovirus 11), and lack of neutralizing antibody to the infecting serotype *(32–34,36–38,84,85)*.

Risk factors for acquisition of EVs in the nursery include prematurity, low birth weight, intensive care, and instrumentation of the nasopharynx or oropharynx *(70,71,73)*. Nosocomially acquired infections tend to cause milder disease with lower mortality rates than do vertical infections *(34)*.

DIAGNOSTIC ASSAYS

The mainstay of diagnosis for EV infections is viral isolation in cell culture. A variety of cell lines support EVs, including monkey kidney cells and human fibroblast, epithelial, and rhabdomyosarcoma cell lines. No single line is optimal for all EVs, so diagnostic laboratories typically use a combination of cell types, such as a monkey kidney line and a fibroblast line *(1)*.

Tissue culture has significant limitations. It requires expertise and is relatively expensive to perform. Not all EV serotypes grow in culture; this is especially true for coxsackie A viruses. The sensitivity of culture is further limited by neutralizing antibody in diagnostic specimens, inadequate collection or processing of specimens, and insensitivity of some cell lines for some serotypes. Finally, growth in culture can be relatively slow, ranging from 3 to more than 8 days. More rapid detection of EVs would be more likely to guide clinical management, including decreasing unnecessary diagnostic evaluations, eliminating unneeded therapies, and providing potential treatment *(1)*.

A variety of antibody and antigen detection assays have been developed, but their sensitivity is limited by the lack of an antigen shared by the majority of EVs *(1)*. Techniques that have been applied to neonatal EV infections include enzyme immunoassay, counterimmunoelectrophoresis, and neutralization assays for antibody to a variety of EVs. Assays to detect IgG, IgM, and IgA antibodies have been developed *(31,86)*. In general, their utility has been restricted by limited sensitivity. Antigen detection assays have been developed and used for study of stool samples and tissues from infants dying in the neonatal period *(87,88)*. As with the antibody tests, sensitivity is generally limited with antigen detection assays.

The application of the PCR to diagnosis of EV infections has been very promising. PCR assays target detection of conserved RNA sequences and therefore detect most EV serotypes, including most of those implicated in neonatal disease. PCR is more sensitive than cell culture and, in the absence of laboratory contamination, is highly specific. Rapid formats have been developed, yielding results in as little as 5 hours. PCR has proven useful for diagnosis of pediatric viral meningitis and nonspecific fever illnesses *(1)*. Testing of cerebrospinal fluid, serum, and throat specimens from children with acute illnesses has sensitivities greater than 90% and high specificity; urine testing is somewhat less sensitive *(89,90)*.

PRENATAL EVALUATION

In the presence of an illness suggestive of an EV infection in a pregnant woman, virologic diagnosis may be sought from maternal throat and rectal swabs and, in the presence of meningitis, cerebrospinal fluid. Viral cultivation may be attempted, or if available and if rapid diagnosis is required, PCR may be performed. Maternal serology is generally not helpful for acute diagnosis unless the likely infecting serotype is known from epidemiologic circumstances, such as an infection in the midst of a community epidemic caused by a known serotype, and an IgM assay for that serotype is available.

EVs have been isolated from amniotic fluid in association with maternal chorioamnionitislike symptoms, fetal demise, or subsequent neonatal illness *(11,12,36,61)*. The sensitivity and predictive value with respect to fetal or neonatal outcome of recovery of an EV from amniotic fluid is unknown. Similarly, EVs have been cultivated from placental tissue and fetal blood from pregnancies terminating in spontaneous abortions or stillbirths, but the sensitivity and predictive value of prenatal culturing of placental tissue or fetal blood for EVs is not known *(9,10,13,14,46,62)*. PCR of amniotic fluid, placenta, or fetal specimens can also be considered for prenatal diagnosis. PCR was performed on amniotic fluid specimens in a study that linked central nervous system and cardiac abnormalities to EV infection *(21)*. In that study, only a small number of control patients was included. As with viral culture, the sensitivity and predictive value of PCR testing of prenatal specimens with respect to fetal or neonatal outcome are unknown.

Currently, the most sound approach to prenatal diagnosis is application of standard obstetrical vigilance, including ultrasound evaluation as indicated. If an abnormality is detected and EV infection is suspected, virologic diagnosis can be attempted by culture or PCR of maternal or fetal specimens. Diagnosis of maternal EV infection might assist management by ruling out alternative diagnoses such as chorioamnionitis or placental abruption. Although detection of an EV in amniotic fluid, placenta, or fetal blood is concerning, data are currently unavailable to make conclusions regarding the likelihood of adverse fetal or neonatal outcome.

EVALUATION OF THE NEONATE

Evaluation of a newborn in whom EV infection is a possible cause of illness should include a thorough history with specific attention to maternal symptoms suggestive of EV infection (e.g., fever and abdominal pain) as well as viral-like symptoms in other close contacts. Examination should include global assessment of well-being, with special attention to organ systems targeted by EVs, including the cardiovascular system (blood pressure, heart rate, perfusion, cyanosis, heart tones, edema); respiratory system (respiratory distress, apnea); central nervous system (lethargy, irritability, bulging fontanelle, focal abnormalities, hypotonia or hypertonia); liver (jaundice, hepatomegaly, liver tenderness, splenomegaly, abdominal distension); and coagulation system (petechiae; ecchymoses; or bleeding from the umbilicus, mucosa, or phlebotomy sites). Presence of a macular or maculopapular rash may be a clue to an EV infection.

Minimum laboratory evaluation should include a complete blood cell count and lumbar puncture, as well as bacterial cultures of blood, urine, and cerebrospinal fluid to rule out bacterial infection. Cerebrospinal fluid analysis, in both nonpoliovirus EV and poliovirus infections, may show a pleocytosis suggestive of viral meningitis (usually <500 white blood cells/mm^3). Occasionally, the cerebrospinal fluid profile may mimic that of bacterial meningitis, with up to several thousand white blood cells/cubic millimeter. A neutrophil predominance is frequently present, and in a minority, increased protein or decreased glucose levels may occur. Conversely, cerebrospinal fluid may be positive by culture or PCR despite a normal cytologic and chemical profile *(33,36,37)*. Central nervous system imaging should be considered if an infant is very lethargic or has focal neurological findings or if there is a neurological deterioration in the presence of significant thrombocytopenia or coagulopathy.

If a newborn appears ill or if there are findings suggestive of hepatic involvement (e.g., hepatomegaly or jaundice) or bleeding, liver function tests should be obtained. Transaminase elevation or increased bilirubin suggests the presence of hepatitis. Ammonia levels may need to be monitored in the presence of severe hepatic involvement, especially if profound lethargy is present. In an infant with hepatitis or evidence of bleeding or in any newborn who appears clinically ill, the platelet count and coagulation profile should be monitored. A chest radiograph is indicated in the presence of respiratory or cardiac symptoms. Infiltrates may indicate pneumonia or heart failure, and cardiac enlargement suggests myocarditis or pericarditis.

Microbiologic evaluation should be targeted at EVs and other pathogens that can cause similar disease manifestations. The latter include herpes simplex virus, adenovirus, bacteria such as group B streptococcus and *Escherichia coli*, and depending on the clinical situation, congenital infections by cytomegalovirus, rubella virus, syphilis, and *Toxoplasma gondii (33,37)*. Viral culture specimens with the highest yield for diagnosis of neonatal EV infections are rectum or stool (91–93% positive), cerebrospinal fluid (62–83% positive), and nasopharyx or throat (52–67% positive). Yields of serum and urine culture are lower (24–47%); however, cultures of serum specimens may grow more rapidly than those of other body fluids/sites *(33,37,91)*. Positive serum cultures are more likely with echoviruses, low serum-neutralizing antibody titer, and onset of illness within the first 5 days of life *(85,91)*.

PCR of serum and urine specimens is more sensitive in neonates than culture of these specimens, with a yield approaching 90%. High sensitivity is maintained for the first several days of illness and provides more rapid diagnosis than achieved with culture *(33,37,92)*. Sensitivity also appears high with PCR assay of cerebrospinal fluid *(93)*. PCR has been used to detect EV infection in neonatal tissue *(94)*, and PCR of serum, cerebrospinal fluid, and stool have been used to identify EV spread in neonatal units and guide infection control efforts *(95–97)*. Serology is generally not useful for acute diagnosis unless the likely infecting serotype is known from epidemiologic circumstances and an IgM assay for that serotype is available.

Viral culture or PCR of maternal rectal or cervical specimens will often yield the same virus as that causing neonatal illness. Maternal serum may also have a significant titer of neutralizing antibody to the causative viral serotype *(37,40,85)*. However, in most cases, diagnosis of a neonatal infection can be made directly from neonatal specimens.

INTERPRETATION OF DIAGNOSTIC EVALUATIONS

In general, positive cultures and PCR assays of mucosal sites such as throat or rectum may reflect asymptomatic infection or presence of virus that is causing symptoms. Positive culture and PCR tests of body fluids such as serum and cerebrospinal fluid more specifically suggest disease causation *(35,91)*. Nevertheless, a positive culture or PCR from a mucosal site in the first month of life (even in the absence of positive testing of normally sterile body fluids) in the presence of an EV-compatible illness and in the absence of another viral (e.g., herpes simplex virus, cytomegalovirus, or adenovirus) or bacterial (e.g., group B *Streptococcus* or *E. coli*) pathogen or noninfectious condition (e.g., metabolic disorder or structural cardiac disease) that can produce the constellation of clinical findings likely signifies that an EV is the etiologic agent.

Herpes simplex virus infection of the newborn can closely mimic findings of neonatal EV infection; surface viral cultures and PCR testing of cerebrospinal fluid and serum for herpes simplex virus and EV usually should be done concomitantly when evaluating a sick newborn *(33)*. Co-infection by EVs and bacteria may occur, so bacterial infection should be ruled out by appropriate cultures before ascribing an illness solely to EV infection *(33,37,98)*. Likewise, for meningitis, evaluation may be indicated for other congenital infections such as syphilis, toxoplasmosis, or rubella. It should be remembered that, after the neonatal period, receipt of live attenuated (oral) poliovirus vaccine can result in a positive viral culture or PCR assay of throat or rectum and occasionally of serum or cerebrospinal fluid.

The primary causes of neonatal EV infections are the coxsackie B viruses and the echoviruses; coxsackie A viruses are implicated less often *(37)*. An association has been observed between EV subgroup and disease pattern, with coxsackie B viruses associated with meningoencephalitis and myocarditis and echoviruses associated with hepatitis and coagulopathy, but significant overlap exists *(34,36,38)*. Coxsackie B virus-associated hepatitis and coagulopathy have been increasingly reported *(99)*. Coxsackieviruses B2–B5 and echoviruses 6, 11, and 19 are frequently the causes of severe neonatal disease *(34,36–38)*. Many other EV serotypes have also been reported to cause severe neonatal disease, however. In the absence of an epidemic situation or the occurrence of a unique disease manifestation, identification of the EV subgroup and serotype is generally not necessary and does not have an impact on clinical management.

REFERENCES

1. Abzug MJ, Rotbart HA. Enterovirus infections of neonates and infants. Semin Pediatr Infect Dis 1999;10:169–176.
2. Baker ME, Baker IG. Acute poliomyelitis in pregnancy. Report of thirty cases. Minn Med 1947;30:729–758.
3. Bates T. Poliomyelitis in pregnancy, fetus, and newborn. Am J Dis Child 1955;90:189–195.
4. Bowers VM, Danforth DN. The significance of poliomyelitis during pregnancy. Am J Obstet Gynecol 1953;65:34–39.
5. Fox MJ, Belfus FH. Poliomyelitis in pregnancy. Am J Obstet Gynecol 1950;59:1134–1139.
6. Horn P. Poliomyelitis in pregnancy. A 20-year report from Los Angeles County, California. J Am Acad Obstet Gynecol 1955;6:121–137.
7. Wyatt HV. Poliomyelitis in the fetus and the newborn. A comment on the new understanding of the pathogenesis. Clin Pediatr 1979;18:33–38.

8. Siegel M, Greenberg M. Poliomyelitis in pregnancy: effect on fetus and newborn infant. J Pediatr 1956;49:280–288.

9. Basso NGS, Fonseca MEF, Garcia AGP, Zuardi JAT, Silva MR, Outani H. Enterovirus isolation from foetal and placental tissues. Acta Virol 1990;34:49–57.

10. Garcia AGP, Basso NGDS, Fonseca MEF, Outani HN. Congenital echo virus infection—morphological and virological study of fetal and placental tissue. J Pathol 1990;160:123–127.

11. Nielsen JL, Berryman GK, Hankins GDV. Intrauterine fetal death and the isolation of echovirus 27 from amniotic fluid. J Infect Dis 1988;158:501–502.

12. Skeels MR, Williams JJ, Ricker FM. Perinatal echovirus infection. N Engl J Med 1981;305:1529.

13. Brady WK, Purdon A. Intrauterine fetal demise associated with enterovirus infection. South Med J 1986;79:770–772.

14. Batcup G, Holt P, Hambling MH, Gerlis LM, Glass MR. Placental and fetal pathology in coxsackie virus A9 infection: a case report. Histopathology 1985;9:1227–1235.

15. Baker DA, Phillips CA. Maternal and neonatal infection with coxsackievirus. Obstet Gynecol 1980;55:12S–15S.

16. Bates HR. Coxsackie virus B3 calcific pancarditis and hydrops fetalis. Am J Obstet Gynecol 1970;106:629–630.

17. Burch GE, Sun SC, Chu KC, Sohal RS, Colcolough HL. Interstitial and coxsackievirus B myocarditis in infants and children. JAMA 1968;203:1–8.

18. Brown GC, Karunas RS. Relationship of congenital anomalies and maternal infection with selected enteroviruses. Am J Epidemiol 1971;95:207–217.

19. Koskimies O, Lapinleimu K, Saxén L. Infections and other maternal factors as risk indicators for congenital malformations: a case-control study with paired serum samples. Pediatrics 1978;61:832–837.

20. Gauntt CJ, Gudvangen RJ, Brans YW, Marlin AE. Coxsackievirus group B antibodies in the ventricular fluid of infants with severe anatomic defects in the central nervous system. Pediatrics 1985;76:64–68.

21. Petitjean J, Tron-Laporte F, Dommerques M, et al. Involvement of enteroviruses in fetal infections. Program Abstr Prog Clin Virol 1994;200.

22. Baetz-Greenwalt B, Ratliff NB, Moodie DS. Hypoplastic right-sided heart complex: a cluster of cases with associated congenital birth defects. A new syndrome? J Pediatr 1983;103:399–401.

23. Kleinman H., Prince JT, Mathey WE, Rosenfield AB, Bearman JE, Syverton JT. ECHO 9 virus infection and congenital abnormalities: a negative report. Pediatrics 1962;29:261–269.

24. Landsman JB, Grist NR, Ross CAC. Echo 9 virus infection and congenital malformations. Br J Prev Soc Med;1964;18:152–156.

25. Peterson JC, Glicklich L. The effect of ECHO 9 infection on the fetus. Am J Dis Child 1960;100:779–780.

26. Rantasalo I, Penthinen K, Saxen L, Ojala A. Echo 9 virus antibody status after an epidemic period and the possible teratogenic effect of the infection. Ann Paediatr Fenn 1960;6:175–184.

27. Overall JC. Intrauterine virus infections and congenital heart disease. Am Heart J 1972;84:823–833.

28. Eagles JM. Are polioviruses a cause of schizophrenia? Br J Psychiatry 1992;160:598–600.

29. Squires RF. Are polioviruses a cause of schizophrenia? Br J Psychiatry 1992;161:427.

30. Rantakallio P, Jones P, Moring J, Von Wendt L. Association between central nervous system infections during childhood and adult onset schizophrenia and other psychoses: a 28-year followup. Int J Epidemiol 1997;26:837–843.

31. Dahlquist GG, Boman JE, Juto P. Enteroviral RNA and IgM antibodies in early pregnancy and risk for childhood-onset IDDM in offspring. Diabetes Care 1999;22:364–365.

32. Lonnrot M, Knip M, Roivainen M, Koskela P, Akerblom HK, Hyoty H. Onset of type 1 diabetes mellitus in infancy after enterovirus infections. Diabet Med 1998;15:431–434.

33. Abzug MJ, Levin MJ, Rotbart HA. Profile of enterovirus disease in the first 2 weeks of life. Pediatr Infect Dis J 1993;12:820–824.
34. Modlin JF. Perinatal echovirus infection: insights from a literature review of 61 cases of serious infection and 16 outbreaks in nurseries. Rev Infect Dis 1986;8:918–926.
35. Jenista JA, Powell KR, Menegus MA. Epidemiology of neonatal enterovirus infection. J Pediatr 1984;104:685–690.
36. Kaplan MH, Klein SW, McPhee J, Harper RG. Group B coxsackievirus infections in infants younger than 3 months of age: a serious childhood illness. Rev Infect Dis 1983;5:1019–1032.
37. Lake AM, Lauer BA, Clark JC, Wesenberg RL, McIntosh K. Enterovirus infections in neonates. J Pediatr 1976;89:787–791.
38. Modlin JF. Fatal echovirus 11 disease in premature neonates. Pediatrics 1988;66:775–780.
39. Birenbaum E, Handsher R, Kuint J, et al. Echovirus type 22 outbreak associated with gastro-intestinal disease in a neonatal intensive care unit. Am J Perinatol 1997;14:469–473.
40. Kibrick S, Benirschke K. Severe generalized disease (encephalohepatomyocarditis) occurring in the newborn period and due to infection with coxsackie virus, group B. Evidence of intrauterine infection with this agent. Pediatrics 1958;22:857–874.
41. Rorabaugh ML, Berlin LE, Heldrich F, et al. Aseptic meningitis in infants younger than 2 years of age: acute illness and neurologic complications. Pediatrics 1993;92:206–211.
42. Haddad J, Messer J, Gut JP, Chaigne D, Christmann D, Willard D. Neonatal echovirus encephalitis with white matter necrosis. Neuropediatrics 1990;21:215–217.
43. Goren A, Kaplan M, Glaser J, Isacsohn M. Chronic neonatal coxsackie myocarditis. Arch Dis Child 1989;64:404–406.
44. Hornung TS, Bernard EJ, Howman-Giles RB, Sholler GF. Myocardial infarction complicating neonatal enterovirus myocarditis. J Paediatr Child Health 1999;35:309–312.
45. Shah SS, Hellenbrand WE, Gallagher PG. Atrial flutter complicating neonatal coxsackie B2 myocarditis. Pediatr Cardiol 1998;19:185–186.
46. Boyd MT, Jordan SW, Davis LE. Fatal pneumonitis from congenital echovirus type 6 infection. Pediatr Infect Dis J 1987;6:1138–1139.
47. Cheeseman SH, Hirsch MS, Keller EW, Keim DE. Fatal neonatal pneumonia caused by echovirus type 9. Am J Dis Child 1977;131:1169.
48. Abzug MJ. Prognosis for neonates with enterovirus hepatitis and coagulopathy. Pediatr Infect Dis J 2001;20:758–763.
49. Abzug MJ, Johnson SM. Catastrophic intracranial hemorrhage complicating perinatal viral infections. Pediatr Infect Dis J 2000;19:556–559.
50. Barre V, Marret S, Mendel I, Lesesve JF, Fessard CI. Enterovirus-associated haemophagocytic syndrome in a neonate. Acta Paediatr 1998;87:469–471.
51. Spector SA, Straube RC. Protean manifestations of perinatal enterovirus infections. West J Med 1983;138:847–851.
52. Farmer K, MacArthur BA, Clay MM. A follow-up study of 15 cases of neonatal meningoencephalitis due to coxsackie virus B5. J Pediatr 1975;87:568–571.
53. Sells CJ, Carpenter RL, Ray CG. Sequelae of central-nervous-system enterovirus infections. N Engl J Med 1975;293:1–4.
54. Wilfert CM, Thompson RJ, Sunder TR, O'Quinn A, Zeller J, Blacharsh J. Longitudinal assessment of children with enteroviral meningitis during the first three months of life. Pediatrics 1981;67:811–815.
55. Bergman I, Painter MJ, Wald ER, Chiponis D, Holland AL, Taylor HG. Outcome in children with enteroviral meningitis during the first year of life. J Pediatr 1987;110:705–709.
56. Rantakallio P, Saukkonen AL, Krause U. Follow-up study of 17 cases of neonatal coxsackie B5 meningitis and one with suspected myocarditis. Scand J Infect Dis 1970;2:25.
57. Rorabaugh ML, Berlin LE, Heldrich F, et al. Aseptic meningitis in infants younger than 2 years of age: acute illness and neurologic complications. Pediatrics 1993;92:206–211.

58. Rorabaugh ML, Berlin LE, Rosenberg L, Rossman M, Allen M, Modlin JF. Absence of neurodevelopmental sequelae from aseptic meningitis. Abstr Soc Pediatr Res 1992:177A.
59. Baskin JL, Soule EH, Mills SD. Poliomyelitis of the newborn. Am J Dis Child 1950;80:10–21.
60. Ogilvie MM, Tearne CF. Spontaneous abortion after hand-foot-and-mouth disease caused by coxsackie virus A16. Br Med J 1980;2:1527–1528.
61. Strong BS, Young SA. Intrauterine coxsackievirus, group B type 1, infection: viral cultivation from amniotic fluid in the third trimester. Am J Perinatol 1995;55:509–512.
62. Jones MJ, Kolb M, Votava HJ, Johnson RL, Smith TF. Intrauterine echovirus type 11 infection. Mayo Clin Proc 1980;55:509–512.
63. Philip AGS, Larson EJ. Overwhelming neonatal infection with ECHO 19 virus. J Pediatr 1973;82:391–397.
64. Berkovich S, Smithwick EM. Transplacental infection due to ECHO virus type 22. J Pediatr 1968;72:94–96.
65. Garcia AGP, Basso NGDS, Fonseca MEF, Zuardi JAT, Outanni HN. Enterovirus associated placental morphology: a light, virological, electron microscopic and immunohistologic study. Placenta 1991;12:533–547.
66. Amstey MS, Miller RK, Menegus MA, di Sant 'Agnese PA. Enterovirus in pregnant women and the perfused placenta. Am J Obstet Gynecol 1988;158:775–782.
67. Reyes MP, Ostrea EM, Roskamp J, Lerner AM. Disseminated neonatal echovirus 11 disease following antenatal maternal infection with a virus-positive cervix and virus-negative gastrointestinal tract. J Med Virol 1983;12:155–159.
68. Reyes MP, Zalenski D, Smith F, Wilson FM, Lerner AM. Coxsackievirus-positive cervices in women with febrile illnesses during the third trimester in pregnancy. Am J Obstet Gynecol 1986;155:159–161.
69. Cherry JD, Soriano F, Jahn CL. Search for perinatal viral infection. A prospective, clinical, virologic, and serologic study. Am J Dis Child 1968;116:245–250.
70. Brightman VJ, McNair Scott TF, Westphal M, Boggs TR. An outbreak of coxsackie B-5 virus infection in a newborn nursery. J Pediatr 1966;69:179–192.
71. Kinney JS, McCray E, Kaplan JE, et al. Risk factors associated with echovirus 11' infection in a hospital nursery. Pediatr Infect Dis J 1986;5:192–197.
72. Nagington J, Wreghitt TG, Gandy G, Roberton NRC, Berry PJ. Fatal echovirus 11 infections in outbreak in special-care baby unit. Lancet 1978;2:725–728.
73. Rabkin CS, Telzak EE, Ho MS, et al. Outbreak of echovirus 11 infection in hospitalized neonates. Pediatr Infect Dis J 1988;7:186–190.
74. Jankovic B, Pasic S, Kanjuh B, et al. Severe neonatal echovirus 17 infection during a nursery outbreak. Pediatr Infect Dis J 1999;18:393–394.
75. Pasic S, Jankovic B, Abinun M, Kanjuh B. Intravenous immunoglobulin prophylaxis in an echovirus 6 and echovirus 4 nursery outbreak. Pediatr Infect Dis J 1997;16:718–720.
76. Aycock WL. The frequency of poliomyelitis in pregnancy. N Engl J Med 1941;225:405–408.
77. Sever JL, Huebner RJ, Costellano GA. Serologic diagnosis "en masse" with multiple antigens. Am Rev Resp Dis 1963;88:342.
78. Freedman PS. Echovirus 11 infection and intrauterine death. Lancet 1979:96–97.
79. Bell EJ, Ross CAC, Grist NR. ECHO 9 infection in pregnant women with suspected rubella. J Clin Pathol 1975;28:267–269.
80. Jenista JA, Prather SA, Menegus MA. Determinants of severity of neonatal enterovirus infection. Am J Dis Child 1983;137:532.
81. Dagan R, Hall CB, Powell KR, Menegus MA. Epidemiology and laboratory diagnosis of infection with viral and bacterial pathogens in infants hospitalized for suspected sepsis. J Pediatr 1989;115:351–356.
82. Rosenlew M, Stenvik M, Roivainen M, Jarvenpaa AL, Hovi T. A population-based prospective survey of newborn infants with suspected systemic infection: occurrence of sporadic enterovirus and adenovirus infections. J Clin Virol 1999;12:211–219.

83. Shattuck KE, Chonmaitree T. The changing spectrum of neonatal meningitis over a 15-year period. Clin Pediatr 1992;31:130–136.
84. Modlin JF, Polk BF, Horton P, Etkind P, Crane E. Perinatal echovirus infection: risk of transmission during a community outbreak. N Engl J Med 1981;305:368–371.
85. Abzug MJ, Keyserling HL, Lee ML, Levin MJ, Rotbart HA. Neonatal enterovirus infection: virology, serology, and effects of intravenous immune globulin. Clin Infect Dis 1995;20:1201–1206.
86. Terletskaia-Ladwig E, Metzger C, Schalasta G, Enders G. Evaluation of enterovirus serological tests IgM-EIA and complement fixation in patients with meningitis, confirmed by detection of enteroviral RNA by RT-PCR in cerebrospinal fluid. J Med Virol 2000;61:221–227.
87. Terletskaia-Ladwig E, Metzger C, Schalasta G, Enders G. A new enzyme immunoassay for the detection of enteroviruses in faecal specimens. J Med Virol 2000;60:439–445.
88. Bourlet T, Gharbi J, Omar S, Aouni M, Pozzetto B. Comparison of a rapid culture method combining an immunoperoxidase test and a group specific anti-VP1 monoclonal antibody with conventional virus isolation techniques for routine detection of enteroviruses in stools. J Med Virol 1998;54:204–209.
89. Rotbart HA, Ahmed A, Hickey S, et al. Diagnosis of enterovirus infection by polymerase chain reaction of multiple specimen types. Pediatr Infect Dis J 1997;16:409–411.
90. Ahmed A, Brito F, Goto C, et al. Clinical utility of the polymerase chain reaction for diagnosis of enteroviral meningitis in infancy. J Pediatr 1997;131:393–397.
91. Dagan R, Jenista JA, Prather SL, Powell KR, Menegus MA. Viremia in hospitalized children with enterovirus infections. J Pediatr 1985;106:397–401.
92. Abzug MJ, Loeffelholz M, Rotbart HA. Diagnosis of neonatal enterovirus infection by polymerase chain reaction. J Pediatr 1995;26:447–450.
93. Yoshio H, Yamada M, Yokoi Y, Iwamoto A, Nakamura M, Mizoguchi. Diagnosis of neonatal enterovirus meningitis by reverse transcription-polymerase chain reaction. J Jpn Assoc Infect Dis 1997;71:1046–1050.
94. Chambon M, Delage C, Bailly JL, et al. Fatal hepatic necrosis in a neonate with echovirus 20 infection: use of the polymerase chain reaction to detect enterovirus in liver tissue. Clin Infect Dis 1997;24:523–524.
95. Austin BJ, Croxson MC, Powell KF, Gunn TR. The successful containment of coxsackie B4 infection in a neonatal unit. J Paediatr Child Health 1999;35:102–104.
96. Chambon M, Bailly JL, Beguet A, et al. An outbreak due to echovirus type 30 in a neonatal unit in France in 1997: usefulness of PCR diagnosis. J Hosp Infect 1999;43:63–68.
97. Takami T, Kawashima H, Takei Y, et al. Usefulness of nested PCR and sequence analysis in a nosocomial outbreak of neonatal enterovirus infection. J Clin Virol 1998;11:67–75.
98. Dronkert ML, Ketel AG, de Groot R. Simultaneous occurrence of group B *Streptococcus* and echovirus 20. Eur J Pediatr 1996;155:915.
99. Isacsohn M, Eidelman AI, Kaplan M, et al. Neonatal coxsackievirus group B infections: experience of a single department of neonatology. Isr J Med Sci 1994;30:371–374.

14

Human Immunodeficiency Virus Type 1

David Berman and Gwendolyn B. Scott

INTRODUCTION

Most children infected with human immunodeficiency virus type 1 (HIV-1) acquire infection by mother-to-child transmission. Progress in understanding HIV-1 transmission, its diagnosis, and its treatment has led to strategies that are remarkably effective in the prevention of perinatal HIV-1 transmission in the United States and other countries with adequate resources. There have been reports of rates of perinatal transmission of between 1 and 4% (1–3). Prophylaxis trials in countries with limited resources using short courses of antiretroviral drugs to interrupt perinatal transmission have provided promising results (4–8). Despite these results, there continue to be large numbers of infants born every year in these countries who are HIV-1 infected. The World Health Organization estimated that, worldwide, as many as 640,000 HIV-1-infected infants were born in 2004 (9). Significant obstacles, many of which are economic, have prevented the implementation of strategies that could be effective in decreasing perinatal transmission in these countries.

HIV-1 STRUCTURE AND LIFE CYCLE

HIV-1 is a member of the lentivirus genus of the Retroviridae family (10,11). HIV-1 is a spherical retrovirus with a cylindrical core that is contained within a lipid bilayer. The virus is composed of several different proteins. It most commonly infects CD4$^+$ lymphocytes and cells of the monocyte-macrophage series. Entry into the CD4 lymphocyte occurs by the interaction of the viral cell glycoprotein and the CD4 cell receptor on the cell surface, resulting in fusion. Once inside the cell, the single-stranded ribonucleic acid (RNA) from the virus is transcribed into linear double-stranded deoxyribonucleic acid (DNA) using an enzyme called reverse transcriptase. This viral DNA is then integrated into the host cell DNA, establishing a chronic infection.

Diversity is characteristic of HIV-1 strains (12). There are three major categories of HIV-1 strains, which are based on the envelope gene coding sequence: M, O, and N (non-M, non-O) (13). The majority of infecting strains belong to the M group. This group is further subdivided into subtypes, and there are 10 subtypes identified at this time (14,15). Subtype B is the most common type in North America.

HIV-2 is another human lentivirus. It is very similar to HIV-1 in genetic composition and disease manifestations. HIV-2 is endemic in western Africa and is only occa-

From: *Infectious Disease: Congenital and Perinatal Infections: A Concise Guide to Diagnosis*
Edited by: C. Hutto © Humana Press Inc., Totowa, NJ

sionally seen in the United States. HIV-1 has accounted for the great majority of disease caused by human lentivirus worldwide.

EPIDEMIOLOGY AND TRANSMISSION OF HIV-1 IN WOMEN

The World Health Organization estimated that approx 38 million people were living with HIV-1 at the end of 2003, including 17 million women representing almost 50% of infected adults *(9)*.

HIV-1 and AIDS occur in women in most areas of the world, but some areas are substantially more affected by this epidemic. The population of countries in sub-Saharan Africa accounts for only 2% of the world's population, but 30% of the cases of HIV-1 occur in these countries. Among countries in southern Africa, the prevalence among pregnant women varies, with countries like Botswana and Zambia having rates of 25% or greater, and other countries having median prevalence rates of about 10% *(9)*. Although less extensive than in southern Africa, the epidemic has continued to increase in Asian countries, including China, Indonesia, Thailand, and Vietnam, some central Asian republics, and the Baltic states *(9)*.

In the United States at the end of 2000, an estimated 350,000 people were living with AIDS *(16)*. Of these, 41% were black, 38% white, and 20% Hispanic. The prevalence in Asians/Pacific Islanders and American Indians or Alaskan Natives was 1% and less than 1%, respectively. Almost 21% of individuals older than 13 years were female. In comparison to the total adult population living with HIV-1 and AIDS in 2002, a substantially greater proportion of women with AIDS, 82%, was African American or Hispanic *(17)*.

Almost 80% of women with HIV-1 or AIDS are 20–44 years of age, and 26% were older than 45 years of age. During the last decade, the rate of increase in new cases was higher for women than men. The proportion of cases among women increased from 7 to 26% between 1985 and 2002. Women also represented about 32% of new cases of HIV-1 infection in 2002 *(17)*.

The routes of transmission for women are primarily through heterosexual contact, intravenous drug use, and, in countries where there are inadequate methods of screening blood, transfusion with infected blood or blood products. Heterosexual transmission is the route by which at least 90% of women are infected worldwide. Transmission by intravenous drug use accounted for 21% of the new HIV-1 infections among women in the United States in 2002 *(17)*. Among the youngest women, those 13–24 years of age, intravenous drug use is less common (<21%) as a route of transmission than heterosexual contact.

EPIDEMIOLOGY AND TRANSMISSION OF HIV-1 IN CHILDREN

At the close of 2003, there were an estimated 2.1 million children younger than 15 years worldwide who were infected with HIV-1 *(9)*. Because children are infected predominantly through perinatal transmission, the demographic characteristics of infected children are similar to those of women.

The epidemiology of HIV-1 in children in the United States has changed over the past few years because of recommendations for universal screening of pregnant women and the use of antiretroviral therapy to interrupt perinatal transmission. Transmission rates of 2% or less are common in many centers providing care for large numbers of

HIV-1-infected pregnant women. The number of infected infants in the United States has declined significantly. In 2001, only 101 children with AIDS were reported to the Centers for Disease Control and Prevention, in comparison to 954 in 1992 *(18)*. This does not include all infected infants, however, and recent estimates are that 230–370 infected infants are born with HIV-1 infection yearly despite current intervention strategies *(19)*.

In the United States and other countries, a small number of children are infected through sexual abuse. In some countries with inadequate methods of screening of the blood supply, contact or use of infected blood or blood products or reuse of contaminated syringes are routes of infection for some children. The predominant transmission route, however, for children in the United States and other countries is perinatal transmission.

TIMING OF HIV-1 TRANSMISSION

Infants may be infected *in utero* through transplacental spread, during labor and delivery through contact with infected blood or secretions in the birth canal, and postnatally through breast-feeding. In countries where women are counseled not to breast-feed, most transmission occurs at the time of delivery. In countries where safe alternatives to breast-feeding are not available for infant nutrition, many infants are infected through breast-feeding. The timing of transmission is defined by the time that HIV-1 is detected in the infant using a standard diagnostic test *(20,21)*. Cord blood should not be used for HIV-1 testing of the infant at birth because of the potential for contamination with maternal blood. If tests that detect the HIV-1 virus, such as an HIV-1 culture or HIV-1 DNA polymerase chain reaction (PCR) assay, are positive within the first 48 hours of life and subsequent tests are also positive, the transmission is considered to have occurred *in utero*. However, if the HIV-1 culture or HIV-1 DNA PCR assays are negative within the first week of life but become positive within the first few weeks of life, then the transmission is considered to have occurred intrapartum.

In utero transmission occurs when HIV-1 passes across the placenta during gestation *(22,23)*. It has been demonstrated that both the placenta and amniotic fluid may contain HIV-1 *(24,25)*. Intrapartum infection occurs when the infant has significant or prolonged contact with maternal secretions during delivery. Prolonged rupture of membranes places the baby at an increased risk for transmission of HIV-1 *(26)*. Elective cesarean section prior to the onset of labor has been shown to decrease perinatal transmission rates significantly *(27,28)*. Transmission to the newborn has occurred at different maternal plasma HIV-1 RNA levels *(29,30)*, and these levels may not always reflect the amount of virus outside the plasma, especially in other compartments, including the genital tract. In a population of infants who are not breast-fed, the proportion of infections that occur *in utero* ranges between 25 and 40%. The remainder are presumed to be infected during the intrapartum period *(31)*. Postpartum transmission occurs through breast-feeding *(32,33)*.

RISK FACTORS FOR TRANSMISSION OF HIV-1

Rates of transmission of HIV-1 from mother to child are presently less than 2% in most major HIV-1 centers throughout the United States. Prior to the use of zidovudine (ZDV) chemoprophylaxis for reduction of perinatal transmission, perinatal transmission rates ranged between 15 and 39%. In the adult female population, risk factors for

Table 1
Factors Affecting Vertical Transmission of HIV-1

Maternal factors
    Viral load
    CD4 lymphocyte count
    Maternal stage of disease
    Primary HIV infection during pregnancy
    Sexually transmitted diseases
Obstetrical factors
    Prolonged rupture of membranes
    Invasive procedures
    Placenta previa
    Chorioamnionitis
    Mode of delivery
Infant factors
    Prematurity
    Birth order of twins
Postnatal factors important to transmission
    Breast-feeding

acquiring HIV-1 include intravenous drug abuse, unprotected sexual intercourse, needle-stick injuries, and significant exposure to HIV-1-infected blood. Factors that are associated with transmission of HIV-1 from mother to infant are listed in Table 1.

Maternal risk factors associated with perinatal transmission of HIV-1 infection include an elevated maternal HIV-1 RNA viral load, severe immune suppression, AIDS-defining illness, and lack of use of ZDV during pregnancy (29,30,34–36). Several obstetrical practices, such as amniocentesis or use of a scalp electrode, may expose the infant to HIV-1-infected blood (37,38). The presence of chorioamnionitis (39) and prolonged rupture of membranes (26,38) are also associated with a higher risk of transmission.

Infant factors include prematurity (<37 weeks of gestation) (40) and birth order of twins, with twin A more likely to be infected (41). In developing countries, additional risk factors include anemia, malnutrition, and vitamin A deficiency (42). Postnatally, HIV-1 can be transmitted by ingestion of human milk from HIV-1-infected women (32,33). HIV-1 has been identified in breast milk (43,44). In a meta-analysis of several published studies, the estimated risk of transmission of HIV-1 through breast milk was 29% (95% confidence interval [CI] 16–42%) in women who acquired HIV-1 postnatally and 14% (95% CI 7–22%) in women who were chronically infected with HIV-1 (45). In the United States and developed countries, where safe, affordable, and accessible alternative feeding methods are available, it is recommended that HIV-1-infected women avoid breast-feeding (46).

MATERNAL HIV-1 TESTING AND COUNSELING

The US Public Health Service recommends that HIV-1 testing and counseling be offered to *all* pregnant women regardless of risk factors and the prevalence rates in the community (19,47). Offering of HIV-1 testing in the hospital, clinic, or private office should be universal and a routine part of prenatal care. Laws regarding HIV-1 testing are not uniform from state to state, and health care providers should be familiar with and follow local and state laws, regulations, and policies regarding HIV-1 screening of pregnant women and their infants *(48)*. In some states, the offering of HIV-1 testing is mandated, and in others, such as New York, there is mandatory HIV-1 testing of all newborns.

In most states, pregnant women receive pre-HIV-1 test counseling and must specifically consent to an HIV-1 antibody test, usually in writing. Pretest counseling should include information about HIV-1 and the risks and benefits of HIV-1 testing presented orally or in writing (such as a pamphlet) and in a language the client understands.

Other states have adopted an Opt-out approach by which pregnant women are notified that an HIV-1 test will be routinely included in the standard battery of prenatal tests for all pregnant women, but they can decline HIV-1 testing *(47)*. This approach allows women to decline testing if they feel it is not in their best interest and simplifies the testing process by eliminating the need for extensive pretest counseling. Accepting or refusing testing must not have detrimental consequences to the quality of prenatal care offered. The woman should be made aware that test results are confidential, but positive results are reported to the state health department in those states that have HIV-1 reporting laws. Under no circumstance are test results disclosed over the phone, through mail, or by facsimile. The mother should be given a date to return for posttest counseling once results are available. Counseling should be done for both positive and negative results. If a woman has a positive HIV-1 enzyme-linked immunosorbent assay (ELISA) with confirmatory Western blot, then she should receive the appropriate posttest counseling and be referred to an obstetrician who has experience in the care of the HIV-1-infected pregnant woman. If an obstetrician is not available, then an internist with knowledge of HIV-1 treatment should be consulted. If the woman tests negative for HIV-1, she should be counseled on how HIV-1 is transmitted and how to avoid contracting HIV-1 infection.

The standard test for diagnosis of HIV-1 in adults is the HIV-1 ELISA combined with a confirmatory test, either the HIV-1 Western blot or immunofluorescent assay (IFA). Of these two confirmatory tests, the Western blot is more commonly used. The HIV-1 ELISA test detects immunoglobulin G antibodies to HIV-1 in the blood. If an HIV-1 ELISA test is positive, the test is repeated using the same blood sample; if it is repeatedly reactive, then a Western blot test is done to determine which viral proteins the antibodies are directed against. Although the result of the HIV-1 ELISA is usually available within 24 hours, the Western blot will take longer to complete.

Both the ELISA and the Western blot must be positive to confirm HIV-1 infection *(49)*. In some cases, an ELISA may be positive, but the Western blot is negative, resulting in a false-positive ELISA. This person is not considered to be HIV-1 infected. If the ELISA is positive and the Western blot is indeterminate, then this may represent either early HIV-1 infection or a person without HIV-1 infection. In this case, the test needs to be repeated; in addition, an HIV-1 DNA PCR assay should be done. This test detects the presence of virus directly and, if positive, would diagnose HIV-1 infection. It is important to have both results before counseling a woman regarding her HIV-1 status. HIV-1 testing should be offered to the pregnant woman early in pregnancy so appropriate therapy can be initiated if the woman is HIV-1 infected. Retesting in the third trimester, preferably before 36 weeks of gestation, is recommended *(50,51)*.

For the woman who does not receive prenatal care or comes to labor and delivery without knowledge of her HIV-1 status, rapid HIV-1 testing can be offered *(52,53)*.

There are four rapid HIV-1 tests approved by the Food and Drug Administration for use in the United States: the OraQuick Rapid HIV-1 Antibody test, the Reveal Rapid HIV-1 Antibody Test, the Uni-Gold Recombigen HIV-1 Test, and the Murex-SUDS-Single Use Diagnostic System HIV-1 Antibody Test (manufacture of this test was discontinued in 2003). All have good sensitivity and specificity. As with other HIV-1 testing, consent is required for the rapid test, and if positive, a follow-up HIV-1 ELISA and Western blot or IFA test needs to be done to confirm the HIV-1 infection. The advantages of this test are that results are available within 30–60 minutes, and the results can be immediately given to the individual tested. A reactive result from a rapid test is considered to be a preliminary positive test result. Thus, if a pregnant woman does not know her HIV-1 status and is late in gestation, a positive rapid HIV-1 test can be used to institute antiretroviral therapy, or if she is in labor, she should be counseled and have the option to receive intravenous ZDV during labor and give ZDV to the newborn within the first 12 hours of life *(54)*. Observational studies and clinical trials have shown that when antiretroviral prophylaxis is administered during labor or within the first 12 hours after birth, the risk of perinatal HIV-1 transmission is reduced from 25 to 9–13% *(55,56)*.

The majority of HIV-1 infection in the United States is caused by HIV-1 subtype B. Standard HIV-1 ELISA screening tests may be negative in 20–30% of patients infected with HIV-2. HIV-2 infection is predominately found in western sub-Saharan Africa. Detection in these cases may require specific testing for HIV-2. These screening tests may also fail to detect the O subtype, which is very rare in the United States. Another rare subtype, N, is not detected with the HIV-1 ELISA but may be positive by Western blot tests *(57)*.

GENERAL CARE ISSUES DURING PREGNANCY

Women should be monitored to assess the status of their HIV-1 infection. The CD4 number and percentage will assess the degree of immune deficiency present, and a viral load determines the risk for disease progression. These studies should be done during each trimester of pregnancy with the goal of reducing the viral load to undetectable and maintaining the CD4 count and percentage within a normal range. Other laboratory tests or blood tests should be done to assess for toxicity of the medications and include a complete blood cell count with platelets, amylase, lipase, and hepatic function studies.

The goal of antiretroviral therapy in pregnancy is to optimize the health of the mother and to prevent transmission of HIV-1 to the infant. The US Public Health Service Task Force has developed *Recommendations for Use of Antiretroviral Drugs in Pregnant HIV-1 Infected Women for Maternal Health and Interventions to Reduce Perinatal HIV-1 Transmission in the United States (53)*. These guidelines are updated on a regular basis and are available on the AIDSinfo Web site (http://AIDSinfo.nih.gov) *(58)*.

DIAGNOSIS OF HIV-1 IN THE INFANT

A diagnosis of HIV-1 infection in an infant is made by tests that can directly detect the virus. HIV-1 antibody tests are not useful for detection of HIV-1 infection in the infant under 18 months of age. Maternal HIV-1 immunoglobulin G antibody is passively transferred across the placenta during late pregnancy, and most infants will be

Table 2
Schedule of Infant Monitoring

Clinical/laboratory studies	Birth	2 weeks	6 weeks	4 months	6 months	12 months	15 months	18 months
History	X	X	X	X	X	X		
Physical examination	X	X	X	X	X	X		
Zidovudine (ZDV)	X	X	Stop					
Trimethoprim-sulfamethoxazole			Start	Stop (if two negative HIV DNA PCR, normal T cells)				
Complete blood cell count and differential	X	X	X	X	X	X		
Lymphocyte subsets, including CD4 count and % CD4			X		X		X	
HIV DNA PCR	X	X	X	X[a]	X[a]			
HIV ELISA/ Western blot						X	X[b]	
Quantitative immuno-globulins				X		X		

[a]Document two negative DNA PCR tests between 1 and 6 months of age.
[b]Document two negative ELISA tests from different specimens after 12 months of age.

HIV-1 antibody positive using the standard assays of HIV-1 ELISA with either the Western blot or the IFA used as a confirmatory test.

The standard assays for diagnosis of HIV-1 in infants under 2 years of age include viral culture, HIV-1 DNA PCR, and HIV-1 RNA PCR *(59)*. Of these tests, the HIV-1 DNA PCR is preferred *(60,61)*. The HIV-1 RNA has good sensitivity and specificity, but there is limited experience with this test as a diagnostic test for infants *(62–64)*. The viral culture is not commercially available, is more work intensive, and requires several days for completion of the test *(65)*. These tests detect the presence of HIV-1 virus in the blood or body fluid. They have good specificity and sensitivity and are readily available in the United States *(66)*. Other tests such as the P24 antigen test and the immune complex dissociated P24 antigen test are not widely used in the United States. Although the P24 tests have good specificity, their sensitivity is much lower *(65)*.

The first HIV-1 DNA PCR test should be done within the first 48 hours of life. If the infant is infected *in utero*, then this will allow an early diagnosis of HIV-1 and early initiation of treatment, which will result in a better overall prognosis for the infant. The schedule for subsequent follow-up of the infant and diagnostic testing is given in Table 2. The DNA PCR should be done at birth, at 4–8 weeks of age, and between 4 and 6 months of age. If all tests are negative after 4 or 6 months of age, then the infant is tested beginning at 12 months of age using the HIV-1 ELISA test. This test is done to determine whether the maternal antibody has disappeared. If the test remains positive at 12 months of age, repeat testing should be done at 15 and 18 months of age. If the ELISA is negative at one of these time points, then the ELISA is repeated one more time to confirm the negative result.

Thus, a child with two negative HIV-1 DNA PCR assays done between 1 and 6 months of age and disappearance of the maternal antibody before the age of 18 months is considered not infected *(67)*. A child who has a positive HIV-1 DNA PCR should have the test repeated as soon as possible. An infant who has been perinatally exposed to HIV-1 would be considered infected if HIV-1 is detected on two blood specimens taken at different times using one or a combination of the acceptable methods for viral detection. These would include two HIV-1 DNA PCR tests, two viral cultures, two HIV-1 RNA PCR tests, or a combination of two of these tests yielding positive results *(67)*. If a child is diagnosed with HIV-1, a pediatric HIV-1 specialist should be consulted regarding the diagnosis, care, and treatment of the child.

THE MANAGEMENT OF THE INFANT

The infant born to an HIV-1-infected mother will need close follow-up throughout the first year of life. The infant should receive diagnostic testing for HIV-1 according to the schedule outlined in Table 2. ZDV will be administered for the first 6 weeks of life with clinical and laboratory monitoring for adverse effects *(68,69)*. Prophylaxis using trimethaprim-sulfamethoxazole to prevent *Pneumocystis carinii* pneumonia will be started at 6 weeks of age and continue until two HIV-1 DNA PCR assays done after 1 month of life are negative, one of which is performed after 4 months of age *(70,71)*. The infant should receive routine newborn care and immunizations. At 12 months of age, the first HIV-1 ELISA/Western blot assay can be done to determine if maternal antibody has disappeared and if further testing is required.

If an infant is determined to be infected with HIV-1, then the child should be referred to an HIV-1 specialist for assistance in the child's care and treatment with antiretroviral agents *(68,69)*. *Guidelines for the Use of Antiretroviral Agents in Pediatric HIV-1 Infection* have been developed by a working group on antiretroviral therapy and medical management of HIV-1-infected children and are found at the AIDSinfo Web site (http://AIDSinfo.nih.gov) *(72,73)*.

The goal of HIV-1 testing during pregnancy is to identify women with HIV-1 so antiretroviral therapy can be instituted for their own health and to reduce the risk for transmission from mother to infant. HIV-1 is a preventable disease in the infant. Identification and appropriate management of the HIV-1-infected pregnant woman will ensure optimal health for both mother and infant.

REFERENCES

1. Dorenbaum A, Cunningham CK, Gelber RD, et al. Two-dose intrapartum/newborn nevirapine and standard antiretroviral therapy to reduce perinatal HIV transmission: a randomized trial. JAMA 2002;288:189–198.
2. Garcia PM, Kalish LA, Pitt J, et al. Maternal levels of plasma human immunodeficiency virus type 1 RNA and the risk of perinatal transmission. Women and Infants Transmission Study Group. N Engl J Med 1999;341:394–402.
3. Ioannidid JP, Abrams EJ, Ammann A, et al. Perinatal transmission of human immunodeficiency virus type 1 by pregnant women with RNA virus loads < 1000 copies/mL. J Infect Dis 2001;183:539–545.
4. Lallemant M, Jourdain G, LeCoeur S, et al. for the Perinatal HIV Prevention Trial (Thailand) Investigators. A trial of shortened zidovudine regimens to prevent mother-to-child transmission of HIV. N Engl J Med 2000;343:982–991.

5. Guay L, Musoke P, Fleming T, et al. Intrapartum and neonatal single-dose nevirapine compared with zidovudine for prevention of mother-child transmission of HIV-1 in Kampala, Uganda: HIVNET 012 randomized trial. Lancet 1999;354:795–802.

6. Petra Study team. Efficacy of three short-course regimens of zidovudine and lamivudine in preventing early and late transmission of HIV-1 from mother to child in Tanzania, South Africa, and Uganda (Petra Study): a randomized, double blind, placebo controlled trial. Lancet 2002:359:1178–1186.

7. Moodley D, Moodley J, Coovadia H, et al. A multicenter randomized controlled trial of nevirapine vs a combination of zidovudine and lamivudine to reduce intrapartum and early postpartum mother to child transmission of human immunodeficiency virus type 1. J Infect Dis 2003;187:725–735.

8. Taha TE, Kumwenda NI, Gibbons A, et al. Short post exposure prophylaxis in newborn babies to reduce mother-to-child transmission of HIV-1: NVAZ randomized clinical trial. Lancet 2003;362:1171–1177.

9. UNAIDS. AIDS Epidemic Update, December 2004:1–91. Available at http://www.UNAIDS.org/en/default.asp.

10. Wain Hobson S, Sonigo P, Danos O, et al. Nucleotide sequence of the AIDS virus, LAV. Cell 1985;40:9–17.

11. Ratner, L, Haseltine W, Patarca R, et al. Complete nucleotide sequence of the AIDS virus, HTLV III. Nature 1985;313:277–284.

12. McCutchan FE. Understanding the genetic diversity of HIV-1. AIDS 2000;14(Suppl 3):S31–S44.

13. Simon F, Mauclere P, Roques P, et al. Identification of a new human immunodeficiency virus type 1 distinct from group M and group O. Nat Med 1998;4:1032–1037.

14. Louwagie J, McCutchan FE, Peeters M, et al. Phylogenetic analysis of gag genes from 70 international HIV-1 isolates provides evidence for multiple genotypes. AIDS 1993;7:769–780.

15. Apetrei CA, Marx PA, Smith SS, The evolution of HIV and its consequences. Infect Dis Clin North Am 2004;18:369–394.

16. Centers for Disease Control and Prevention. Update: AIDS United States 2000. MMWR Morb Mortal Wkly Rep 2002;51;592–595.

17. Centers for Disease Control and Prevention. Cases of HIV infection and AIDS in the United States. HIV/AIDS Surveill Rep 2002;14:1–40. Also available at: http://www.cdc.gov/hiv/stats/hasrlink.htm.

18. Centers for Disease Control and Prevention. US HIV and AIDS cases reported through December 2001. HIV/AIDS Surveill Rep 2001;13:1 44.

19. Centers for Disease Control. Revised recommendations for HIV screening of pregnant women. MMWR Morb Mortal Wkly Rep 2001;50:59–86.

20. Bryson YJ, Luzuriaga K, Sullivan JL, et al. Proposed definitions for *in utero* vs intrapartum transmission of HIV-1. N Engl J Med 1992;327:1246–1247.

21. Kalish LA, Pitt J, Lew JF, et al. Defining the time of fetal or perinatal acquisition of human immunodeficiency virus type 1 infection on the basis of age at first positive culture. J Infect Dis 1997;175:712–715.

22. Sprecher S, Soumenkoff G, Puissant F, Degueldre M. Vertical transmission of HIV in 15-week fetus. Lancet 1986;2:288–289.

23. Jovaisas E, Koch MA, Schafer A, et al. LAV/HTLV-III in a 20-week fetus [letter]. Lancet 1985;2:1129.

24. Di Maria H, Courpotin C, Rouzioux C, et al. Transplacental transmission of human immunodeficiency virus. Lancet 1986;2:215–216.

25. Mundy DC, Schinazi RF, Gerber AR, et al. Human immunodeficiency virus isolated from amniotic fluid. Lancet 1997;2:459.

26. The International Perinatal HIV Group. Duration of ruptured membranes and vertical transmission of HIV-1: a meta-analysis from 15 prospective cohort studies. AIDS 2001;15:357–368.

27. The European Mode of Delivery Collaboration. Elective caesarean section vs vaginal delivery in prevention of vertical HIV-1 transmission: a randomized clinical trial. Lancet 1999;353:1035–1039.
28. The International Perinatal HIV Group. Mode of delivery and vertical transmission of HIV-1: a meta analysis from fifteen prospective cohort studies. N Engl J Med 1999;340:977–987.
29. Dickover RE, Garratty EM, Herman SA, et al. Identification of levels of maternal HIV-1 RNA associated with risk of perinatal transmission: effect of maternal zidovudine treatment on viral load. JAMA 1996;275:599–605.
30. Sperling RS, Shapiro DE, Coombs RW, et al. Maternal viral load, zidovudine treatment, and the risk of transmission of human immunodeficiency virus type 1 from mother to infant. N Engl J Med 1996;335:1621–1629.
31. Dunn DT, Brandt CD, Krivine A, et al. The sensitivity of HIV-1 DNA polymerase chain reaction in the neonatal period and the relative contributions of intra-uterine and intra-partum transmission. AIDS 1992;9:F7–F11.
32. Ziegler JB, Cooper DA, Johnson RO, Gold J. Postnatal transmission of AIDS-associated retrovirus from mother to infant. Lancet 1985;1:896–897.
33. Nduati R, John CG, Richardson BA, et al. Human immunodeficiency virus type 1-infected cells in breast milk: association with immunosuppression and vitamin A deficiency. J Infect Dis 1995;172:1461–1468.
34. Connor E.M., Sperling R.S, Gelber R, et al. Reduction of maternal-infant transmission of human immunodeficiency virus type-1 with zidovudine treatment. N Eng J Med 1994;331:1173–1180.
35. Boyer PJ, Dillon M, Navaie M, et al. Factors predictive of maternal-fetal transmission of HIV-1: Preliminary analysis of zidovudine given during pregnancy and/or delivery. JAMA 1994;271:1925–1930.
36. Mayaux MJ, Blanche S, Rouzioux C, et al. Maternal factors associated with perinatal HIV-1 transmission: the French Cohort Study: 7 years of follow-up observation. J AIDS Hum Retrovirol 1995;8:188–194.
37. Mandelbrot L, Mayaux MJ, Bongain A, et al. Obstetric factors and mother-to-child transmission of human immunodeficiency virus type 1: the French perinatal cohorts. Am J Obstet Gynecol 1996;175:661–667.
38. Landesman SH, Kalish LA, Burn DN, et al. Obstetrical factors and the transmission of human immunodeficiency virus type 1 from mother to child. N Engl J Med 1996;334:1617–1623.
39. St. Louis ME, Kamenga M, Brown C, et al. Risk for perinatal HIV-1 transmission according to maternal immunologic, virologic and placental factors. JAMA 1993;269:2853–2859.
40. Goedert JJ, Mendez H, Drummond JE, et al. Mother-to-infant transmission of human immunodeficiency virus type 1: association with prematurity or low anti-gp120. Lancet 1989;2:1351–1354.
41. Goedert JJ, Duliege AM, Amos CI, Felton S, Biggar RJ. High risk of HIV-1 infection for first-born twins. The International Registry of HIV-exposed Twins. Lancet 1991;338:1471–1475.
42. Semba RD, Miotti PG, Chiphangwi JD, et al. Maternal vitamin A deficiency and mother-to-child transmission of HIV-1. Lancet 1994;343:1593–1597.
43. Thiry L, Sprecher-Goldberger S, Jonckheer T, et al. Isolation of AIDS virus from cell-free breast milk of three healthy virus carriers. Lancet 1985;2:891–892.
44. Van de Perre P, Simonon A, Hitimana D, et al. Infective and anti-infective properties of breast milk from HIV-1 infected women. Lancet 1993;341:914–918.
45. Dunn DT, Newell ML, Ades AE, Peckham CS. Risk of human immunodeficiency virus type 1 transmission through breastfeeding. Lancet 1992:340:585–588.
46. American Academy of Pediatrics. Committee on Pediatrics AIDS. Human milk, breastfeeding, and transmission of human immunodeficiency virus in the United States. Pediatrics 1995;96:977–979.

47. Centers for Disease Control and Prevention. HIV testing among pregnant women—United States and Canada, 1998–2001. MMWR Morb Mortal Wkly Rep 2002;51:1013–1016.
48. American College of Obstetricians and Gynecologists. Survey of State Laws on HIV and Pregnant Women, 1999–2000. Moore KG, ed. Washington, DC: American College of Obstetricians and Gynecologists, 2000.
49. Centers for Disease Control. Interpretation of the use of the Western blot essay for serodiagnosis of human immunodeficiency virus type 1 infections. MMWR Morb Mortal Wkly Rep 1989;38:1–7.
50. Sansom SL, Jamieson DJ, Farnham PG, Bulterys M, Fowler MG. Human immunodeficiency virus retesting during pregnancy: costs and effectiveness in preventing perinatal transmission. Obstet Gynecol 2003;102:782–790.
51. Centers for Disease Control and Prevention. Prenatal HIV testing and the antiretroviral prophylaxis at an urban hospital—Atlanta, Georgia, 1997–2000. MMWR Morb Mortal Wkly Rep 2004;52:1245–1250.
52. Minkoff H, O'Sullivan MJ. The case for rapid HIV testing during labor. JAMA 1998;279:1743–1744.
53. Centers for Disease Control and Prevention. US Public Health Service Task recommendations for use of antiretroviral drugs in pregnant HIV-1 infected women for maternal health and interventions to reduce perinatal HIV-1 transmission in the United States. MMWR Morb Mortal Wkly Rep 2002;51:1–38.
54. Centers for Disease Control and Prevention. Rapid point-of-care testing for HIV-1 during labor and delivery—Chicago, Illinois, 2002. MMWR Morb Mortal Wkly Rep 2003;53:866–868.
55. Wade NA, Birkhead GS, Warren BL, et al. Abbreviated regimen of zidovudine prophylaxis and perinatal transmission of the human immunodeficiency virus. N Engl J Med 1998;339:1409–1414.
56. Frenkel LM, Cowles MK, Shapiro DE, et al: Analysis of the maternal components of the AIDS clinical trial group 076 zidovudine regimen in the prevention of mother-to-infant transmission of human immunodeficiency virus type 1. J Infect Dis 1997;175:971–974.
57. Haas J, Geiss M, Bohler T. False negative polymerase chain reaction-based diagnosis of human immunodeficiency virus (HIV) type 1 in children infected with HIV strains of African origin [letter]. J Infect Dis 1996;174:244–245.
58. Public Health Service Task Force Recommendations for Use of Antiretroviral Drugs in Pregnant HIV-1-Infected Women for Maternal Health and Interventions to Reduce Perinatal HIV-1 Transmission in the United States—February 24, 2005. Available at: http://AIDSinfo.nih.gov. Accessed April 6, 2005.
59. Husson RN, Comeau AM, Hoff R. Diagnosis of human immunodeficiency virus infection in infants and children. Pediatrics 1990;86:1–10.
60. Bremer JW, Lew JF, Cooper E. Diagnosis of infection with human immunodeficiency virus type 1 by a DNA polymerase chain reaction assay among infants enrolled in the Women and Infants' Transmission Study. J Pediatr 1996;129:198–207.
61. Owens DK, Holodniy M, McDonald TW, et al. A meta-analytic evaluation of the polymerase chain reaction for the diagnosis of HIV infection in infants. JAMA 1996;275:1342–1348.
62. Simonds RJ, Brown TM, Thea DM, et al. Sensitivity and specificity of a qualitative RNA detection assay to diagnose HIV infection in young infants. AIDS 1998;12:1545–1549.
63. Delamare C, Burgard M, Mayaux MJ, et al. HIV-1 RNA detection in plasma for the diagnosis of infection in neonate. J Acquir Immune Defic Syndr Hum Retrovirol 1997;15:121–125.
64. Cunningham CK, Charbonneau TT, Song K, et al. Comparison of human immunodeficiency virus 1 DNA polymerase chain reaction and qualitative RNA polymerase chain reaction in human immunodeficiency virus 1-exposed infants. Pediatr Infect Dis J 1999;18:30–35.

65. Burgard M, Mayaux MJ, Blanche S, et al. The use of viral culture and p24 antigen testing to diagnose human immunodeficiency virus infection in neonates. N Engl J Med 1992;327:1192–1197.
66. Dunn DT, Brandt CD, Krivine A, et al. The sensitivity of HIV-1 DNA polymerase chain reaction in the neonatal period and the relative contributions of intra-uterine and intra-partum transmission. AIDS 1995;9:F7–F11.
67. Centers for Disease Control and Prevention. 1994 Revised classification system for human immunodeficiency virus infection in children less than 13 years of age. MMWR Morb Mortal Wkly Rep 43:1–10.
68. Laufer M, Scott GB. Medical management of HIV disease in children. Pediatr Clin North Am 2000;47:127–133.
69. King SM. Committee on Pediatrics AIDS, and Infectious Diseases and Immunizations Committee. Evaluation and treatment of the human immunodeficiency virus 1-exposed infant. Pediatrics 2004;114:497–505.
70. Simonds RJ, Oxtoby MJ, Caldwell MB, et al. *Pneumocystis carinii* pneumonia among US children with perinatally acquired HIV infection. JAMA 1993;270:470–473.
71. Centers for Disease Control and Prevention. 1995 revised guidelines for prophylaxis against *Pneumocystis carinii* pneumonia for children infected with or perinatally exposed to human immunodeficiency virus. MMWR Morb Mortal Wkly Rep 1995;44:1–11.
72. Centers for Disease Control and Prevention. Working Group on Antiretroviral Therapy and Medical Management of HIV-Infected Children—guidelines for the use of antiretroviral agents in pediatric HIV infection. MMWR Morb Mortal Wkly Rep 1998;47(RR-4):1–31.
73. Working Group on Antiretroviral Therapy and Management of HIV-Infected Children. Guidelines for the Use of Antiretroviral Agents in Pediatric HIV Infection, March 24, 2005:1–50. Available at: http://AIDSinfo.nih.gov.

15

Hepatitis Viruses

Ravi Jhaveri and Yvonne Bryson

INTRODUCTION

The hepatitis viruses are a diverse group that has as their common feature the liver as their primary target of infection. They come from several families of viruses, cause infection via different mechanisms, and have a variety of clinical manifestations. The differential diagnosis for hepatitis in pregnancy includes other viruses (cytomegalovirus, Epstein-Barr virus), toxic exposures (acetaminophen), autoimmune disease (e.g., systemic lupus erythematosus), and other entities unique to pregnancy (e.g., HELLP [hemolysis, elevated liver enzymes, and low platelet count]).

This chapter reviews basic information regarding the five known major hepatitis viruses and their clinical presentation and management during pregnancy. The essential features of each virus are discussed in Table 1.

HEPATITIS A VIRUS

Basic Virology and Epidemiology

Hepatitis A virus (HAV) is a member of the Picornavirus family. It is a single-stranded, plus sense (directly translated into protein) ribonucleic acid (RNA) virus approx 30 μm in diameter. The HAV RNA has 7500 nucleotides and is translated to a single polyprotein that is cleaved by its own protease to yield individual viral proteins.

HAV is spread via contamination by infected human excrement *(1)*. The virus may be found in contaminated water or fish that have been in infected water or food handled by infected persons. The virus can also infect subhuman primates when HAV is acquired in captivity in the same manner as humans. HAV is seen primarily in endemic areas where sanitation is poor and has a much lower prevalence in population groups with a higher socioeconomic status. In HAV-prevalent areas, most people are exposed and develop immunity to the virus at a young age. In areas where HAV is less prevalent, disease is seen in older individuals, who have more symptoms related to infection *(2)*. Risk factors for acquiring HAV include living in or traveling to an endemic area, contact with an infected individual, working in a day care or health care facility, and anal intercourse.

HAV has a high attack rate, which means the majority (approx 70%) of those exposed to HAV will become infected. This is the basis for the recommendations for

From: *Infectious Disease: Congenital and Perinatal Infections: A Concise Guide to Diagnosis*
Edited by: C. Hutto © Humana Press Inc., Totowa, NJ

Table 1
Essential Features of Hepatitus Viruses

Viral agent	Type of virus	Main route of acquisition	Acute/chronic infection	Vertical transmission	Worse in pregnancy	Diagnostic markers
Hepatitis A (HAV)	Plus sense, single-stranded RNA virus	Fecal-oral transmission	Acute only	Yes (not significant)	No, worse	Serum HAV IgM
Hepatitis B (HBV)	DNA virus	Blood-borne contact, sexual transmission	**Acute and chronic**	**Yes**	No, worse	Serum HBsAg, HBsAb (IgG), HBeAg, HBcAb
Hepatitis C (HCV)	Plus sense RNA virus	Blood-borne contact	**Acute and chronic**	**Yes**	No, worse	Serum HCV IgG, serum HCV RNA (qualitative and quantitative)
Hepatitis D (HDV)	Replication-defective DNA virus	Blood-borne contact	Acute and chronic	No	No	Serum HDV IgM worse
Hepatitis E (HEV)	Plus sense, single-stranded RNA virus	Fecal-oral transmission	Acute only	Yes	**Worse**	Serum HEV IgM, serum and stool HEV PCR (experimental)

Distinguishing features of each virus in **bold**.

prophylaxis with immune globulin previously and HAV vaccine currently of household contacts or others at high risk of exposure *(1)*.

Course of Infection

After exposure, the virus invades the host's intestinal tissue and spreads via the blood to the liver. The typical incubation period is 7–14 days but can be as long as 6 weeks. During this time, excretion of HAV in the stool is at its highest level. HAV continues to be excreted for approx 7 days after onset of illness.

Symptoms of acute HAV infection include fever, malaise, jaundice, and abdominal pain. Conversely, many patients may be asymptomatic. In general, symptomatology in children is less frequent than in adulthood. HAV leads to fulminant liver failure in 1% of cases and does not establish chronic infection or a carrier state *(1–3)*.

Infection During Pregnancy and Vertical Transmission

HAV can cause disease during pregnancy, but the illness is similar to that in other adults. Pregnant mothers are at no greater risk of fulminant hepatic failure than the general population *(2,3)*.

Vertical Transmission

HAV has been shown to cross the placenta, but intrauterine infection has not been shown to be clinically significant. Infants are at risk of acquiring HAV postnatally through direct contact with the mother if the mother is still excreting virus *(2,3)*. Breastfeeding has not been shown to be a route of transmission.

Prenatal Evaluation

Prenatal visit should include history and physical exam to assess for any risk factors or manifestations of HAV infection. History should include questions regarding the conditions of the home, persons in the household who may be at increased risk of infection, foreign travel, and food intake. Physical exam should include inspection for jaundice, palpation for enlargement of the liver, or other findings of liver disease.

Postnatal Evaluation of the Infant

Examination of the infant should include the routine elements of a newborn exam. Jaundice may be seen early in life but of course could be caused by other factors. Fulminant failure in the neonatal period is very rare. Outbreaks have occurred in hospitals among staff exposed to infants born to HAV-infected mothers.

Laboratory Studies of Mother and Infant

If HAV infection is suspected in the mother, the definitive test is for the presence of HAV-specific immunoglobulin (Ig) M in the serum. This antibody should be present by the time a patient has symptoms of disease and will persist for several months. An IgG response is usually detectable by 10–12 weeks after the exposure *(1)*. Liver enzymes during acute illness will be elevated, with the aspartate aminotransferase and alanine aminotransferase ranging from 200 to 5000 in most cases. Levels that significantly exceed the usual may indicate fulminant hepatic failure and require urgent attention.

Infants who demonstrate signs of hepatitis in the newborn period with a symptomatic mother may be tested for IgM antibody to HAV. Proper precautions to limit the exposure of others should be taken.

HEPATITIS B VIRUS

Basic Virology and Epidemiology

Hepatitis B virus (HBV) is a member of the Hepadnavirus family. It is a large deoxyribonucleic acid (DNA) virus with a circular chromosome that undergoes an RNA stage in the host cell during its replicative cycle. It subsequently produces viral DNA, which ultimately leads to synthesis of the viral proteins. The major proteins involved in HBV infection are the surface antigen (HBsAg), core antigen (HBcAg), and the e antigen (HBeAg). The HBsAg is an element of the outer surface of the virus; HBcAg and HBeAg are different forms of the same polyprotein. HBcAg is made up of subunit proteins that form the genomic core of the full virus; HBeAg is a truncated form of this protein that is thought to play a role in signaling for viral replication *(4)*.

HBV infection occurs only in humans and is passed from person to person by sexual and blood-borne contact, as well as vertical transmission. HBV is a worldwide public health concern. It is estimated that 350 million people are carriers of the virus, with prevalence rates in Africa and Asia of greater than 8%. In developing nations, the major route of acquisition of HBV is by vertical transmission from mother to child at birth; in the Western Hemisphere, most individuals acquire infection in adolescence and adulthood via sexual or parenteral routes *(2–4)*.

Course of Infection

Incubation of HBV after exposure averages 70 days before the onset of symptoms. Acute HBV infection is subtle in most adult cases but may be symptomatic in about 30% of patients. Symptoms include fever, jaundice, malaise, and abdominal pain, with a clinical course identical to HAV. HBV may have some extrahepatic manifestations that are characteristic: Gianotti-Crosti skin eruption, also known as papular acrodermatitis of childhood, and acute glomerulonephritis. Symptoms appear after HBsAg levels have peaked in the bloodstream *(4)*.

About 90% of patients with acute HBV infection will have spontaneous resolution of their infection. A very small percentage of patients develop fulminant hepatic failure after acute infection. Of patients, 5–10% develop a chronic carrier state in which the virus remains active at a low level. These carriers are at high risk for end-stage liver disease and, ultimately, hepatocellular carcinoma. Patients with chronic HBV infection may also present with glomerulonephritis secondary to immune complex deposition. In addition to their own morbidity, HBV carriers represent the largest reservoir for transmission of HBV *(4)*.

Infection During Pregnancy

HBV can infect pregnant women but does not cause more severe disease than seen in the general population. Chronic carriers of the virus usually have uncomplicated pregnancies unless evidence of liver failure is present. The importance of HBV infection during pregnancy is the significant risk of transmission to the infant *(2,3,5)*. If the mother is known to be HBV infected and is acutely infected or a chronic carrier, the infant is at risk not only for infection, but also to become a chronic HBV carrier.

Vertical Transmission

HBV can be passed from mother to infant during a maternal acute infection, or if the mother is a chronic carrier. The risk of transmission is greater in acute infections when the virus is acquired by the mother later in pregnancy, presumably because of lack of adequate protective antibody passed from mother to child. It has been estimated that 85% of transmission occurs during blood exposure at delivery, and only 15% of transmission is *in utero*. Mothers with evidence of active viral replication by detection of viral and immunologic markers have a much higher incidence of vertical transmission *(2,3)*.

Breast-feeding in infected mothers has been studied and found not to pose a risk for transmission *(8)*. Presumably, maternal antibody is transmitted in enough quantity to neutralize any virus present.

Prenatal Evaluation

Mothers who exhibit symptoms of acute hepatitis, including fever, jaundice, abdominal pain, and who by history engaged in high-risk behaviors for acquisition of HBV (e.g., promiscuous sexual practices, sex with a known HBV carrier, or intravenous drug use) should be screened for viral markers of infection. Most states require that all mothers be tested for laboratory evidence of hepatitis B infection.

HBsAg is a marker of either early acute infection or ongoing chronic replication. HBsAb is a marker of the immune response to the virus. Mothers who are HBsAg positive are at high risk for transmitting the virus to their offspring *(7)*.

HBeAg is a marker used to estimate the amount of active viral replication. Studies have shown that patients who are HBeAg positive transmit the virus at a much higher rate (90%) to their offspring than do mothers who are HBeAg negative (40%) *(3)*.

Postnatal Evaluation of the Infant

Physical examination of infants in the postnatal period will usually be unremarkable. HBV can cause symptoms at birth if the mother has active replication of HBV, including fulminant hepatic failure, but they are rare.

Infants born to mothers with active HBV infection or who are chronic carriers of the virus should receive prophylaxis with the hepatitis B immunoglobulin within the first 12 hours of life, as well as prompt initiation of the hepatitis B vaccine series.

Laboratory Evaluation of Mother and Infant

As discussed, the mother should have as part of her routine prenatal evaluation testing for HBsAg and HBsAb. If the mother is HBsAg positive, it is recommended that she should have further assessment with HBeAg for activity of her infection.

Babies receiving prophylaxis should have follow-up testing for HBsAg and HBsAb at 6 months to confirm that the infant has not developed a carrier state but rather is protected against HBV infection. If the HBsAg is negative and HbsAb is positive, the infant is considered immune, and no further testing is necessary *(7)*.

HEPATITIS C VIRUS

Basic Virology and Epidemiology

Hepatitis C virus (HCV) is a flavivirus that was determined in 1989 to be the major cause of transfusion-related "non-A, non-B" hepatitis. It is a single-stranded, plus sense RNA virus with a genome size of approx 9500 bp. It encodes for a single large polyprotein that is cleaved to form individual viral proteins. The virus displays marked heterogeneity, with six distinct genotypes, and numerous quasi-species attributable to "hypervariable" regions of the two envelope proteins that readily mutate. Currently, there is no established cell culture system for HCV, and chimpanzees are the only available laboratory animal model, so little is still known about the mechanisms of infection *(2,3,8)*.

HCV is spread primarily by blood-borne contact with infected blood. The most common risk factors identified are intravenous drug use and blood transfusion or transplantation prior to 1992. Sexual acquisition of the virus is a very inefficient form of transmission and has not been proven definitively in the absence of confounding risk factors. The prevalence of HCV infection in the United States is approx 2%, and in 1999 chronic HCV infection and subsequent liver failure were the leading indications for liver transplantation *(8,9)*.

Course of Infection

HCV, when transmitted via blood-borne contact, usually causes an acute subclinical hepatitis. HCV then commonly progresses to chronic hepatitis that is also relatively asymptomatic. Symptoms are indolent when they do occur, sometimes months to years later, and include fever, fatigue, and jaundice. Patients may present with only signs of end-stage liver disease. Fulminant hepatic failure with HCV is exceedingly rare *(8)*.

Extrahepatic manifestations of HCV can occur and are primarily the result of immune complex deposition. These include mixed cryoglobulinemia, a chronic purpuric rash concentrated on the lower extremities, and porphyria cutanea tarda, which consists of bullous skin lesions and ulceration on sun-exposed areas coupled with elevated urinary porphyrin levels *(8,10)*.

Infection During Pregnancy

Acute HCV infection can occur during pregnancy. It is more common to see a pregnant patient who either has a known chronic HCV infection or has chronic infection diagnosed during her prenatal evaluation. HCV infection has not been shown to be more severe during pregnancy or to more rapidly progress during pregnancy *(2,3)*.

Vertical Transmission

HCV is transmitted vertically, but the rate is low in the absence of other risk factors. Most studies have shown 5–10% of infants acquire the virus from infected mothers *(11–13)*. Mothers with HIV co-infection have a much higher rate of vertical transmission of HCV, but the mechanism for this is not known. HIV co-infection leads to an HCV transmission rate of approx 20% in some studies *(11–13)*. The mode of delivery has not been shown to affect transmission rates in HCV-infected mothers, but data indicate that cesarean section may protect against transmission in the HCV and HIV co-infected mother *(14)*.

HCV infection in the newborn behaves differently from that in adults. Newborns establish chronic infection at a much lower rate than do older children and adults. It is not uncommon to see an infant who has detectable HCV RNA at birth that resolves spontaneously several months later. The reasons for this observation have not been explained *(13,15–17)*.

Studies of the potential of breast-feeding transmission have found a very low rate of infection to date *(15–18)*. Discussions about the nonnutritional benefits of breast-feeding should take place before recommending for or against breast-feeding in an HCV-infected mother *(11,19,20)*.

Prenatal Assessment

Testing for HCV currently is not offered routinely. Prenatal assessment for HCV should include a thorough social history to assess for possible risk factors. Questions regarding intravenous drug use, transfusion history prior to 1992, or any other potential blood-borne contact should raise concern *(9)*. Physical exam, in addition to examination of the abdomen for liver size or tenderness, should also include inspection of the skin for other manifestations of HCV infection.

Laboratory assessment should include liver function tests if indicated by history or physical exam and if abnormal in the absence of symptoms should raise suspicion for HCV. Patients already infected with HIV should be tested for HCV because many of the risk factors overlap. The opposite is also true.

Postnatal Evaluation of the Infant

At birth, infants born to HCV-infected mothers should have no detectable symptoms or abnormalities on physical exam. Disease in the newborn period from HCV is uncommon.

Laboratory Evaluation of Mother and Infant

Laboratory studies should begin with an assay for anti-HCV antibody in the mother. Anti-HCV antibody should begin to appear 2–3 weeks after acute illness. If the infection is acute, PCR for HCV RNA in plasma can be obtained and is positive early in the infection. If the mother is a chronically infected patient, a quantitative level of HCV RNA may be helpful. Studies have shown that very high levels of maternal plasma HCV RNA correlate with vertical transmission.

At this time, there are no established guidelines for testing infants born to HCV-positive mothers *(2,3)*. PCR for HCV RNA is the most useful assay in the first year of life because maternal antibody may be present for several months. Some studies indicate that the best time for the first PCR for HCV RNA is at 1 month of age *(21)*. If the HCV RNA is negative at 1 month, the infant should be followed, and repeat testing should be done at later points, such as 6 months and 1 year. Infected infants may have elevations of alanine aminotransferase and high levels of plasma HCV RNA. These values, however, do not necessarily correlate with ultimate chronic infection. There are no current established predictive laboratory evaluations to distinguish infants in whom infections will resolve from those who will develop chronic infections. Acute infection may resolve in infants, as indicated by absence of detectable HCV RNA. If the infant is still positive for HCV RNA after 1 year of age, it is likely that chronic infection has been established. Children with positive HCV RNA assays after 1 year of age should be followed by a specialist experienced in management of HCV-infected children.

HEPATITIS D VIRUS

Basic Virology and Epidemiology

Hepatitis D virus (HDV) is replication-defective RNA virus. HDV requires co-infection with HBV to complete assembly of new HDV viral particles *(22)*.

Infection with HDV can occur as an initial co-infection with HBV or as a superinfection in a previously infected patient with HBV. In the case of initial co-infection, symptoms usually resolve without incident, and immunity is long lasting. If a patient with chronic HBV infection acquires HDV, chronic infection is likely, and symptoms may be more severe (22).

Course of Infection

HDV infection presents as acute symptoms of hepatitis, with jaundice, fever, and abdominal pain. It can also present with acute signs of hepatitis in a chronic carrier of HBV who was previously well (2,22).

Infection During Pregnancy and Vertical Transmission

HDV does not have any clinical bearing on the pregnant patient. HBV should be the main concern in a patient with evidence of HDV infection during pregnancy. HDV is not transmitted vertically from mother to infant. Breast-feeding is not a risk.

Evaluation of the pregnant patient at risk should include a thorough history and physical. Evaluation of the infant born to an infected mother should include a proper physical examination, but no specific workup is necessary.

Laboratory Evaluation of Mother and Infant

Primary emphasis in these patients should be on coexisting HBV infection, not on HDV. However, a serologic assay for anti-HDV antibody is available to establish the diagnosis in the mother. The infant needs no laboratory studies (22).

HEPATITIS E VIRUS

Basic Virology and Epidemiology

Hepatitis E virus (HEV) is still a relatively newly discovered virus. HEV is a small, nonenveloped, single-stranded plus sense RNA virus. The viral genome includes 7500 bp that code for three sets of genes. HEV is genetically related to the Calicivirus family. It has two distinct geographic subtypes, the Asian and Mexican strains (23,24).

HEV is transmitted by fecal-oral contact. It occurs primarily in outbreaks in underdeveloped countries but can also occur sporadically. The source of the outbreaks is contaminated water, and in endemic areas, HEV accounts for most cases of acute hepatitis. Most patients diagnosed with HEV in the United States are travelers who acquired the virus in a foreign country. The attack rate of HEV appears to be about 50 times less than that of HAV in infected households (1 vs 50–75%) (23,24).

Course of Infection

HEV usually causes acute hepatitis in approx 75% of patients infected. The incubation period ranges from 15 to 65 days, and symptoms vary from mild to severe. Fulminant hepatic failure is rare with HEV in the nonpregnant host.

HEV RNA can be detected in stool for 1 week prior to symptoms and more than 2 weeks after the onset. HEV RNA can be detected for 2 weeks in the blood after the onset of symptoms.

Symptoms of acute hepatitis with HEV include jaundice, fever, and abdominal pain. The syndrome is identical to that of acute HAV or HBV. In general, as with HAV, symptoms increase in frequency with age in the general population.

HEV has not been shown to establish chronic infection. It has no known association with cirrhosis or hepatocellular carcinoma (23,24).

Infection During Pregnancy

Pregnant women can develop severe illness with HEV. The rate of fulminant hepatic failure is approx 20 times higher in the pregnant patient than her nonpregnant counterparts. Studies showed the risk of fulminant hepatic failure increases as pregnancy advances, with third trimester infection associated with a 50% rate of maternal demise. The reasons for the devastating effects of HEV during pregnancy are not currrently understood *(2,3,5)*.

Vertical Transmission

Vertical transmission of HEV does occur and can cause symptoms that range from mild hepatitis to severe fulminant failure, with hepatic necrosis and death. The details of viral transmission and replication perinatally have not been elucidated, although the virus is passed *in utero* because several cases have described infants with severe HEV disease at birth who died within 24 hours *(25)*.

Breast-feeding has not been shown to be a risk factor for transmission, likely for the same reasons as HAV.

Prenatal Evaluation

Evaluation of the pregnant patient should include a history of foreign travel. Clues to the diagnosis are exposure to contaminated food or water from an area endemic for HEV or an area with a recent HEV outbreak. Physical exam will be significant for jaundice and hepatomegaly.

As part of prenatal counseling, pregnant women should be advised not to travel to countries where HEV is endemic. In countries endemic for HEV, precautions should be taken to avoid contaminated water and food (boiling water before drinking, peeling fruits and vegetables, avoiding ice in beverages).

Postnatal Evaluation of the Infant

Evaluation of an infant suspected of HEV exposure should include a full physical exam at birth. Special attention should be paid to liver size and the appearance of jaundice. Blood glucose and body temperature may also be low. Proper supportive care should be provided.

Laboratory Evaluation of Mother and Infant

HEV can be detected by testing either for viral RNA or antibody response to the virus. PCR for HEV RNA is available on a research basis for detection of viral genetic material. Testing for IgM antibody against HEV is available at several referral laboratories *(23,24)*.

OTHER HEPATITIS VIRUSES

There are several other newly discovered viruses that have been added to the hepatitis alphabet of viruses, although subsequent research has shown not all of them belong in the group. This section briefly describes some of those viruses that may be shown in the future to be transmitted *in utero* or perinatally.

GB Virus C or Hepatitis G Virus

GB virus C (GBV-C) or hepatitis G virus was initially discovered using PCR-based techniques on stored blood specimens from patients with non-A to E hepatitis but was dismissed as a pathogen. However, GBV-C is a subtype of the GB viruses, which were shown to cause elevations in liver enzymes in animal models of infection *(26)*.

The clinical relevance of GBV-C has yet to be determined. Seroprevalence rates in the overtly healthy blood donor population tested yielded rates between 1 and 10%, depending on the region tested. Serum viral levels were also shown to be very high (10^7 copies per milliliter) in asymptomatic patients. Vertical transmission of GBV-C has been documented. After review of the data, GBV-C has generally been thought to be a "passenger" virus that is highly prevalent but is not thought to be a cause of significant disease *(26–28)*.

TT Virus

TT virus (named after patient initials) was discovered using PCR-based testing on samples from patients who developed elevated liver enzymes posttransfusion. Genetic analysis placed the virus in a new group of viruses called the Circinoviruses. The virus appears to be very diverse, with a large "hypervariable" region in its genome *(26)*.

Infection with TT virus appears to be very common. Seroprevalence studies of TT virus vary from 30% in the United States to 90–100% in areas of Asia and the Middle East. Studies have shown TT virus DNA in stool specimens, leading to the belief that it is enterically transmitted as well. Data on vertical transmission are somewhat conflicting *(28)*. It appears that TT virus is also ubiquitous and possibly a member of our normal flora. Its link with actual disease has yet to be proven *(26)*.

CONCLUSION

The hepatitis viruses are a diverse group. Appropriate evaluation of the pregnant patient and her newborn coupled with knowledge of the important characteristics of each virus can help prevent many of the adverse outcomes associated with infection.

REFERENCES

1. Kemmer NM, Miskovsky EP. Hepatitis A. Infect Dis Clin North Am 2000;14:605–615.
2. Dinsmoor MJ. Hepatitis in the obstetric patient. Infect Dis Clin North Am 1997;11:77–91.
3. Reinus JFL, Enid L. Pregnancy and Liver Disease. Clinics in Liver Disease 1999;3:115–130.
4. Befeler AS, Di Bisceglie AM. Hepatitis B. Infect Dis Clin North Am 2000;14:617–632.
5. Jaiswal SP, Jain AK, Naik G, Soni N, Chitnis DS. Viral hepatitis during pregnancy. Int J Gynaecol Obstet 2001;72:103–108.
6. Beasley RP, Stevens CE, Shiao IS, Meng HC. Evidence against breast-feeding as a mechanism for vertical transmission of hepatitis B. Lancet 1975;2:740–741.
7. Control CFD. Recommendations of the Immunization Practices Advisory Committee Prevention of Perinatal Transmission of Hepatitis B Virus: prenatal screening of all pregnant women for hepatitis B surface antigen. MMWR Morb Mortal Wkly Rep 1988;37:341–351.
8. Cheney CP, Chopra S, Graham C. Hepatitis C. Infect Dis Clin North Am 2000;14:633–667.
9. Hepatitis C fact sheet. Centers for Disease Control. www.cdc.gov/incidod/diseases/hepatitis/c/fact.htm.
10. Bonkovsky HL, Mehta S. Hepatitis C: a review and update. J Am Acad Dermatol 2001;44:159–182.
11. Jonas MM. Treatment of chronic hepatitis C in pediatric patients. Clin Liver Dis 1999;3:855–867.
12. Granovsky MO, Minkoff HL, Tess BH, et al. Hepatitis C virus infection in the mothers and infants cohort study. Pediatrics 1998;102:355–359.

13. Ceci O, Margiotta M, Marello F, et al. Vertical transmission of hepatitis C virus in a cohort of 2,447 HIV-seronegative pregnant women: a 24-month prospective study. J Pediatr Gastroenterol Nutr 2001;33:570–575.
14. European Pediatric Hepatitis C Virus Network. Effects of mode of delivery and infant feeding on the risk of mother-to-child transmission of hepatitis C virus. European Paediatric Hepatitis C Virus Network. BJOG 2001;108:371–377.
15. Ketzinel-Gilad M, Colodner SL, Hadary R, Granot E, Shouval D, Galun E. Transient transmission of hepatitis C virus from mothers to newborns. Eur J Clin Microbiol Infect Dis 2000;19:267–274.
16. Vogt M, Lang T, Frosner G, et al. Prevalence and clinical outcome of hepatitis C infection in children who underwent cardiac surgery before the implementation of blood-donor screening. N Engl J Med 1999;341:866–870.
17. Fujisawa T, Komatsu H, Inui A, et al. Spontaneous remission of chronic hepatitis C in children. Eur J Pediatr 1997;156:773–776.
18. Tajiri H, Miyoshi Y, Funada S, et al. Prospective study of mother-to-infant transmission of hepatitis C virus. Pediatr Infect Dis J 2001;20:10–14.
19. Polywka S, Schroter M, Feucht HH, Zollner B, Laufs R. Low risk of vertical transmission of hepatitis C virus by breast milk. Clin Infect Dis 1999;29:1327–1329.
20. Ruiz-Extremera A, Salmeron J, Torres C, et al. Follow-up of transmission of hepatitis C to babies of human immunodeficiency virus-negative women: the role of breast-feeding in transmission. Pediatr Infect Dis J 2000;19:511–516.
21. Dunn DT, Gibb DM, Healy M, et al. Timing and interpretation of tests for diagnosing perinatally acquired hepatitis C virus infection. Pediatr Infect Dis J 2001;20:715–716.
22. Hadziyannis SJMD. Hepatitis D. Clin Liver Dis 1999;3:309–325.
23. Krawczynski K, Aggarwal R, Kamili S. Hepatitis E. Infect Dis Clin North Am 2000;14:669–687.
24. Aggarwal R, Krawczynski K. Hepatitis E: an overview and recent advances in clinical and laboratory research. J Gastroenterol Hepatol 2000;15:9–20.
25. Khuroo MS, Kamili S, Jameel S. Vertical transmission of hepatitis E virus. Lancet 1995;345:1025–1026.
26. Bowden S. New hepatitis viruses: contenders and pretenders. J Gastroenterol Hepatol 2001;16:124–131.
27. Tillmann HL, Heiken H, Knapik-Botor A, et al. Infection with GB virus C and reduced mortality among HIV-infected patients. N Engl J Med 2001;345:715–724.
28. Williams CF, Klinzman D, Yamashita TE, et al. Persistent GB virus C infection and survival in HIV-infected men. N Engl J Med 2004;350:981–990.

16

Lymphocytic Choriomeningitis Virus

Kevin A. Cassady

INTRODUCTION

There has been an upsurge of interest in lymphocytic choriomeningitis virus (LCMV) as a human pathogen and specifically as an underdiagnosed congenital infection (1,2). LCMV is a member of the Arenaviridae family of viruses. Arenaviruses have a complex life cycle involving chronic infection and shedding of the virus in rodents and episodic infections in humans (3,4). Six of the arenaviruses (Lassa, Junin, Machupo, Guanarito, Sabia, and Whiteater Arroyo virus) produce an acute and highly fatal hemmorhagic disease in humans (mortality rates 15–30%) (4). LCMV, unlike the arenoviral hemorrhagic fever viruses, produces a flulike illness and aseptic meningitis with a mortality rate of less than 1% in infected adults (2).

Epidemiology studies have shown that between 7 and 11.5% of sampled rodents in varied geographic locales have serologic evidence of LCMV infection (5–8). The virus was initially recognized in the 1930s as a cause of aseptic meningitis, was implicated in approx 10% of cases of aseptic meningitis in the winter season in the 1950s, and was identified as a congenital pathogen in 1955 in Great Britain (2,9). Recent serologic studies demonstrated that between 1.7 and 5.4% of individuals tested had been infected with LCMV (antibody against LCMV at a titer >1:16 dilutions) (8,10,11). Occupational exposure, age, and lower socioeconomic status are associated with a greater likelihood of a positive test (11). Our current understanding of congenital LCMV infection is based on a limited number (26) of published case reports; therefore, the pathogen csis, incidence, attack rate, and outcome are not fully understood (1) The current understanding of congenital LCMV infection may be biased toward more clinically apparent and severe disease.

PATHOGENESIS AND CLINICAL MANIFESTATIONS

Arenaviruses are segemented ambisense ribonucleic acid (RNA) viruses that cause chronic infections in rodents in Europe, Africa, and the Americas (4). Chronically infected animals shed the virus in urine, feces, saliva, and other mucosal secretions (11,12). The virus can attach, enter, and replicate in numerous cell types and species. Humans are infected either by inhalation of the infected aerosols or after contact with infected fomites (12). After local replication at the site of inoculation, reticuloendothelial spread and viremia follow (2).

From: *Infectious Disease: Congenital and Perinatal Infections: A Concise Guide to Diagnosis*
Edited by: C. Hutto © Humana Press Inc., Totowa, NJ

An estimated one-third of acquired LCMV infections are asymptomatic or mild *(2)*. The disease is classically a biphasic illness consisting of an initial systemic flu-like illness characterized by sore throat, adenopathy, fever, headache, myalgias, cough, chest pain, nausea, and vomiting. In an estimated 10–30% of patients, these systemic symptoms abate and are followed by meningitis symptoms consisting of photophobia and headache and occasionally progressing to encephalitis with altered mental status and focal neurologic changes *(2)*. The virus has been reported as a rare cause of transverse myelitis, sensorineural hearing loss, and hydrocephalus *(2)*. Although LCMV can produce persistent infection in rodents, chronic infection in humans has not been demonstrated *(1)*.

Like most congenital infections, the organism is thought to infect the baby transplacentally, during the initial maternal viremia *(1)*. In the limited number of cases reported, 52–63% of pregnant women had an illness consistent with LCMV infection during the second and third trimester, and 24–46% reported contact with rodents *(1,2)*. Intrauterine infection has been associated with spontaneous abortion; however, the role of gestational age and viral load is not known.

The clinical manifestations provide some insight into the pathogenic mechanism of infection in the baby. The virus likely enters the brain through the choroid plexus and replicates in the ependymal and periventricular germinal matrix, producing a necrotizing ependymitis *(13)*. Consequently, periventricular calcification and hydrocephalus are two of the clinical manifestations of congenital LCMV. A hallmark of congenital LCMV infection is chorioretinitis, which occurs in 92% of affected children *(1,2,14)*. Ocular manifestations of LCMV infection are also seen experimentally in congenitally infected rats *(15)*. Although animal studies suggest that the host immune response may contribute significantly to the retinal damage, it is not known if this mechanism is responsible for chorioretinitis in humans.

Maternal and Neonatal Disease

Acquired LCMV infection is usually entertained as a diagnosis in cases of aseptic meningitis; however, two-thirds of cases are either subclinical infections or present as nonspecific systemic illness. About one-third of infected individuals will develop meningitis or meningoencephalitis. The illness is described classically as a biphasic illness with the central nervous system (CNS) symptoms developing after resolution of the systemic symptoms. Laboratory findings during the initial systemic phase of the illness consist of mildly elevated transaminases (aspartase aminotransferase and lactate dehydrogenase) and thrombocytopenia and leukopenia.

Although a biphasic clinical pattern is the classic presentation, the disease can also manifest as isolated CNS disease with no prodrome. In patients with CNS disease, a significant cerebrospinal fluid (CSF) pleocytosis occurs, with white blood cell counts in the 30–8000 cells/mm^3 range and mononuclear cell predominance. The CSF protein is elevated, and the glucose levels are modestly decreased, similar to the CSF profile with other viral meningitides. The nonspecific clinical and laboratory findings can delay the diagnosis as other infectious and noninfectious etiologies are pursued.

Congenital LCMV infection resembles congenital human cytomegalovirus (CMV) or toxoplasmosis, with severe ocular and CNS manifestation in infected infants. The majority of infants (92%) exhibit chorioretinitis. The scarring usually occurs peripherally, but in 36% the scarring was macular, similar to CMV or toxoplasmosis. LCMV can also produce CNS lesions with periventricular calcifications, hydrocephalus, or microcephaly in the congenitally infected infant. Neurologic sequelae (mental retardation, cerebral palsy, seizures, or decreased visual acuity) occur in 84% of the reported cases. Unlike children with congenital CMV or toxoplasmosis, LCMV-infected infants rarely (2 of the 38 reported cases) exhibit hepatosplenomegaly, systemic manifestations of disease, or hearing deficits.

Outcome

Acquired LCMV infection in adults usually produces a self-limited illness; however, in congenitally infected children the prognosis is poor. In a review of 23 cases of congenital LCMV, one-third of the children died, and the majority (63%) of survivors exhibited severe neurologic sequelae, including spastic quadriplegia, seizures, mental retardation, and visual loss *(1)*.

DIAGNOSIS

Although the virus can be cultured during the viremic stage, most clinicians do not entertain the diagnosis at this stage of the illness; furthermore, many laboratories are not equipped to identify LCMV in cell culture. Instead, serology is the mainstay of diagnosis in adults. In congenitally infected children, diagnosis has been confirmed based on the presence of immunoglobulin (Ig) G and IgM antibodies against LCMV and the absence of cultures or serologic evidence for the other more common congenital or perinatal infections (CMV, toxoplasmosis, syphilis, enterovirus, herpes simplex virus, and rubella).

Of the three serologic tests reported in the literature, the immunofluorescent antibody-based study exhibits greater sensitivity than the complement fixation assay or neutralizing antibody tests. An enzyme-linked immunosorbent assay, which measures the titer of IgG and IgM antibody to LCMV, is also available through the Centers for Disease Control and Prevention. In some cases, diagnosis of congenital LCMV infection was confirmed by detection of antibodies in the CSF from children with CNS disease. Nucleic acid detection and reverse transcriptase polymerase chain reaction have been used in isolated cases and may become more prevalent in the future. Primers exist for many of the Arenaviruses and have been used to diagnose LCMV, Lassa fever, and Venezuelan and Argentine hemorrhagic fever *(16–21)*. It is unknown how effective nucleic acid-based tests are in the diagnosis of congenital LCMV infection.

CONCLUSION

LCMV infection should be considered as a potential etiology of congenital infection in babies with CNS disease (micro- or macrocephaly, hydrocephalus) and chorioretinitis. The disease most closely resembles congenital toxoplasmosis or CMV infection in babies with the exception that LCMV-infected newborns rarely exhibit hepatosplenomegaly or hearing loss. Diagnosis of congenital LCMV infection is based on compatible clinical findings, serologic evidence of LCMV infection (IgM and IgG against LCMV), and negative diagnostic studies for other congenital infections (CMV culture, toxoplasmosis serology, syphilis, enterovirus, rubella, and herpes simplex virus).

REFERENCES

1. Wright R, Johnson D, Neumann M, et al. Congenital lymphocytic choriomeningitis virus syndrome: a disease that mimics congenital toxoplasmosis or cytomegalovirus infection. Pediatrics 1997;100:E9.

2. Barton LL, Mets MB. Congenital lymphocytic choriomeningitis virus infection: decade of rediscovery. Clin Infect Dis 2001;33:370–374.

3. Ciurea A, Klenerman P, Hunziker L, et al. Persistence of lymphocytic choriomeningitis virus at very low levels in immune mice. Proc Natl Acad Sci U S A 1999;96:11,964–11,969.

4. Buchmeier MJ, Bowden MD, Peters CJ. Arenaviridae: the viruses and their replication. In: Fields BN, Knipe DM, Howley PM, et al., eds. Fields Virology, Vol. 2. Philadelphia: Lippincott, Williams, Wilkins, 2001:1635–1668.

5. el Karamany RM, Imam IZ. Antibodies to lymphocytic choriomeningitis virus in wild rodent sera in Egypt. J Hyg Epidemiol Microbiol Immunol 1991;35:97–103.

6. Morita C, Matsuura Y, Kawashima E, et al. Seroepidemiological survey of lymphocytic choriomeningitis virus in wild house mouse (*Mus musculus*) in Yokohama Port, Japan. J Vet Med Sci 1991;53:219–222.

7. Childs JE, Glass GE, Korch GW, Ksiazek TG, Leduc JW. Lymphocytic choriomeningitis virus infection and house mouse (*Mus musculus*) distribution in urban Baltimore. Am J Trop Med Hyg 1992;47:27–34.

8. Lledo L, Gegundez MI, Saz JV, Bahamontes N, Beltran M. Lymphocytic choriomeningitis virus infection in a province of Spain: analysis of sera from the general population and wild rodents. J Med Virol 2003;70:273–275.

9. Komrower GM, Williams BL, Stones PB. Lymphocytic choriomeningitis in the newborn; probable transplacental infection. Lancet 1955;268:697–698.

10. Stephensen CB, Blount SR, Lanford RE, et al. Prevalence of serum antibodies against lymphocytic choriomeningitis virus in selected populations from two US cities. J Med Virol 1992;38:27–31.

11. Park JY, Peters CJ, Rollin PE, et al. Age distribution of lymphocytic choriomeningitis virus serum antibody in Birmingham, Alabama: evidence of a decreased risk of infection. Am J Trop Med Hyg 1997;57:37–41.

12. Dykewicz CA, Dato VM, Fisher-Hoch SP, et al. Lymphocytic choriomeningitis outbreak associated with nude mice in a research institute. JAMA 1992;267:1349–1353.

13. Lehmann-Grube F. Portraits of viruses: arenaviruses. Intervirology 1984;22:121–145.

14. Mets MB. Childhood blindness and visual loss: an assessment at two institutions including a "new" cause. Trans Am Ophthalmol Soc 1999;97:653–696.

15. del Cerro M, Grover D, Monjan AA, Pfau C, Dematte J. Congenital retinitis in the rat following maternal exposure to lymphocytic choriomeningitis virus. Exp Eye Res 1984;38:313–324.

16. Lunkenheimer K, Hufert FT, Schmitz H. Detection of Lassa virus RNA in specimens from patients with Lassa fever by using the polymerase chain reaction. J Clin Microbiol 1990;28:2689–2692.

17. Lozano ME, Ghiringhelli PD, Romanowski V, Grau O. A simple nucleic acid amplification assay for the rapid detection of Junin virus in whole blood samples. Virus Res 1993;27:37–53.

18. Demby AH, Chamberlain J, Brown DW, Clegg CS. Early diagnosis of Lassa fever by reverse transcription-PCR. J Clin Microbiol 1994;32:2898–2903.

19. Park JY, Peters CJ, Rollin PE, et al. Development of a reverse transcription-polymerase chain reaction assay for diagnosis of lymphocytic choriomeningitis virus infection and its use in a prospective surveillance study. J Med Virol 1997;51:107–114.

20. Enders G, Varho-Gobel M, Lohler J, Terletskaia-Ladwig E, Eggers M. Congenital lymphocytic choriomeningitis virus infection: an underdiagnosed disease. Pediatr Infect Dis J 1999;18:652–655.
21. Drosten C, Gottig S, Schilling S, et al. Rapid detection and quantification of RNA of Ebola and Marburg viruses, Lassa virus, Crimean-Congo hemorrhagic fever virus, Rift Valley fever virus, dengue virus, and yellow fever virus by real-time reverse transcription-PCR. J Clin Microbiol 2002;40:2323–2330.

17

Dengue Virus

Enid J. García-Rivera and José G. Rigau-Pérez

INTRODUCTION

Dengue is the most frequently reported human viral disease transmitted by arthropod vectors. The disease is endemic in most tropical and subtropical areas; over half of the world's population lives in locations that are at risk for transmission (Fig. 1). Worldwide, there are an estimated 50–100 million cases of dengue and 250,000–500,000 cases of dengue hemorrhagic fever (DHF) annually. During the last few decades, dengue epidemics have been reported in countries that had not previously been considered endemic (1). This chapter provides a brief review of the clinical and laboratory features of dengue and DHF, a detailed discussion of dengue infection during pregnancy, and specific characteristics of dengue during the perinatal period.

DISEASE TRANSMISSION

Dengue is an acute viral disease transmitted by *Aedes* mosquitoes and caused by one of four dengue virus serotypes (DEN-1, DEN-2, DEN-3, and DEN-4). These arthropod-borne viruses (arboviruses) are composed of single-stranded ribonucleic acid (RNA) and belong to the genus *Flavivirus*, family Flaviviridae, which includes other well-known viruses, such as yellow fever, St. Louis encephalitis, Japanese encephalitis, and West Nile virus. The four dengue virus serotypes are antigenically related but distinct enough that infection with one serotype provides lifelong immunity to that serotype but not to the others. Short-term cross-immunity against the other serotypes develops but lasts only several months. Therefore, a person can theoretically have up to four dengue infections, one with each serotype (2).

The most common vector of dengue in the world is *Aedes aegypti*, a species closely associated with human habitation. In some regions, other *Aedes* species, such as *Aedes albopictus* and *Aedes polynesiensis* are also involved. The bite of an infectious female mosquito transmits dengue to humans. The *Ae. aegypti* mosquito usually rests in dark, indoor sites such as closets and under beds and is primarily a daytime feeder, biting mainly in the morning or late in the afternoon. The female mosquito lays its eggs preferentially in artificial containers. Larvae are commonly found in containers with relatively clean water, such as discarded tires, buckets, flowerpots, wading pools, and blocked rain gutters. Larvae can also be found in natural sites such as bromeliads and tree holes.

From: *Infectious Disease: Congenital and Perinatal Infections: A Concise Guide to Diagnosis*
Edited by: C. Hutto © Humana Press Inc., Totowa, NJ

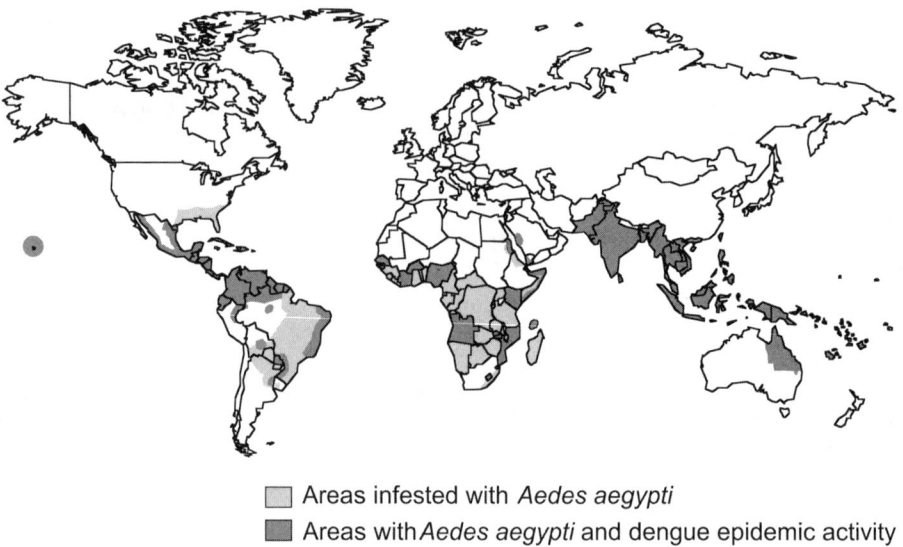

Areas infested with *Aedes aegypti*

Areas with *Aedes aegypti* and dengue epidemic activity

Fig. 1. World distribution of dengue, 2003.

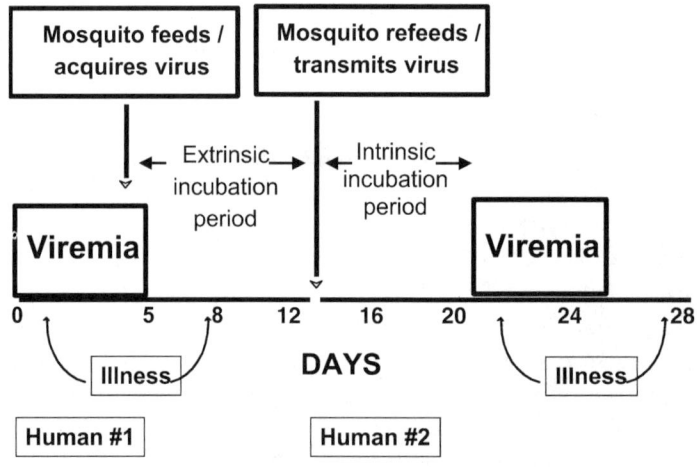

Fig. 2. Transmission of dengue virus by *Aedes aegypti*.

The transmission cycle of dengue virus begins when the female mosquito bites a viremic person. Eight to 12 days (extrinsic incubation period) must elapse before the mosquito becomes infective. It can then transmit the virus throughout its lifetime whenever it bites or even probes the skin of another person. Once the virus is inoculated into the susceptible human, it replicates in the local lymph nodes and the liver *(3)*. The virus is then released from these tissues and infects white blood cells (WBCs) and distant lymphatic tissue, circulates in the blood, and is eventually cleared by the host immune response. The incubation period for disease in humans (intrinsic incubation period) may range from 3 to 14 days and most often lasts between 4 and 7 days (Fig. 2). No carrier state ensues, and no viral recrudescence occurs.

CLINICAL MANIFESTATIONS OF DENGUE INFECTION

The clinical manifestations of dengue infection include a wide spectrum of syndromes, from asymptomatic infection or minimally symptomatic disease to severe illness and sometimes death. There are at least four categories of disease severity: undifferentiated fever, dengue fever (the classic "breakbone fever"), DHF (which includes dengue shock syndrome [DSS]), and "unusual manifestations," including severe gastrointestinal hemorrhage, hepatic failure, cardiomyopathy, and encephalopathy or encephalitis.

Dengue Fever

Dengue fever is characterized by sudden onset of fever, frontal headache, retro-orbital pain, general malaise, generalized myalgias and arthralgias, nausea, vomiting, and rash. One characteristic feature of dengue fever is the severity of body pain, which can be incapacitating and explains why the disease is sometimes called breakbone fever. Other nonspecific symptoms may be present, such as anorexia, mild conjunctival injection, diarrhea, pruritus, and changes in taste sensation. Leukopenia and thrombocytopenia are frequent, and liver enzymes may be mildly elevated. The febrile period lasts 5–7 days, but the patient may remain symptomatic for several more days. The disappearance of fever correlates with the disappearance of viremia. Convalescence may be marked by a period of lassitude. There have been reports of severe depression after the acute period of illness *(4,5)*.

Skin eruptions may be more common in primary infections *(6)*. The rash may be present in different ways, including flushing of the face, neck, or chest during the febrile period; an erythematous or maculopapular rash after the third or fourth day; a confluent petechial rash with round pale areas of normal skin; or a combination of these. Less frequent than rash but not rare are mild hemorrhagic manifestations, such as petechiae, epistaxis, gingival hemorrhage, gastrointestinal hemorrhage, and microscopic hematuria. Hemorrhage is more commonly associated with a platelet count below $50,000/mm^3$, although hemorrhage does not necessarily occur with a low platelet count *(7)*. The tourniquet test, a method for the assessment of capillary fragility or platelet function, may be positive in more than one-third of patients with dengue fever. To perform the tourniquet test, the blood pressure cuff is inflated to a point midway between the systolic and diastolic blood pressures and maintained for 5 minutes. After deflating the cuff and waiting for the skin to return to its normal color, the number of petechiae in a 1-in.^{2} area on the ventral surface of the forearm is counted. Twenty or more petechiae in the patch constitutes a positive test *(8)*.

Clinical findings alone are not very helpful for distinguishing dengue fever from other febrile illnesses, such as influenza, measles, rubella, mild leptospirosis, typhoid, or malaria. If symptoms start more than 2 weeks after the patient has left a dengue-endemic area or if the fever lasts more than 2 weeks, dengue can probably be ruled out.

Risk Factors for Severe Disease

Several risk factors have been associated with severe disease, including virus strain, the presence of preexisting anti-dengue antibodies, factors related to host genetics, and age. The risk for developing DHF is higher in locations with two or more virus serotypes circulating simultaneously, especially when the second infecting serotype is of Southeast Asian origin *(9)*. The presence of circulating anti-dengue antibodies, acquired actively (by prior infection) or passively (by transplacental passage of maternal dengue immunoglobulin [Ig] G antibody in infants) is the most frequently reported of the multiple contributing causes of a severe response to dengue *(10,11)*.

Several studies have demonstrated the transplacental passage of anti-dengue IgG antibodies to the fetus *(12–17)*. Infants with maternal antibodies may be at risk of developing DHF/DSS *(18)*.

The course of the disease provides warnings of an increased probability of DHF. The first (and easiest) information for the physician to ascertain is the time elapsed since the onset of symptoms. DHF/DSS usually develops around days 3–7 of illness, near the time of defervescence, a period when intensified observation of the patient should occur. A progressive drop in platelet count and a concurrent increase in hematocrit are indicators of the onset of excessive capillary leakage and increased probability of impending shock. The less-frequent but severe complications of dengue infection (abrupt gastrointestinal hemorrhage, hepatic failure, cardiomyopathy, and encephalopathy or encephalitis) may not follow the course of DHF/DSS and are associated with a high risk of death.

Dengue Hemorrhagic Fever/Dengue Shock Syndrome

DHF is defined by the World Health Organization as an acute febrile illness with minor or major hemorrhage, thrombocytopenia of 100,000 platelets/mm^3 or less, and evidence of excessive plasma leakage documented by hemoconcentration (hematocrit increased by 20% or more or decreased by the same amount after intravenous fluid therapy), evidence of pleural or other effusions, or hypoalbuminemia or hypoproteinemia. The severity of DHF is classified into four grades, all of which must also fulfill the above criteria:

> Grade I: A hemorrhagic manifestation is provoked, that is, a positive tourniquet test.
> Grade II: The patient has spontaneous hemorrhage, the most common is skin hemorrhages.
> Grade III: The patient shows signs of circulatory failure, manifested by rapid and weak pulse, narrowing of pulse pressure (20 mmHg or less), or hypotension, with the presence of cold, clammy skin and restlessness.
> Grade IV: Profound shock with undetectable blood pressure and pulse.

DHF grades III and IV are considered DSS, the most severe presentation of dengue infection, which is characterized by rapid onset of shock, generally occurring near the time of defervescence. Prognosis depends on the anticipation and early recognition and treatment of shock, which may have a short duration but is life-threatening. In hospitals with experience in DSS management, the case fatality rate in DHF can be as low as 0.2%. Once shock has set in, the fatality rate may be over 10% *(19)*.

RISK OF MATERNAL INFECTION DURING PREGNANCY

With the reemergence of dengue as an important cause of morbidity in many tropical and subtropical countries, pregnant women are more frequently exposed to the virus. With increased transmission, factors related to increased disease severity may occur more frequently. The probability for genetic changes in the virus is increased as well as the probability of greater virulence and greater epidemic potential for the virus. As the frequency of previous infections increases in a community, the risk of severe disease also increases. The only published report of the incidence of dengue infection during pregnancy is a seroepidemiologic study conducted in the Dominican Republic in 1973. Evidence of recent dengue infection was found in 52 of 139 (37%) pregnant women, all of whom were asymptomatic *(20)*. The incidence of 37% was surprising because the dengue transmission period was described as "nonepidemic." That 100% of the women were asymptomatic was also surprising. In spite of the lack of other studies, it is clear that dengue virus infection among pregnant women may be a common event in dengue-endemic areas.

No studies have been published regarding the risk of exposure for pregnant travelers in dengue endemic areas, and reported cases are rare. Among the 1275 cases of suspected dengue imported to the United States and reported to the Centers for Disease Control and Prevention (CDC) Dengue Branch from 1994 to 2000, only one pregnant patient was reported (CDC, unpublished data, 2003). The patient had traveled to the Caribbean and developed anti-dengue IgM antibodies, but serologic results to rule out dengue infection in the newborn were indeterminate.

DENGUE INFECTION IN THE PREGNANT WOMAN

Although many arboviruses are known to cause fetal death, premature birth, and teratogenic changes in humans and animals, the few reports of fetal malformation or wastage from dengue infection are poorly documented, and the evidence is contradictory. Despite the small number of reported cases during the perinatal period (9 reports that included 20 mother-infant pairs), it is nevertheless evident that there is potential for severe disease with dengue infection in the mother and the newborn *(21–29)*.

The paucity of documented patients with dengue during pregnancy suggests that the most common clinical result in the mother is an asymptomatic or minimally symptomatic infection. It is also possible that most cases do not result in reportable complications. In the last four decades after laboratory diagnostic methods became more generally available, case reports of pregnant patients during the perinatal period with hemorrhage and probable or confirmed dengue infection have been published. Hemorrhagic manifestations are usually mild and include mucocutaneous (e.g., petechiae in buccal cavity and in subconjuntivas, nose or gum bleeding) or subcutaneous bleeding (e.g., petechiae in skin, easy bruising). Severe bleeding has also been documented.

In 1970, Moreau and colleagues described a 25-year-old Tahitian patient with gum bleeding, uterine hemorrhage, and spontaneous abortion *(21)*, and in 1989, Taechakraichana and Limpaphayom described a 20-year-old Thai patient with DHF at 23 weeks of gestation with satisfactory recovery *(22)*. Among patients during the perinatal period, a 32-year-old mother with serologic evidence of acute dengue infection at term was reported from Thailand in 1994. She required cesarean section because of previous cesarean intervention and developed continuous bleeding from the surgical wound, resulting in a large blood collection in the lower uterine segment *(23)*. In 1997, Chye et al. reported two laboratory-positive dengue patients at 36 and 38 weeks of gestation in Malaysia *(24)*. One patient developed DHF with severe preeclampsia and required induction of labor. The other patient only developed petechiae and epistaxis. In the same year, Bunyavejchevin et al. reported two mothers from Thailand with dengue infection during the perinatal period. Both of these had mild hemorrhagic manifestations, and one case developed DHF also complicated by severe preeclampsia *(25)*. In 1999, Carles also reported four mothers in French Guiana with dengue infection within 1 week of delivery *(26)*. Although low platelet counts were reported, no hemorrhagic complication was recorded.

Reports of dengue infections have come from Guadeloupe (one mother developed severe thrombocytopenia, giving birth via cesarean section, and the other had preterm labor; mothers and infants recovered without complications) and from Thailand (thrombocytopenia with and without hemorrhagic complications) *(27–29)*.

In a review of laboratory-positive cases of mother–infant pairs in Puerto Rico from 1994 to 2003, four cases of maternal–fetal transmission were documented. All mothers were positive for anti-dengue IgM antibody, and infants were diagnosed by virus isolation, polymerase chain reaction, or anti-dengue IgM detection (CDC, unpublished data, 2003). In three of the four cases, the disease in the mother was only suspected following occurrence of symptoms in the newborn. All mothers showed fever, and as in other groups with dengue, leukopenia and thrombocytopenia were present in the four pregnant women.

Preeclampsia and eclampsia postpartum have been reported in 3 (13%) of the 24 cases of maternal dengue infection reported during the perinatal period. Of the three cases, two also fulfilled the diagnostic criteria for DHF. Because DHF is associated with thrombocytopenia and elevated liver enzymes, it must be differentiated from the HELLP syndrome, in which hemolysis, elevated liver enzymes, and low platelet count are characteristic features. Although hemolysis does not occur in DHF, early diagnosis and differentiation of DHF and HELLP syndrome are critical. Any pregnant woman with a history of exposure to dengue virus who presents in the third trimester with clinical findings compatible with a suspected dengue case should be evaluated with a CBC, liver function tests, and specific tests for dengue infection.

In the evaluation of a pregnant woman with suspected dengue, the medical history must elicit information about international travel history to tropical or subtropical areas and past exposure to dengue infection. The physical examination should include the search for hemorrhage (including tourniquet test), hypotension, or increased vascular permeability (ascites or pulmonary effusions, hypoalbuminemia, or hypoproteinemia). Peripheral edema is not a useful indicator of increased vascular permeability because swelling may be present in up to 30% of normal pregnancies. Close follow-up of blood pressure and hydration status are mandatory. Evaluation of fetal well-being is also required in all cases. Fetal movements, nonstress test, or uterine biophysical profile could be useful measures of fetal well-being.

DENGUE IN THE NEWBORN

Three mechanisms of dengue-related illness in the fetus can be postulated:

1. Maternal infection during pregnancy may result in hematogenous spread of the virus to the placenta and subsequent passage to the fetus.
2. Maternal viremia during labor could result in viral transmission and infection of the fetus or the newborn because of blood exchange during the delivery process.
3. Severe maternal illness during pregnancy or labor could alter placental function and injure the fetus in the absence of actual fetal infection.

Close monitoring is needed for newborns whose mothers present symptoms compatible with dengue infection from 14 days before delivery to 14 days postpartum because symptoms in the newborn may appear immediately after delivery or several days later. The newborns may show the effects of maternal infection or may develop dengue fever or DHF. In a review of 18 reported cases of laboratory-positive dengue infection among newborns, 8 neonates were diagnosed as dengue fever, and 10 fulfilled the criteria for DHF *(23–31)*.

Dengue Fever in the Newborn

High temperature (38–39°C) was documented in the eight cases of dengue fever in term newborns and lasted from 24 to 48 hours. Flushed skin or an erythematous rash in the face also occurred in five patients while they were febrile, and the rash subsequently became generalized or localized in the arms and legs. Nonspecific signs, such as poor sucking, irritability, diarrhea, and pallor, were also present. Acrocyanosis or cyanosis of the perioral and periorbital area was reported in two of the five patients. The symptoms were present for 3–5 days, with an uneventful recovery in all cases.

Hepatomegaly was present at the onset of symptoms in two of the eight dengue fever cases, with mild elevations of hepatic enzymes. Jaundice was not documented, and bilirubin levels were within normal limits. Splenomegaly was not reported. The WBC count was normal in three cases; two showed mild leukopenia. Hemoglobin and hematocrit were within normal limits. Thrombocytopenia was present in all newborns with classic dengue fever, with the lowest reported values ranging from 18,000 to 50,000 platelets/mm^3. None showed evidence of bleeding, and all recovered uneventfully.

DHF in the Newborn

DHF in the newborn may begin as a severe, nonspecific illness. Hypoactivity and irritability were the initial changes noted in the majority of the cases *(31)*. Other symptoms documented included hypotonia, mottled skin, tachypnea, and bradycardia during or after the febrile period. Acrocyanosis or cyanosis of the perioral and periorbital areas was present in 4 patients. Among 10 neonatal DHF cases, the febrile period extended from 24 to 48 hours. Severe respiratory distress was present in 3 of the 10 reported cases of neonatal DHF, 2 of whom required mechanical ventilation. Changes in chest radiographs were compatible with respiratory distress syndrome, and 1 of the 3 also developed a pleural effusion. In neonatal cases of DHF, mucocutaneous or subcutaneous bleeding was the most common hemorrhagic manifestation. Evidence of gastrointestinal bleeding was reported, and 1 newborn developed massive intracerebral hemorrhage and severe respiratory distress and died 6 days after delivery *(30)*.

Of the 10 newborns diagnosed with DHF, WBC counts and hematocrit levels were available for only 2 cases. Mild leukopenia (WBCs <5000) was present in both, with leukocytosis (WBCs >15,000) occurring after defervescence in 1 newborn. An increase in hematocrit greater than 20% was documented in 5 cases. All neonatal DHF cases had thrombocytopenia as required by the case definition, with 5 of the 8 newborns showing platelet levels below 20,000 platelets/mm^3.

Hepatic involvement was also a common finding in newborns with DHF. Hepatomegaly was present in five of the seven DHF cases. Liver enzymes were elevated in the four cases in which liver enzymes were documented. Indirect and direct bilirubin were usually normal, and jaundice was not documented. In one newborn, a prolonged prothrombin and partial thromboplastin time were present.

Clinical Evaluation of the Newborn

The physical examination of newborns of mothers with suspected dengue or DHF must include assessment of changes in temperature, hydration status, peripheral perfusion, respiratory rate, cardiac rate, hemodynamic status, evidence of increased vascular permeability, and any evidence of hemorrhage or effusions. The sensitivity and specificity of the tourniquet test for the assessment of bleeding in the newborn have not been reported. If the mother is ill at delivery, close observation of the general status of the newborn is required for 4–6 days after delivery because symptoms may not be present immediately after birth. Because symptoms in the newborn may be nonspecific, a high degree of suspicion is needed, and the maternal history, especially a recent travel history, gives important information for the appropriate diagnosis.

LABORATORY EVALUATION OF THE MOTHER AND THE NEWBORN

The laboratory evaluation of both mother and newborn with a suspected case of dengue must include a variety of diagnostic tests, including specific tests for dengue. A complete blood cell count (CBC) with differential should be ordered for evaluation of the WBC count, hemoglobin and hematocrit levels. Serial CBCs are needed during the first days of illness to evaluate the disease progression, especially for hemoconcentration, an important marker of increased capillary permeability. Serial platelet count measurements are also needed. A continuous, marked decline in platelet level could be the first sign of the development of DHF.

Other tests needed for patient evaluation include liver function tests (aspartate aminotransferase and alanine aminotransferase), blood chemistries, urine analysis, prothrombin time, and partial thromboplastin time. Hepatic involvement is common, with a relatively higher increase of aspartate aminotransferase than alanine aminotransferase. Hypoalbuminemia or hypoproteinemia can be evidence of increased capillary permeability. Urinalysis is needed to assess the presence of gross or microscopic hematuria. Coagulation abnormalities can be present in DHF but are not common in dengue fever.

Laboratory Diagnosis of Dengue Infection

Knowledge of the periods for viremia and antibody response is necessary for the appropriate diagnosis of dengue infection. Dengue virus circulates in blood for an average of 5 days after the onset of symptoms, and the virus isolation rate has been found to parallel the fever curve *(32,33)*. Isolation of the virus can be accomplished if a serum sample is taken soon after the onset of illness and processed without delay (Table 1). Virus isolation and RNA detection are considered confirmatory evidence of dengue infection *(34)*.

Serological diagnosis depends on the presence of antidengue IgM antibody or a rise in IgG antibody titer in paired (acute and convalescent phase) sera. Neither of these serologic techniques can be used to routinely identify the infecting virus serotype because broad cross-reactivity exists among flaviviruses. Currently, the most widely used IgM assay is the IgM capture enzyme-linked immunosorbent assay. Because of its

Table 1
Collecting and Processing Specimens for Laboratory Diagnosis of Dengue Infection

Type of specimen	Type of analysis	Time of collection	Clot retraction	Storage	Shipment
Acute phase blood (S1)	Virus isolation and/or serology	0–5 days after onset	2–6 hours, 4°C	Serum –70°C	Dry ice
Convalescent phase blood (S2)	Serology	6–21 days after onset	2–13 hours, ambient	Serum –20°C	Frozen or ambient
Tissue	Immunohisto- chemistry or virus isolation	As soon as possible after death		–70°C or in formalin	Dry ice or ambient

Adapted from ref. *35.*

simplicity, this test is useful for testing a large number of samples in a single test. IgM antibody becomes detectable during the acute phase of illness, and 90% of infected persons are IgM positive by the 6th day after the onset of symptoms *(35)*. Specimens collected less than 6 days after the onset of symptoms will have a variable percentage of samples without IgM antibodies because of insufficient time to produce antidengue antibodies. For this reason, negative results in samples obtained during the acute period are considered indeterminate, and a second sample, drawn during the convalescent period (6–21 days after onset), should be requested (Table 1). Negative results in samples obtained in this period may be considered true negatives *(34)*. The presence of antidengue IgM antibodies is considered as only probable evidence of recent dengue infection because it may be detectable for a median of about 60 days.

The laboratory diagnosis of dengue also depends on the quality of the specimens received. Serum is the specimen of choice for both virological and serological studies. The types of specimens required and their storage and shipment requirements are shown in Table 1.

The CDC provides reference laboratory service and accepts samples of suspected dengue cases for laboratory confirmation. Samples must be identified and accompanied with a dengue case investigation form (provided by the CDC), which collects the necessary demographic and clinical data to guide laboratory analyses. For more information contact the Dengue Branch, Centers for Disease Control and Prevention, at 1324 Calle Cañada, San Juan, PR 00920-3860, or phone 787-706-2399. All samples are processed free of charge.

CONCLUSIONS

The appropriate diagnosis of dengue infection during the perinatal period could be a challenge for health care providers. The disease is rare, the differential diagnosis is broad, and the nonspecific nature of many symptoms in dengue requires a high level of suspicion for early recognition of the disease.

REFERENCES

 1. Gubler DJ. Dengue and dengue hemorrhagic fever: its history and resurgence as a global public health problem. In: Gubler DJ, Kuno G, eds. Dengue and Dengue Hemorrhagic Fever. Wallingford, UK: CAB International, 1997:1–22.

2. Rigau-Pérez JG, Clark GG, Gubler DJ, Reiter P, Sanders EJ, Vorndam AV. Dengue and dengue hemorrhagic fever. Lancet 1998:352:971–977.
3. Gubler DJ, Suharyono W, Sumarmo, Wulur H, Jahja E, Sulianti-Saroso J. Virological surveillance for dengue hemorrhagic fever in Indonesia using the mosquito inoculation technique. Bull WHO 1979;57:932–936.
4. Siler J F, Hall M W, Hitchens A P. Dengue: its history, epidemiology, mechanism of transmission, etiology, clinical manifestations, immunity, and prevention. Philippine J Sci 1926;29:1–304.
5. George R, Lum LCS. Clinical spectrum of infection. In: Gubler DJ, Kuno G, eds. Dengue and Dengue Hemorrhagic Fever. Wallingford, UK: CAB International, 1997:89–113.
6. Cobra C, Rigau-Pérez J, Kuno G, Vorndam V. Symptoms of dengue fever in relation to host immunologic response and virus serotype, Puerto Rico, 1990–1991. Am J Epidemiol 1995;142:1204–1211.
7. Dietz V, Gubler DJ, Ortiz S, et al. The 1986 dengue and dengue hemorrhagic fever epidemic in Puerto Rico: epidemiologic and clinical observations. P R Health Sci J 1996;15:201–210.
8. Wintrobe MM. Clinical Hematology. Philadelphia: Lea and Febiger, 1961:299.
9. Gubler DJ, Trent DW. Emergence of epidemic dengue/dengue hemorrhagic fever as a public health problem in the Americas. Infect Agents Dis 1993;2:383–393.
10. Halstead SB. Pathogenesis of dengue: challenges to molecular biology. Science 1988;239:476–481.
11. Halstead SB. Epidemiology of dengue and dengue hemorrhagic fever. In: Gubler DJ, Kuno G, eds. Dengue and dengue hemorrhagic fever. Wallingford, UK: CAB International, 1997:23–44.
12. Kliks SC, Nimmanitya S, Nisalak A, Burke D. Evidence that maternal antibodies are important in the development of dengue hemorrhagic fever in infants. Am J Trop Med Hyg 1988;38:411–419.
13. Figueiredo LT, Carlucci RH, Duarte G. Prospective study with infants whose mother had dengue during pregnancy. Rev Inst Med Trop Sao Paulo 1994;136:417–421.
14. Carey D, Myers R, Wilson E, Manoharan A. Transplacentally-acquired group-B HI antibody and dengue infection among infants in Vellore, South India. Ind J Med Res 1968;56:1468–1477.
15. Cantelar FN, Molina AL. Dengue: estudio clinicoserológico en madres y recién nacidos. Rev Cubana Med Trop 1981;33:96–105.
16. Molina AL, Cantelar FN, García-Santana C. Dengue: respuesta serológica e inmunológica en recién nacidos. Rev Cub Hig Epid 1981;19:346–350.
17. Martínez E, Guzmán M, Valdés M, Soler M, Kourí G. Dengue fever and hemorrhagic dengue in infants with a primary infection. Rev Cubana Med Trop 1993;45:97–101.
18. Halstead S, Nimmammitya S, Margiotta M. Dengue and chinkungunya virus infection in man in Thailand, 1962–1964. Am J Trop Med Hyg 1969;18:972–983.
19. Tassniyom S, Vasanawathana S, Chirawatkul A, Rojanasuphot S. Failure of high dose methylprednisolone in established dengue shock syndrome: a placebo-controlled, double blind study. Pediatrics 1993;92:111–115.
20. Ventura A, Ehrenkranz J, Rosenthal D. Placental passage of antibodies to dengue virus in persons living in a region of hyperendemic dengue virus infection. J Infect Dis 1975;131(Suppl):S62–S68.
21. Moreau JP, Rosen L, Saugrain J, Lagraulet J. An epidemic of dengue on Tahiti associated with hemorrhagic manifestations. Am J Trop Med Hyg 1973;22:237–241.
22. Taechakraichana N, Limpaphayom K. Dengue hemorrhagic fever in pregnancy. Chula Med J 1989;33:213–218.

23. Thaithumyanon P, Thisyakorn U, Deerojnawong J, Innis DL. Dengue infection complicated by severe hemorrhage and vertical transmission in a parturient woman. Clin Infect Dis 1994;18:248–249.
24. Chye JK, Lim CT, Kwee BN, Lim JMH, George R, Lam SK. Vertical transmission of dengue. Clin Infect Dis 1997;25:1374–1377.
25. Bunyavejchevin S, Tanawattanacharoen S, Taechakraichana N, Thisyakorn U, Tannirandirn Y, Limpaphayom K. Dengue hemorrhagic fever during pregnancy: antepartum, intrapartum and postpartum management. J Obstet Gynaecol Res 1997;23:445–448.
26. Carles G, Peiffer H, Talarmin A. Effects of dengue fever during pregnancy in French Guiana. Clin Infect Dis 1999;28:637–649.
27. Boussemart T, Babe P, Sibille G, Neyret C, Berchel C. Prenatal transmission of dengue: two new cases. J Perinatol 2001;21:255–257.
28. Kerdpanich A, Watanaveradej V, Samakoses R, et al. Perinatal dengue infection. Southeast Asian J Trop Med Public Health 2001;32:488–493.
29. Chotigeat U, Kalayanarooj S, Nisalak A. Vertical transmission of dengue infection in Thai infants: two cases reports. J Med Assoc Thai 2003;86(Suppl 3):S628–S632.
30. Watanaveeradej V, Kerdpanich A, Chulyamitporn T, Nisalak A, Endy P. Perinatal transmission of dengue viral infection. Am J Trop Med Hyg 2000;62(3 Suppl):S342.
31. Poli L, Chungue E, Soulignac O, Gestas P, Kuo P, Papouin-Rauzy M. Dengue materno-foetale. Bull Soc Path Exot 1991;84:513–521.
32. Gubler DJ, Suharyono W, Tan R, Abidin M, Sie A. Viremia in patients with naturally acquired dengue infection. Bull WHO 1981;59:623–630.
33. Vaughn DW, Green S, Kalayanarooj S, et al. Dengue in the early febrile phase: viremia and antibody responses. J Infect Dis 1997;176:322–330.
34. Vorndam AV, Kuno G. Laboratory diagnosis of dengue virus infections. In: Gubler DJ, Kuno G, eds. Dengue and dengue hemorrhagic fever. Wallingford, UK: CAB International, 1997:313–333.
35. Gubler DJ, Sather GE. Laboratory diagnosis of dengue and dengue hemorrhagic fever. In: Fonseca da Cunha F, ed. Simposio Internacional sobre Febre Amarela e Dengue, 1988. Rio de Janeiro: Fundaçao Oswaldo Cruz/Bio-Manguinhos, 1988:291–322.

18
Syphilis

Sithembiso Velaphi and Pablo J. Sanchez

INTRODUCTION

The incidence of congenital syphilis in the United States has decreased significantly in recent years largely because of successful efforts by the Centers for Disease Control and Prevention (CDC) and local health departments to control syphilis in adults (1,2). Worldwide, however, syphilis continues to have a major impact on public health, and congenital syphilis remains an important cause of fetal and neonatal mortality (3). Congenital syphilis can be prevented by routine prenatal serologic screening and penicillin treatment of infected women and their sexual partners (4–6). All pregnant women should have a nontreponemal serologic test for syphilis performed at the first prenatal visit and in high-risk areas, at the beginning of the third trimester (28 weeks), and at delivery (7). No infant or mother should be discharged home from the hospital without the maternal serologic status documented at least once during pregnancy and preferably again at delivery. A nonreactive maternal nontreponemal test at delivery, however, may not exclude incubating syphilis or even primary syphilis when nontreponemal and treponemal antibodies have not yet reached detectable levels (8,9). By current methodologies, detection of treponemal infection in the asymptomatic infant of an infected mother with negative serologies is impossible. Infants born to such seronegative women are at risk of developing syphilis in the ensuing 3–14 weeks. In areas where syphilis is prevalent, consideration should be given to screening women again at the first postpartum visit (9). All cases of syphilis must be reported to the local health department for partner notification and identification of core populations and environments (10,11). The clinical signs of syphilis in infants are well known to health care providers, yet its accurate diagnosis in the majority of infants born to mothers with syphilis is problematic. The identification of the infected infant who lacks clinical signs of syphilis remains elusive. The inability to detect or culture the causative agent, *Treponema pallidum*, from neonatal clinical specimens and the difficulty in interpreting serologic tests in the infant because of transplacentally acquired maternal immunoglobulin (Ig) G antibodies has hindered our diagnosis and ultimately our understanding of this disease. Finally, difficulty exists in the identification of infants with central nervous system (CNS) infection caused by *T. pallidum*. These inadequacies in diagnosis have complicated the management of infants born to mothers with syphilis and have limited the available treatment options (12).

From: *Infectious Disease: Congenital and Perinatal Infections: A Concise Guide to Diagnosis*
Edited by: C. Hutto © Humana Press Inc., Totowa, NJ

TRANSMISSION

Vertical transmission of *T. pallidum* occurs transplacentally as a consequence of maternal spirochetemia. Transplacental transmission has been supported by (1) identification of *T. pallidum* in the placenta from pregnancies of mothers infected with syphilis *(13)*, (2) placental changes associated with congenital syphilis *(13,14)*, and (3) identification of *T. pallidum* in amniotic fluid and fetal blood from pregnancies complicated by syphilis *(15–19)*. It also is possible that an infant may be infected through contact with infectious maternal blood or genital lesions at the time of delivery.

Intrauterine infection can occur at any time during pregnancy, but transmission increases with advancing gestation. The risk of an infant acquiring syphilis from his mother is dependent on the stage and duration of maternal infection *(20–22)*. Studies from the 1950s demonstrated that, among women with syphilis of less than 4 years' duration, 41% of their infants were live born and had congenital syphilis, 25% were stillborn, 14% died in the neonatal period, 21% had low birth weight but no evidence of syphilis, and only 18% were normal full-term infants. In contrast, only 2% of infants born to mothers with late disease had congenital syphilis *(20)*.

In a similar study *(21)*, untreated maternal primary or secondary syphilis resulted in 50% of infants having congenital syphilis; the other half either were stillborn, premature, or died in the neonatal period. With early latent infection, 40% of infants had congenital syphilis; with late latent disease, only 10% developed syphilis. More recent data support the high transmission rate associated with early syphilis in mothers, a finding that is probably related to the higher spirochetemia that occurs during early syphilis. Untreated primary, secondary, early latent, and late latent infections were associated with vertical transmission rates of 29, 59, 50, and 13%, respectively *(22)*. These data have important implications for the evaluation and treatment of infants (*see* Evaluation and Treatment section).

The contribution of maternal infection with the human immunodeficiency virus (HIV) to vertical transmission of *T. pallidum* has not been well elucidated. Concern exists that infants born to mothers who are co-infected with HIV and syphilis are more likely to be infected with *T. pallidum* than infants born to HIV-negative mothers with syphilis *(23)*. It also is possible that syphilis during pregnancy may increase the risk of infection of the infant with HIV. Clearly, more studies are needed. Our inability to diagnose congenital syphilis in newborns accurately has hindered our understanding of this complex interaction.

CLINICAL MANIFESTATIONS IN THE FETUS AND NEONATE

Fetal infection with syphilis can be recognized by antenatal ultrasonography. Hydrops fetalis and hepatomegaly are seen in infected fetuses. Bowel dilation also has been described. After birth, the clinical signs of congenital syphilis have been divided arbitrarily into those manifestations that appear in the first 2 years of age, termed *early congenital syphilis*; those that are a result of active infection and inflammation; and those that occur beyond 2 years, designated as *late congenital syphilis (24–26)*. The last represent sequelae of the early manifestations or reaction to ongoing inflammation. The clinical findings of early and late congenital syphilis are provided in Table 1. Many infants with congenital syphilis have no clinical signs of infection, and the diagnosis is often impossible to ascertain.

Table 1
Clinical Findings in Infants With Congenital Syphilis

Early congenital syphilis
    Physical examination findings
        Nonimmune hydrops fetalis
        Intrauterine growth restriction
        Hepatomegaly (Fig. 1)[a]
        Jaundice
        Splenomegaly (Fig. 1)[a]
        Adenopathy
        Rhinitis (snuffles)
        Skin rash (Fig. 2)[a]
        Mucus patch
        Condylomata lata
        Pseudoparalysis of Parrot
        Chorioretinitis
        Cataract
        Central nervous system: asymptomatic invasion, cranial nerve palsies, seizures
    Laboratory findings
        Anemia
        Thrombocytopenia[a]
        Cerebrospinal fluid pleocytosis, elevated protein content
        Liver function abnormalities, including direct hyperbilirubinemia
    Radiographic findings
        Bone abnormalities: periostitis, osteochondritis[a]
        Pneumonia alba
    Other
        Nephrotic syndrome, pancreatitis, myocarditis, fever, gastrointestinal malabsorption,
          hypopituitarism
Late congenital syphilis
    Dentition: Hutchinson's teeth[b], Mulberry molars
    Eye: interstitial keratitis[b], healed chorioretinitis
    Eighth nerve deafness[b]
    Rhagades

Central nervous system: mental retardation, hydrocephalus, seizures, optic nerve atrophy, juvenile general paresis, cranial nerve palsies

Bone/joint: frontal bossing, saddle nose deformity, protuberant mandible, saber shin, sterno-clavicular joint thickening (Higouménaki's sign), Clutton's joints

[a]Prominent feature.
[b]Compose Hutchinson's triad, which is specific for congenital syphilis.

DIAGNOSIS

Methods that are used in the diagnosis of syphilis include (1) direct visualization of the organism by dark-field microscopy or fluorescent antibody technique of infected fluids or lesions *(27)*; (2) demonstration of the organism by special stains on histopathologic examination of tissue such as umbilical cord and placenta *(13,14)*; (3) animal inoculation (rabbit infectivity test) *(19,28–31)*; (4) demonstration of serologic

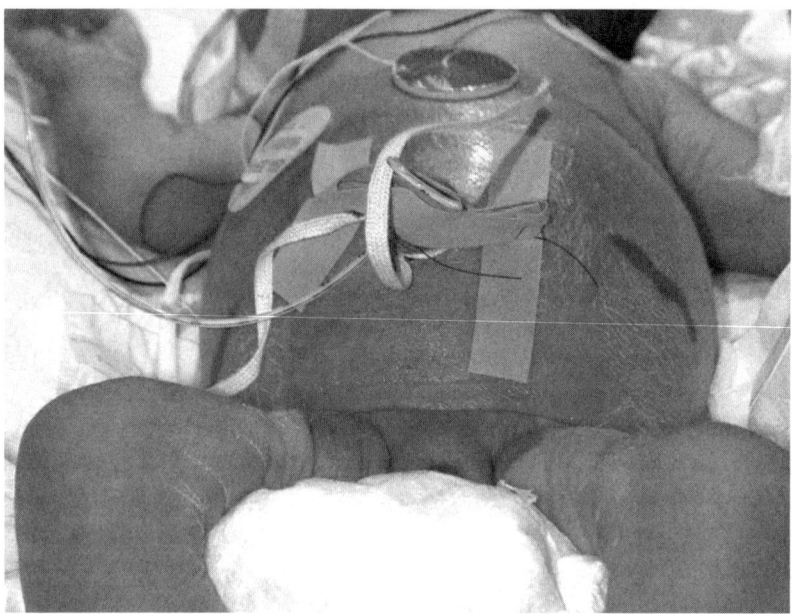

Fig. 1. Newborn with congenital syphilis exhibiting protuberant abdomen indicative of marked hepatosplenomegaly.

reactions typical of syphilis; and (5) detection of *T. pallidum* deoxyribonucleic acid (DNA) in clinical specimens by polymerase chain reaction (PCR) *(29–32)*. Histopathological examination of the placenta or umbilical cord using specific fluorescent antitreponemal antibody staining is recommended. The placenta is abnormally large and pale during congenital syphilis, and histopathology reveals necrotizing funisitis, villous enlargement, and acute villitis. The addition of histological evaluation of the placenta to conventional diagnostic criteria has improved the detection rate for congenital syphilis from 67 to 89% among live-born infants and from 91 to 97% in stillborn infants *(14)*.

The gold standard for diagnosing syphilis is identification of spirochetes in clinical specimens. The sensitivity of dark-field microscopy for visualization of motile spirochetes is poor because the organism is often present in low concentrations. In addition, the majority of infected infants lack lesions on which to perform dark-field microscopy. Because *T. pallidum* cannot be cultured routinely from clinical specimens, animal inoculation using the rabbit infectivity test (RIT) is available as a research tool for identifying the spirochete in a clinical specimen. RIT involves intratesticular rabbit inoculation of clinical specimens such as blood, cerebrospinal fluid (CSF), or amniotic fluid and monitoring the rabbit for evidence of syphilis as manifested by orchitis or seroconversion. Subsequent visualization of motile spirochetes by dark-field microscopy in testicular tissue confirms the diagnosis of syphilis in the patient. PCR has detected *T. pallidum* DNA in clinical specimens such as neonatal blood and CSF. Compared to isolation of the organism by RIT, the sensitivity and specificity of PCR on CSF was 65–71% and 97–100%, respectively *(29–31)*. Among 17 infants who had spirochetes detected in CSF by rabbit inoculation, blood PCR test was the best predic-

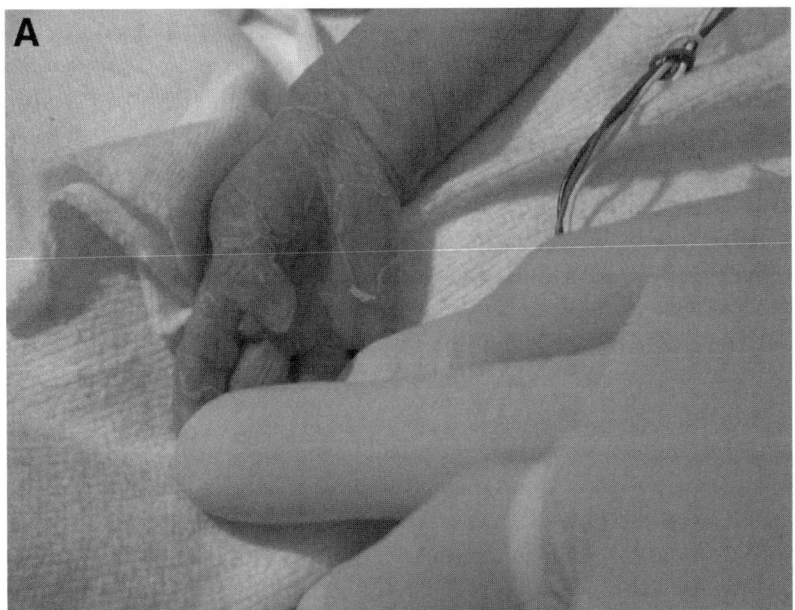

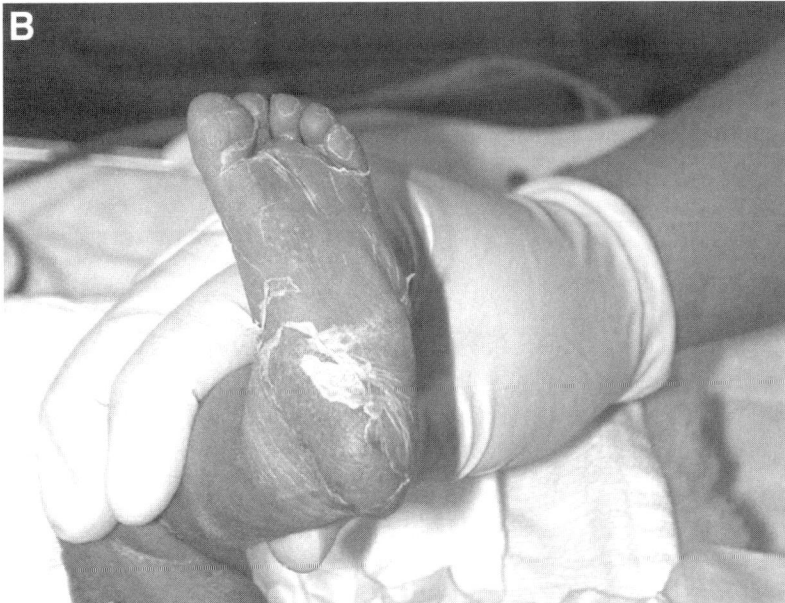

Fig. 2. Rash of hand and foot in infant with congenital syphilis.

tor of CNS infection with *T. pallidum (31)*. This finding further supports the concept that spirochetes gain access to the CNS by a hematogenous route. However, PCR is not commercially available, and its use has not been standardized in congenital syphilis. Therefore, the diagnosis of congenital syphilis is suggested by results of serologic tests performed on the mother and infant and findings on the infant's physical examination, laboratory tests including CSF examination, and radiographs of long bones *(7,24)*.

Serology

Serologic tests form the basis of diagnosis *(33)*. Two types of serologic tests for syphilis are the nontreponemal antibody tests and the treponemal antibody tests. The nontreponemal tests that are used routinely in the clinical setting are the rapid plasma reagin (RPR) test and the Venereal Diseases Research Laboratory (VDRL) test, both of which utilize an antigen composed of lecithin, cholesterol, and cardiolipin (diphosphatidylglycerol) to detect an antibody against cardiolipin that is present in sera of patients with syphilis. These tests measure mostly IgG and some IgM antibodies. Because both assays are quantitative, they are useful to assess adequacy of treatment and to detect reinfection. A fourfold increase in RPR or VDRL titers is indicative of active disease; a fourfold decrease suggests adequate therapy. Both tests usually decrease to nonreactivity or low-titer levels after 6–12 months of treatment. In some patients, the tests remain reactive at low titers, usually less than 1:8, indefinitely despite adequate treatment, and this situation is referred to as the *serofast state*. Such individuals are not infectious.

Because the RPR titer is often one to two dilutions higher than that obtained using the VDRL test, the RPR test is preferred for screening of pregnant women. On the other hand, the VDRL test is recommended for use on CSF. Because titer results may differ when these two tests are performed on serum from the same patient, it is important to perform the same nontreponemal test on the infant that was performed on the mother. A diagnosis of congenital syphilis is supported by an infant's RPR or VDRL titer that is fourfold or greater than that of the corresponding maternal titer. Such infants must be treated and managed as having proven or highly probably congenital syphilis (*see* Evaluation and Treatment section).

A significant difficulty with the nontreponemal tests is the occurrence of a negative reaction caused by the prozone phenomenon. This occurs in 1–2% of individuals usually with secondary syphilis and is caused by an excess amount of reagin antibody present in the patient's undiluted serum that prevents flocculation. Diluting the serum sample before testing overcomes the inhibition and results in the positive reaction. The health care provider must be aware that if congenital syphilis is suspected yet the maternal nontreponemal test result is nonreactive, then the laboratory must be consulted to verify that her specimen was appropriately diluted before the test was performed. The prozone reaction has contributed to misdiagnosed cases of congenital syphilis.

Both the RPR and VDRL tests occasionally produce reactive results in patients for whom there is no other evidence of syphilitic infection. These reactions are called biologic false positives and occur in approx 1% of adults. The serologic titer usually is low, less than 1:8, and in most instances the treponemal test is nonreactive. They occur in patients with other acute illnesses, especially pneumonia, hepatitis, and viral exanthematous disease, or after vaccinations. Conditions associated with chronic biologic false-positive reactions that persist for over 6 months are drug addiction, chronic hepatitis, old age, leprosy, and collagen vascular disease, especially systemic lupus erythematosus. A particularly concerning finding has been a relative increase in biologic false-positive reactions in women who are infected with HIV.

The treponemal tests that are in current use include the fluorescent treponemal antibody absorption (FTA-ABS) tests that use lyophilized *T. pallidum* as antigen and hemagglutination assays such as the *T. pallidum* particle agglutination test, which uses a lysate of *T. pallidum*. Both have similar sensitivity and specificity. These tests detect mostly IgG and some IgM antibodies to *T. pallidum* and are used to confirm reactive nontreponemal test results. The FTA-ABS test, however, is time consuming and expensive; the microhemagglutination assays are more automated and easier to perform technically. For this reason, they have largely replaced the FTA-ABS test as the most efficient specific test for antibody to *T. pallidum*. Recombinant proteins of *T. pallidum* have been used as the antigen source in enzyme-linked immunosorbent assays and optical immunoassays that rapidly detect treponemal IgG antibodies. The use of the optical immunoassay has enabled the early detection of infected pregnant women and has allowed on-site treatment. Its use in the United States, however, remains investigational.

The treponemal tests are nonquantitative tests and therefore are not useful for distinguishing active infection from past infection or assessing adequacy of treatment. Because of transplacental passage of IgG antibodies, all infants born to mothers with a reactive treponemal test also will have a reactive test. Therefore, they are not useful in evaluation of newborns. They also are not helpful in making a diagnosis of syphilis in infants younger than 18 months of age because maternal IgG antibodies may persist for that duration of time. The treponemal tests remain reactive indefinitely unless treatment for syphilis is given early in the disease course. Although these tests indicate experience with a treponemal infection, they may cross-react with the antigen of other treponemal diseases, such as those causing yaws and pinta.

Currently, there is no IgM test that is recommended for routine clinical use in neonates. Total serum IgM levels are insensitive and nonspecific. Rheumatoid factor, that is, fetal IgM antibody directed against maternal IgG antibodies, may cause as many as 35% false-positive test results. Elevations of total serum IgM concentrations have been seen in neonates with noninfectious conditions. In addition, competitive inhibition of IgM antibody by maternal IgG antibodies may result in false-negative test results. When compared with clinical diagnosis of congenital syphilis, the FTA-ABS 19S IgM had a sensitivity of 73% but a specificity of 100% *(12)*. In the same study, the IgM enzyme-linked immunosorbent assay (Captia™) test, which is no longer commercially available in the United States, had a sensitivity of 88% and specificity of 100%. Immunoblotting has been used to detect IgM and IgA antibodies directed against specific *T. pallidum* membrane lipoprotein antigens, particularly against a 47-kDa membrane lipoprotein that is highly immunogenic in adults *(27,29–31,34–39)*. The sensitivity of the IgM immunoblot nears 100%, and it has been shown to be predictive of CNS invasion by *T. pallidum (31)*. However, no IgM immunoblot assay is currently commercially available.

Cerebrospinal Fluid

CNS infection is defined by abnormal CSF findings that consist of a reactive VDRL test, pleocytosis, or elevated protein content. In neonates, elevated CSF white blood cell count and protein content are defined as greater than 25 per mm^3 and greater than 150 mg/dL, respectively. In infants older than 28 days, CSF pleocytosis is defined as greater than 5 per mm^3 and an elevated protein content as greater than 40 mg/dL. Because neonatal CSF often contains numerous red blood cells as a result of a traumatic lumbar puncture, the white blood cell count and protein concentration can be adjusted

Table 2
Treatment Guidelines for Acquired Syphilis During Pregnancy

Stage of infection	Regimen
Primary Secondary Early latent (≤1 year duration)	2.4 mU benzathine penicillin G im × 1[a]
Late latent (>1 year duration) Unknown duration	2.4 mU benzathine penicillin G im weekly × 3
Neurosyphilis	2–4 mU aqueous penicillin G iv every 4 hours × 10–14 days[b] or 2.4 mU procaine penicillin G im and 500 mg probenicid po four times daily × 10–14 days[b]

[a]A second dose 1 week later is recommended by some authorities for secondary syphilis.
[b]Some authorities recommend following this regimen with 2.4 mU benzathine penicillin im weekly × 3.

for blood contamination according to the following formulas: Adjusted white blood cell count = Actual white blood cell count − (Red blood cell count/500), and Adjusted protein content = Actual protein content − (Red blood cell count/1000). The presence of red blood cells in the CSF also could produce a false-positive VDRL test result. It is possible for a reactive CSF VDRL test result to be caused by transplacentally acquired nontreponemal IgG antibodies from the mother because these antibodies pass from the infant's serum to CSF. Nonetheless, a reactive CSF VDRL test, pleocytosis, or elevated protein content mandates treatment for possible CNS infection with *T. pallidum (7)*.

As compared to isolation of spirochetes from infant CSF by RIT, the sensitivity and specificity of a reactive CSF VDRL test, pleocytosis, and elevated protein content were 53 and 90%, 38 and 88%, and 56 and 78%, respectively *(31)*. CNS infection has been documented in 41% of infants who have any abnormality on clinical, laboratory, or radiographic evaluation and in 60% of those who have an abnormal physical examination consistent with a diagnosis of congenital syphilis. Spirochetes also have been isolated from CSF by RIT in three infants with normal CSF indices and nonreactive CSF VDRL test. These results indicate that CNS invasion is common among infected infants, and that once clinical, laboratory, or radiographic evaluation supports a diagnosis of congenital syphilis, then therapy effective against CNS disease is warranted.

EVALUATION AND TREATMENT

The decision to evaluate and ultimately treat an infant for congenital syphilis is based on clinical, laboratory, radiographic, and epidemiological considerations. The evaluation includes an assessment of the mother's serologic status *(40)*. If the mother has been treated, the health care provider must assess the adequacy of therapy (Table 2). At a minimum, all infants born to mothers who have reactive nontreponemal and treponemal test results should be evaluated with a serum quantitative nontreponemal serologic test. Many infants are born to women who have had syphilis in the past, received therapy, and remained seroreactive. Their infants also will be seroreactive. Both the nontreponemal (RPR) and treponemal (*T. pallidum* particle agglutination) tests measure IgG antibodies and therefore do not distinguish disease of the infant from maternally derived antibody. Ensuring that the infant does not have congenital disease in the immediate newborn period may not be possible. Treatment decisions often must be made on the basis of (1) identification of syphilis in the mother; (2) adequacy of maternal treatment; (3) presence of clinical, laboratory, or radiographic evidence of syphilis in the infant; and (4) comparison of maternal (at delivery) and infant nontreponemal serologic titers utilizing the same test and preferably the same laboratory *(7,41)*.

Because of routine serologic screening of pregnant women for syphilis, the pediatric health care provider is often alerted to the possibility of congenital syphilis when the maternal serologic tests are reactive. Otherwise, when a diagnosis of congenital syphilis is entertained in a newborn, one should first obtain a maternal nontreponemal test (Fig. 3). A nonreactive result excludes the diagnosis unless the maternal serum specimen is exhibiting a prozone phenomenon. If the nontreponemal test result is nonreactive even after dilution of the specimen, then the diagnosis of congenital syphilis in an infant who has clinical signs of a congenital infection is excluded, and the possibility of disease caused by other agents such as cytomegalovirus or *Toxoplasma gondii* should be investigated. If the maternal nontreponemal test is reactive, then the specific titer of the assay and a treponemal test are obtained. Maternal syphilis is confirmed if the treponemal test result is reactive; a nonreactive test indicates a biologic false-positive reaction. Testing of all pregnant women with syphilis for co-infection with HIV is strongly recommended, even though infants born to co-infected mothers do not require any different evaluation, therapy, or follow-up for syphilis.

All infants born to mothers with reactive serologic tests for syphilis should have a serum quantitative nontreponemal test performed and a thorough physical examination that focuses on finding evidence of congenital syphilis. The nontreponemal test that is performed on the infant should be the same as the one that was done on the mother to compare serologic titers. Although uncommon, a serum quantitative nontreponemal titer that is fourfold or greater than the corresponding maternal titer is diagnostic of congenital syphilis. Such a finding has been associated with the isolation of spirochetes from blood or CSF by RIT *(29)*. It is important to remember, however, that the majority of infants with congenital syphilis have serum nontreponemal titers that are the same or less than that of the mother.

It has been debated whether the infant's nontreponemal serologic test should be performed on serum obtained from a peripheral vein or artery or an umbilical cord blood specimen *(41,42)*. Both the CDC *(7)* and the American Academy of Pediatrics *(43)* recommend that umbilical cord blood should not be used because it has been associated with false-positive reactions secondary to contamination of the umbilical cord blood specimen with maternal blood or Wharton's jelly. However, umbilical cord blood is readily available and easily collected, and it is an adequate specimen if appropriate care is taken during its collection to minimize contamination with maternal blood. Testing only those infants whose mothers have reactive serologic tests for syphilis can minimize false-positive test results. Umbilical cord blood, however, should not be used to screen all infants for congenital syphilis.

Approach to Infants With Proven or Highly Probable Infection

Infants with proven or highly probable congenital syphilis are those "symptomatic" infants who have (1) an abnormal physical examination that is consistent with congeni-

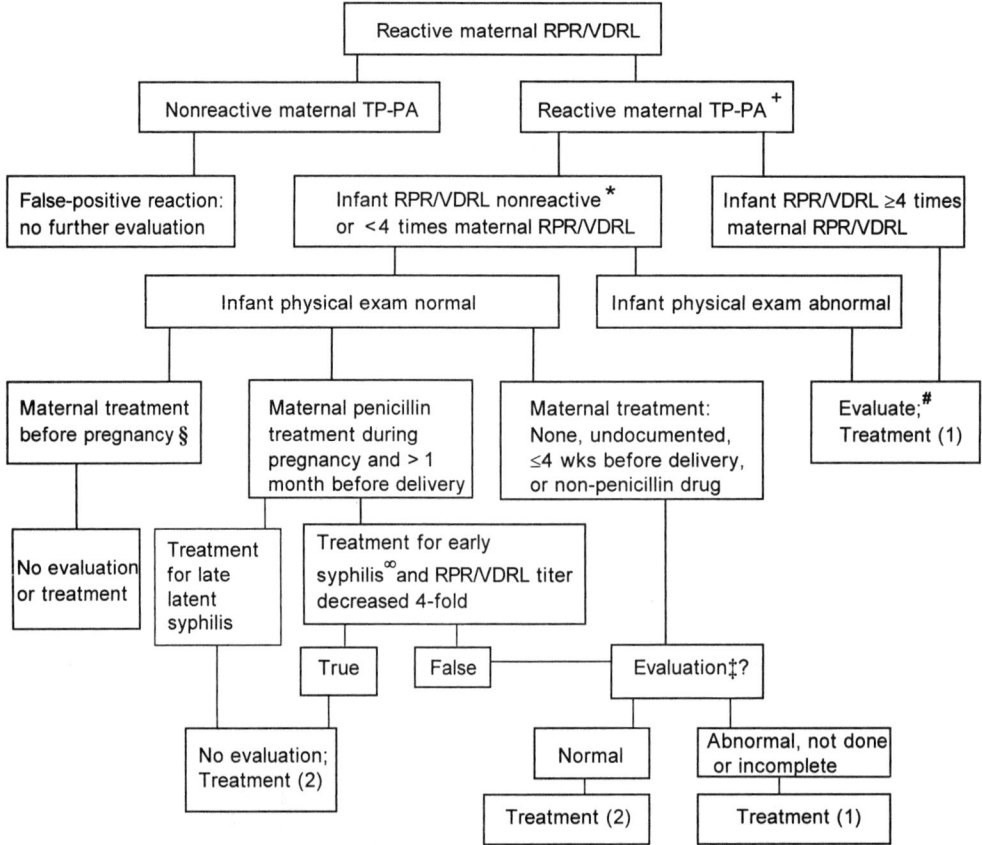

Fig. 3. Algorithm for evaluation and treatment of infants born to mothers with reactive serologic tests for syphilis.

+ Test for HIV-antibody. Infants of HIV-Ab ⊕ mothers do not require different evaluation or treatment.
* Infant's RPR may be nonreactive due to low maternal RPR titer or recent maternal infection. If the mother has untreated or inadequately treated syphilis and infant's physical exam is normal, treat infant with a single IM injection of benzathine penicillin (50,000 U/kg). No further evaluation needed.
\# Evaluation consists of CBC, platelet count; CSF examination for cell count, protein, and quantitative VDRL. Other tests as clinically indicated: long-bone x-rays, cranial ultrasound, auditory brainstem response, eye exam, chest X-ray, liver function tests, urine or meconium toxicology.
§ Women who maintain a VDRL titer ≤1:2 (RPR ≤1:4) beyond 1 year following successful treatment are considered serofast.
∞ Early syphilis: primary, secondary or early latent infection.
‡ CBC, platelet count; CSF examination for cell count, protein, and quantitative VDRL; Long bone x-rays.

TREATMENT:
(1) Aqueous penicillin G 50,000 U/kg IV q 12 hr (≤1 wk of age), q 8 hr (>1 wk), or procaine penicillin G 50,000 U/kg IM single daily dose x 10 days.
(2) Benzathine penicillin G 50,000 U/kg IM x 1 dose.

tal syphilis; (2) a serum quantitative nontreponemal serologic titer that is fourfold or greater than the mother's; or (3) a positive dark-field or fluorescent antibody test of body fluid, lesion, or tissue. The evaluation of theses infants should consist of a complete blood cell count (CBC) and platelet count as well as CSF examination for cell count, protein content, and VDRL test. Anemia and thrombocytopenia may not be detected by routine physical examination. In addition, spirochetemia with invasion of the CNS occurs in approx 40–50% of symptomatic infants *(29,31)*. Although these infants must receive a full course of penicillin therapy that will treat possible neurosyphilis, it is beneficial for follow-up purposes to establish CNS abnormalities at presentation. Other tests such as bone and chest roentgenograms, liver function tests, cranial ultrasound, ophthalmologic examination, and auditory brain stem response should be performed as clinically indicated. The need to perform radiographic studies on symptomatic infants has been debated *(44)*. Bone abnormalities such as osteochondritis and periostitis occur frequently in symptomatic infants. However, abnormal findings do not change therapy in this group of infants. Therefore, the CDC has recommended that bone radiographs be performed if there is a clinical indication such as pseudoparalysis or possible fracture of an extremity. The American Academy of Pediatrics recommends that bone radiographs be performed unless the diagnosis has been otherwise established, which in the case of symptomatic infants, there usually exist other reasons for the diagnosis of congenital syphilis.

The recommended treatment of neonates with proven or highly probable disease is aqueous crystalline penicillin G (50,000 U/kg iv every 12 hours for the first 7 days of age and every 8 hours thereafter up to 1 month of age) or procaine penicillin G (50,000 U/kg im daily) for 10 days *(7,43,45)*. If more than 1 day of therapy is missed, the entire course should be restarted. Whenever possible, a full 10-day course of penicillin is preferred even if ampicillin was initially provided for possible sepsis. There is no alternative therapy because data are lacking on the efficacy of such agents as ampicillin or ceftriaxone. With the recent shortage of aqueous penicillin G in the United States, the CDC recommended that ceftriaxone be used for 10 days at an appropriate dose for weight and gestational age (www.cdc.gov/nchstp/dstd/penicillinG.htm). Infants and children who require treatment for syphilis but who have a history of penicillin allergy or develop an allergic reaction presumed secondary to penicillin should be desensitized, if necessary, and then treated with penicillin *(7,46)*. The use of agents other than penicillin requires close clinical and serologic follow-up to assess adequacy of therapy. The Jarisch-Herxheimer reaction occurs rarely in infected infants. It may be manifested by fever, rash, worsening liver function tests, and hypotension, but there is no prophylaxis.

Approach to Asymptomatic Infant

The management of the "asymptomatic" infant who has a normal physical examination and a serum quantitative nontreponemal test that is the same or less than fourfold the maternal titer is more problematic (Fig. 3). The maternal syphilis and treatment history must be carefully assessed. The likelihood that such an infant is infected with *T. pallidum* is dependent on the maternal stage of syphilis during pregnancy and at the time of delivery, the adequacy of her therapy for syphilis before delivery, and the timing in pregnancy of such therapy. Vertical transmission is related directly to the maternal stage of syphilis, with early syphilis and particularly secondary syphilis, resulting in significantly higher transmission rates than late latent infection.

Other circumstances that place the newborn at high risk of having congenital syphilis despite being asymptomatic include no maternal treatment, inadequate treatment for her stage of syphilis, unknown treatment or treatment with erythromycin or any other nonpenicillin drug, or treatment provided 4 weeks or less before delivery. Maternal treatment with any drug other than penicillin is not adequate therapy for the fetus as numerous treatment failures have been reported following maternal treatment with erythromycin during pregnancy. Maternal treatment for syphilis in the last 4 weeks of pregnancy also is not considered to be adequate fetal therapy *(47)*. Concern exists that increases in renal clearance and plasma volume that occur as pregnancy progresses may result in lower serum and CSF penicillin concentrations in both the mother and fetus *(48)*. Moreover, there may have been insufficient time for the fetus to be adequately treated, thus necessitating penicillin therapy for the newborn.

Other high-risk conditions include maternal reinfection with syphilis during the pregnancy, as evidenced by RPR titer that has increased fourfold and the mother was not retreated. Also, if the mother was treated for early syphilis during pregnancy but her nontreponemal serologic titer did not decrease fourfold, one is unable to evaluate the adequacy of her therapy. In all of these instances, the infant requires treatment *(49,50)*.

Whether to perform a complete evaluation (CSF analysis for VDRL test, cell count, and protein; long-bone radiographs; and CBC and platelet count) on the infant depends on the maternal treatment history and planned treatment of the infant. The recommended treatment options are (1) aqueous crystalline penicillin G (50,000 U/kg iv every 12 hours for the for 7 days of age and every 8 hours thereafter up to 1 month of age) or procaine penicillin G (50,000 U/kg im daily) for 10 days or (2) benzathine penicillin G (50,000 U/kg as a single im dose *[7]*).

Although preferred to help establish a diagnosis of congenital syphilis, a complete evaluation is not necessary if a full 10-day course of parenteral penicillin is provided because such therapy would treat for the possibility of CNS infection with *T. pallidum*. The need to perform a lumbar puncture has been questioned because the yield of abnormal findings from examination of the CSF is low among asymptomatic infants *(51)*. However, a primary benefit of obtaining CSF studies is identification of infants with possible CNS infection who require close serologic and CSF follow-up. Likewise, long-bone radiographs are abnormal in approx 65% of infants with clinical findings of syphilis but only in a minority of asymptomatic infants. The finding of osteochondritis or periostitis in an infant born to a mother with reactive serologic tests for syphilis is indicative of congenital syphilis, and the infant requires a full 10-day course of penicillin therapy for highly probable disease. Such infants with abnormal evaluations are likely to have CNS infection even if there are no clinical signs of neurosyphilis *(31)*.

On the other hand, if a single intramuscular dose of benzathine penicillin G therapy is administered, then the infant must be fully evaluated, the evaluation must be completely normal, and follow-up must be certain. If any part of the infant's evaluation is abnormal or not performed or if the CSF analysis is impossible to interpret because of contamination with blood, then a 10-day course of penicillin is required.

Concern exists about the use of benzathine penicillin G for the treatment of asymptomatic infants born to mothers with syphilis. Three infants have been reported who developed clinical signs of syphilis at 4, 9, and 14 weeks of age after receiving a single intramuscular injection of benzathine penicillin in the newborn period *(52,53)*. All of the infants were assessed as having normal physical examinations at the time of treatment. One mother had untreated early latent syphilis, another had syphilis of unknown duration; the third mother had secondary syphilis that was treated 1 month before delivery. None of the infants, however, had been fully evaluated for evidence of syphilis when they received benzathine penicillin, hence the importance of performing a full evaluation on at-risk infants if benzathine penicillin is used. Of infants who have some abnormality on clinical, laboratory, or radiographic evaluation, 40% have spirochetes detected in CSF by RIT *(31)*, and it is known that benzathine penicillin G does not reach treponemocidal concentrations in CSF *(54)*. However, CNS infection is uncommon among asymptomatic infants with normal evaluations who are born to a mother with untreated or inadequately treated syphilis. In addition, there has been vast clinical experience with benzathine penicillin for syphilis, and its use decreases hospital costs by allowing for earlier discharge with improved maternal-infant interaction. In one small study of 152 asymptomatic infants who were randomly assigned to receive either a single intramuscular injection of benzathine penicillin G or 10 days of daily procaine penicillin G, no treatment failures were reported *(55)*. Overall, it has been estimated that benzathine penicillin G may have a failure rate of approx 2–3% *(56)*.

For infants who have a normal physical examination and a serum quantitative nontreponemal serologic titer that is the same or less than fourfold the maternal titer and (1) maternal treatment was during pregnancy, administered more than 4 weeks before delivery and appropriate for the stage of infection; (2) maternal nontreponemal titers decreased fourfold after appropriate therapy for early syphilis or remained stable and low for late syphilis; and (3) no evidence of reinfection or relapse, then no evaluation is required. Approximately 2–14% of newborns whose mothers received penicillin treatment during pregnancy for syphilis will have clinical, laboratory, or radiographic evidence of congenital syphilis *(47,57–59)*. Because of the possibility of fetal syphilis despite maternal treatment and the fact that these infants were exposed to mothers with active syphilis, a single intramuscular dose of benzathine penicillin G 50,000 U/kg is recommended. Some specialists, however, would not treat but provide close serologic follow-up, preferably monthly, until the infant's RPR test is nonreactive. If such close follow-up is not possible, then a single intramuscular dose of benzathine penicillin G should be provided.

For infants who have a normal physical examination, a serum quantitative nontreponemal serologic titer that is the same or less than fourfold the maternal titer, maternal treatment that was adequate before pregnancy, a nontreponemal serologic titer that has remained low and stable before and during pregnancy and at delivery (e.g., VDRL ≤1:2, RPR ≤1:4), no evaluation or treatment of the infant is recommended. If follow-up is uncertain, a single intramuscular injection of benzathine penicillin G 50,000 U/kg could be administered prophylactically.

After the neonatal period, children who are identified as having congenital syphilis should have a complete evaluation consisting of CSF examination, CBC and platelet count, and testing for HIV infection. Other tests, such as long-bone radiographs, chest radiograph, liver function tests, ophthalmological examination, and auditory brain stem response, should be performed as clinically indicated. In addition, birth and maternal records should be reviewed to assess whether such children have congenital or acquired syphilis. Children with acquired syphilis should be evaluated for the possibility of sexual abuse. Any child who is suspected of having congenital syphilis or who has neurological involvement should be treated with aqueous penicillin G 200,000–300,000 U/kg per day iv, administered as 50,000 U/kg every 4–6 hours for 10 days. Some specialists also suggest giving these patients a single dose of benzathine penicillin G 50,000 U/kg im following the 10-day course of intravenous aqueous penicillin *(7)*.

FOLLOW-UP

Infants who have reactive serologic tests for syphilis should have serial quantitative nontreponemal tests performed until the test becomes nonreactive *(7,24,43)*. Follow-up for these infants can be incorporated into routine pediatric care at 2, 4, 6, 12, and 15 months. Nontreponemal antibody titers should decline by 3 months of age, and the test should become nonreactive by 6 months of age if the infant was not infected or was infected but adequately treated *(60)*. The serologic response after therapy may be slower for infants treated after the neonatal period. If the nontreponemal titer increases four-fold, the infant should be further evaluated with a CSF examination and receive a 10-day course of intravenous aqueous penicillin G. Similarly, infants who maintain persistently low, stable nontreponemal titers beyond 12 months of age should be re-evaluated and treated. A reactive treponemal test after 18 months of age, when the infant has lost all maternal antibody, confirms the diagnosis of congenital syphilis *(61)*. If such a child has not received treatment for syphilis previously, then the child should be evaluated and treated.

Infants who had abnormal CSF findings at presentation should have a repeat lumbar puncture performed every 6 months after therapy until the results are normal. A reactive CSF VDRL, unexplained pleocytosis, or elevated protein content is an indication for retreatment.

The prognosis of infants with congenital syphilis has not been well studied, but it should be excellent if neonates are identified soon after birth and are provided with effective penicillin therapy early in infancy. Infants treated for early congenital syphilis are at risk of developing such late complications or sequelae as hypopituitarism *(62)*, interstitial keratitis, and teeth as well as bone and joint abnormalities *(25)*.

ACKNOWLEDGMENT

This work was supported by grant no. 1R29 AI 34932-01 from the National Institute of Allergy and Infectious Diseases and by contract no. C1000 689 with the Centers for Disease Control and Prevention to P. J. S.

REFERENCES

1. St Louis ME, Wasserheit JM. Elimination of syphilis in the United States. Science 1998;281:353–354.
2. Centers for Disease Control and Prevention. Congenital syphilis—United States, 2000. MMWR Morb Mortal Wkly Rep 2001;50:573–577.
3. Gust DA, Levine WC, St Louis ME, Braxton J, Berman SM. Mortality associated with congenital syphilis in the United States, 1992–1998. Pediatrics 2002;109:e79.
4. Southwick KL, Guidry HM, Weldon MM, et al. An epidemic of congenital syphilis in Jefferson County, Texas, 1994–1995: inadequate prenatal syphilis testing after an outbreak in adults. Am J Public Health 1999;89:557–560.
5. Warner L, Rochat RW, Fichtner RR, Stoll BJ, Nathan L, Toomey KE. Missed opportunities for congenital syphilis prevention in an urban southeastern hospital. Sex Trans Dis 2001;28:92–98.
6. Webber MP, Lambert G, Bateman DA, et al. Maternal risk factors for congenital syphilis: a case-control study. Am J Epidemiol 1993;137:415–422.

7. Centers for Disease Control and Prevention. Sexually transmitted diseases treatment guidelines 2002. MMWR Morb Mortal Wkly Rep 2002;51:18–30.
8. Dorfman DH, Glaser JH. Congenital syphilis presenting in infants after the newborn period. N Engl J Med 1990;323:1299–1302.
9. Sanchez PJ, Wendel GD, Norgard MV. Congenital syphilis associated with negative results of maternal serologic tests at delivery. Am J Dis Child 1991;145:967–969.
10. Centers for Disease Control and Prevention. Congenital syphilis—New York City, 1986–1988. MMWR Morb Mortal Wkly Rep 1989;38:825–829.
11. Zenker PN, Berman SM. Congenital syphilis: reporting and reality. Am J Public Health 1990;80:271–272.
12. Stoll BJ, Lee FK, Larsen S, et al. Clinical and serologic evaluation of neonates for congenital syphilis: a continuing diagnostic dilemma. J Infect Dis 1993;167:415–422.
13. Genest DR, Choi-Hong SR, Tate JE, et al. Diagnosis of congenital syphilis from placental examination: comparison of histopathology, Steiner stain, and polymerase chain reaction for *Treponema pallidum* DNA. Hum Pathol 1996;27:366–372.
14. Sheffield JS, S·nchez PJ, Wendel GD Jr, et al. Placental histopathology of congenital syphilis. Obstet Gynecol 2002;100:126–133.
15. Hollier LM, Harstad TW, Sanchez PJ, Twickler DM, Wendel GD Jr. Fetal syphilis: clinical and laboratory characteristics. Obstet Gynecol 2001;97:947–953.
16. Wendel GD, S·nchez PJ, Peters MT, et al. Identification of *Treponema pallidum* in amniotic fluid and fetal blood from pregnancies complicated by congenital syphilis. Obstet Gynecol 1991;78:890–895.
17. Nathan L, Bohman VR, S·nchez PJ, et al. *In utero* infection with *Treponema pallidum* in early pregnancy. Prenat Diagn 1997;17:119–123.
18. Wendel GD, Maberry MC, Christmas JT, et al. Examination of amniotic fluid in diagnosing congenital syphilis with fetal death. Obstet Gynecol 1989;74:967–970.
19. Nathan L, Twickler DM, Peters MT, et al. Fetal syphilis: correlation of sonographic findings and rabbit infectivity testing of amniotic fluid. J Ultrasound Med 1993;2:97–101.
20. Ingraham NR. The value of penicillin alone in the prevention and treatment of congenital syphilis. Acta Derm Venereol 1951;31(Suppl 24):60–87.
21. Fiumara NJ, Fleming WL, Downing JG, et al. The incidence of prenatal syphilis at the Boston City Hospital. N Engl J Med 1952;247:48–52.
22. Sheffield JS, Wendel GD Jr, Zeray F, et al. Congenital syphilis: the influence of maternal stage of syphilis on vertical transmission [abstract]. Am J Obstet Gynecol 1999;180:S85.
23. Schulte JM, Burkham S, Hamaker D, et al. Syphilis among HIV-infected mothers and their infants in Texas from 1988 to 1994. Sex Transm Dis 2001;28:315–320.
24. Ingall D, S·nchez PJ. Syphilis. In Remington JS, Klein JO, eds. Infectious Diseases of the Fetus and Newborn Infant, 5th ed. Philadelphia: Saunders, 2001:643–381.
25. Fiumara NJ, Lessel S. Manifestations of late congenital syphilis. Arch Dermatol 1970;102:78–83.
26. Sanchez PJ, Wendel GD. Syphilis in pregnancy. Clin Perinatol 1997;24:71–90.
27. Bromberg K, Rawstron S, Tannis G. Diagnosis of congenital syphilis by combining *Treponema pallidum*-specific IgM detection with immunofluorescent antigen detection of *T. pallidum*. J Infect Dis 1993;168:238–242.
28. Lukehart SA, Hook EW III, Baker-Zander SA, et al. Invasion of the central nervous system by *Treponema pallidum*: implications for diagnoses and therapy. Ann Intern Med 1988;109:855–862.
29. Sanchez PJ, Wendel GD, Grimpel E, et al. Evaluation of molecular methodologies and rabbit infectivity testing for the diagnosis of congenital syphilis and central nervous system invasion by *Treponema pallidum*. J Infect Dis 1993;167:148–157.
30. Grimprel E, Sanchez PJ, Wendel GD Jr, et al. Use of polymerase chain reaction and rabbit infectivity testing to detect *Treponema pallidum* in amniotic fluids, fetal and neonatal sera, and cerebrospinal fluid. J Clin Microbiol 1991;29:1711–1718.

31. Michelow IC, Wendel GD Jr, Norgard MV, et al. Central nervous system infection in congenital syphilis. N Engl J Med 2002;346:1792–1798.
32. Burstain JM, Grimprel E, Lukehart SA, et al. Sensitive detection of *Treponema pallidum* by using the polymerase chain reaction. J Clin Microbiol 1991;29:62–69.
33. Larsen SA, Steiner BM, Rudolph AH. Laboratory diagnosis and interpretation of tests for syphilis. Clin Microbiol 1995;8:1–21.
34. Dobson SRM, Taber LH, Baughn RE. Recognition of *Treponema pallidum* antigens by IgM and IgG antibodies in congenitally infected newborns and their mothers. J Infect Dis 1988;157:903–910.
35. Lewis LL. Congenital syphilis: serologic diagnosis in the young infant. Infect Dis Clin North Am 1992;6:31–39.
36. Lewis LL, Taber LH, Baughn RE. Evaluation of immunoglobulin M Western blot analysis in the diagnosis of congenital syphilis. J Clin Microbiol 1990;28:296–302.
37. Sanchez PJ, McCracken GH, Wendel GD, et al. Molecular analysis of the fetal IgM response to *Treponema pallidum* antigens: implications for improved serodiagnosis of congenital syphilis. J Infect Dis 1989;159:508–517.
38. Sanchez PJ, Wendel GD, Norgard MV. IgM antibody to *Treponema pallidum* in cerebrospinal fluid of infants with congenital syphilis. Am J Dis Child 1992;146:1171–1175.
39. Schmitz JL, Gertis KS, Mauney C, et al. Laboratory diagnosis of congenital syphilis by immunoglobulin M (IgM) and IgA immunoblotting. Clin Diagn Lab Immunol 1994;1:32–37.
40. Wendel GD Jr, Sheffield JS, Hollier LM, Hill JB, Ramsey PS, S·nchez PJ. Treatment of syphilis in pregnancy and prevention of congenital syphilis. Clin Infect Dis 2002;35(Suppl 2):S200–S209.
41. Rawstron SA, Bromberg K. Comparison of maternal and newborn serologic tests for syphilis. Am J Dis Child 1991;145:1383–1388.
42. Chhabra RS, Brion LP, Castro M, et al. Comparison of maternal sera, cord blood and neonatal sera for detecting presumptive congenital syphilis: relationship with maternal treatment. Pediatrics 1993;91:88–91.
43. American Academy of Pediatrics. Syphilis. In: Pickering LK, ed. Red Book: 2003 Report of the Committee on Infectious Diseases, 26th ed. Elk Grove Village, IL: American Academy of Pediatrics, 2003:595–607.
44. Moyer VA, Schneider V, Yetman R, Garcia-Sprats J, Parks D, Cooper T. Contribution of long-bone radiographs to the management of congenital syphilis in the newborn infant. Arch Pediatr Adolesc Med 1998;152:353–357.
45. Azimi PH, Janner D, Berne P, et al. Concentrations of procaine and aqueous penicillin in the cerebrospinal fluid of infants treated for congenital syphilis. J Pediatr 1994;124:649–653.
46. Wendel GD Jr, Stark BJ, Jamison RB, et al. Penicillin allergy and desensitization in serious infections during pregnancy. N Engl J Med 1985;312:1229–1232.
47. Benzick AE, Wirthwein DP, Weinberg A, et al. Pituitary gland gumma in congenital syphilis after failed maternal treatment: a case report. Pediatrics 1999;104:e4.
48. Nathan L, Bawdon RE, Sidawi E, et al. Penicillin levels following administration of benzathine penicillin G in pregnancy. Obstet Gynecol 1993;82:338–342.
49. Finelli L, Crayne EM, Spitalny KC. Treatment of infants with reactive syphilis serology, New Jersey. Pediatrics 1998;102:e27.
50. Radcliffe M, Meyer M, Roditi D, Malan A. Single-dose benzathine penicillin in infants at risk of congenital syphilis—results of a randomised study. S Afr Med J 1997;87:62–65.
51. Beeram MR, Chopde N, Dawood Y, et al. Lumbar puncture in the evaluation of possible asymptomatic congenital syphilis in neonates. J Pediatr 1996;128:125–129.
52. Beck-Sague C, Alexander R. Failure of benzathine penicillin and treatment in early congenital syphilis. Pediatr Infect Dis 1987;6:1061–1064.

53. Woolf A, Wilfert CM, Kelsey DB, et al. Childhood syphilis in North Carolina. N C Med J 1980;41:443–449.
54. Speer ME, Taber LH, Clark DB, et al. Cerebrospinal fluid levels of benzathine penicillin in the neonate. J Pediatr 1977;91:996–997.
55. Paryani SG, Vaughn AJ, Crosby M, Lawrence S. Treatment of asymptomatic congenital syphilis benzathine vs procaine penicillin G therapy. J Pediatr 1994;125:471–475.
56. Hardy JB, Hardy PH, Oppenheimer EH. Failure of penicillin in a newborn with congenital syphilis. JAMA 1970;212:1345–1349.
57. Alexander JM, Sheffield JS, Sanchez PJ, Mayfield J, Wendel GD Jr. Efficacy of treatment for syphilis in pregnancy. Obstet Gynecol 1999;93:5–8.
58. Conover CS, Rend CA, Miller GB Jr, Schmid GP. Congenital syphilis after treatment of maternal syphilis with a penicillin regimen exceeding CDC guidelines. Infect Dis Obstet Gynecol 1998;6:134–137.
59. Sheffield JS, S·nchez PJ, Morris G, et al. Congenital syphilis after maternal treatment for syphilis during pregnancy. Am J Obstet Gynecol 2002;186:569–573.
60. Chang SN, Chung KY, Lee MG, Lee JB. Seroreversion of the serological tests for syphilis in the newborns born to treated syphilitic mothers. Genitourin Med 1995;71:68–70.
61. Rawstron SA, Mehta S, Marcellino L, Rempel J, Chery F, Bromberg K. Congenital syphilis and fluorescent treponemal antibody test reactivity after the age of 1 year. Sex Transm Dis 2001;28:412–416.
62. Nolt D, Saad R, Kouatli A, et al. Survival with hypopituitarism from congenital syphilis. Pediatrics 2002;109:e63.

19

Group B Streptococcus

Cecelia Hutto

INTRODUCTION

For three decades, group B streptococcus (GBS) has been the most common cause of bacterial sepsis and meningitis in neonates in the United States *(1,2)*. Prior to 1996, when guidelines for intrapartum antibiotics to prevent early GBS disease in neonates were first published, there were approx 7500 cases of neonatal disease yearly in the United States, and the mortality was almost 50% *(3,4)*. Adoption of prevention guidelines by many hospitals resulted in a 70% decline in the incidence of early-onset GBS disease in neonates by the mid-1990s *(5)*. Despite this remarkable progress, GBS remains a leading cause of neonatal mortality and morbidity *(4)*.

MICROBIOLOGY

Group B streptococci, *Streptococcus agalactiae*, are Gram-positive, cytochrome-negative aerobic diplococci. They cause a thin zone of b-hemolysis when cultured on a blood agar plate. Group B streptococci, like other streptococcal species, have a group-specific capsular carbohydrate antigen that allows differentiation from other streptococci. Nine serotypes of group B streptococcus (Ia, Ib, and II–VIII) are characterized on the basis of differences in their capsular polysaccharides *(6)*. Five serotypes (Ia, Ib, II, III, and V) have accounted for 95% of disease in infants *(7)*. The presence of type-specific antibodies confers resistance to that specific serotype *(6)*.

EPIDEMIOLOGY AND TRANSMISSION

Group B streptococci are primarily inhabitants of the lower gastrointestinal tract, but colonization of the genitourinary tract and pharynx can also occur. Studies from different areas of the world have reported colonization rates in women at delivery ranging from 15 to 40% *(6)*. Differences in rates of colonization have been attributed to differences in the populations studied as well as variation in the culture methods used, including the number of sites cultured in women and the culture process *(6)*.

Among adults, epidemiological studies support sexual activity as a route of spread for GBS *(8)*. Mother-to-infant transmission of GBS can occur either prior to birth by the ascending route through ruptured membranes or at the time of delivery by contact with the organism in the birth canal. Less commonly, infants may acquire GBS through

From: *Infectious Disease: Congenital and Perinatal Infections: A Concise Guide to Diagnosis*
Edited by: C. Hutto © Humana Press Inc., Totowa, NJ

Table 1
Factors Associated With Risk for Early-Onset Group B Streptococcal Disease

	Reference
Maternal colonization at delivery	*10, 12*
Gestational age (<7 weeks)	*13*
Prolonged rupture of membranes (≥18 hours)	*13, 14*
Chorioamnionitis	*10, 15*
Intrapartum fever	*13, 15*
Maternal age	*13*
African American race	*13, 16*
Low level of antibody to infecting serotype	*17*

nosocomial transmission by contact with the hands of hospital personnel or individuals in their homes *(9,10)*.

About 50% of neonates born to mothers colonized with GBS acquire the bacteria and are colonized themselves. Higher rates of colonization have been reported in infants born to mothers with heavy colonization, as defined by colonization at multiple sites and having higher bacterial colony counts at the sites of colonization *(11)*. The sites of colonization in the neonate may include the external auditory canal (especially within the first 24 hours of life), throat, umbilicus, and rectum.

Most colonized neonates remain asymptomatic. In some, GBS causes severe invasive disease beginning either during the first week of life, termed *early-onset disease*, or from 7 days to 3 months of age, termed *late-onset disease*.

Risk Factors for Neonatal Disease

A number of factors, many of which are pregnancy related, have been identified that increase the risk for early-onset disease in the infant *(10–17)*. These are shown in Table 1. Maternal colonization with GBS is probably the most important predictor of early-onset disease in the neonate. Because maternal colonization may be intermittent or transient, the time at which cultures are done during pregnancy is important. Cultures obtained late in gestation are most predictive of colonization at the time of delivery *(11)*. The infants of mothers with heavy colonization have a higher risk for GBS disease *(18)*. Other factors associated with an increased risk of GBS disease are gestational age less than 37 weeks, prolonged rupture of membranes (>18 hours), chorioamnionitis, intrapartum fever, young maternal age, African American race, and low levels of antibody to the infecting serotype.

EVALUATION OF MOTHERS

GBS may be the cause of significant morbidity and mortality among pregnant women. In addition to urinary tract infections (UTIs), women may have chorioamnionitis, postpartum wound infection, bacteremia, or puerperal sepsis. Any pregnant mother with symptoms of a UTI should have a urine culture done, and the culture should be labeled as that of a pregnant woman. Because GBS bacteriuria is considered evidence of heavy colonization in the pregnant woman, any quantity of GBS in the urine of a pregnant woman should be reported by the laboratory to the obstetrician *(19)*. Women who are symptomatic should be treated with standard therapy for the UTI. Whether a woman is symptomatic or asymptomatic, intrapartum antibiotics are recommended during labor for women who have bacteriuria *(19)*. If a wound infection is suspected, cultures of the wound and blood should be obtained, and blood cultures are indicated in women with signs of bacteremia or sepsis. The diagnosis of chorioamnionitis is usually made on the basis of clinical signs, including fever, uterine tenderness, and tachycardia in the mother and tachycardia in the fetus *(20)*. For women with chorioamnionitis, UTI, and bacteremia, the risk of colonization and disease in their infants is significantly increased.

Guidelines for Screening and Intrapartum Antibiotics

Most infants with early-onset disease are born to mothers who are only colonized with GBS and are asymptomatic. Guidelines for screening and providing intrapartum prophylaxis to pregnant women at risk for GBS to prevent early-onset neonatal disease were published in 1996 and 1997 by the American Academy of Pediatrics, American College of Obstetrics and Gynecology, and the Centers for Disease Control and Prevention (CDC) *(21–23)*. Population-based surveillance by the Active Bacterial Core Surveillance/Emerging Infections Program Network found that these prevention efforts were successful in preventing invasive GBS disease and death in many infants *(24)*.

Despite this progress, GBS continues to be an important cause of morbidity and mortality in neonates. The initial prevention strategies have been revised by a working group convened by the CDC in an effort to further decrease GBS disease in neonates *(19)*. A key change in the most recent guidelines, relative to earlier guidelines, is that it is now recommended that all pregnant women have vaginal and rectal GBS screening cultures at 35–37 weeks of gestation to determine the risk of GBS disease in their newborn *(19)*. Previously, one approach had recommended that assessment of a pregnant woman's risk could be based on factors known to increase the risk of neonatal GBS disease, including preterm delivery, rupture of membranes longer than 18 hours, and intrapartum fever *(21)*. However, a population-based multistate surveillance study found that screening women based on cultures was significantly more effective in identifying women with colonization and preventing GBS disease in their infants *(25)*. Now, the risk-based approach is recommended only in specific situations, including women who did not receive prenatal care or for whom results of cultures are not available *(19)*.

For any woman having cultures positive for GBS, unless a planned cesarean section for delivery is performed and there is no labor or rupture of membranes, intrapartum antibiotics are recommended *(19)*. Other recommended indications for intrapartum antibiotics can be found in the revised recommendations published by the CDC *(19)*. The guidelines also provided recommendations for antibiotics for women who are allergic to penicillin and specific recommendations for obtaining cultures to enhance their sensitivity for detecting colonization. Recommendations for obtaining cultures are discussed in the Diagnostic Assays section.

NEONATAL GROUP B STREPTOCOCCUS DISEASE

Based on the infant's age at the time of disease onset, invasive GBS disease in neonates is categorized as early onset or late onset. Early-onset disease is most common and occurs within the first 6 days of life. Almost 90% of infants with early-onset disease have signs of infection within the first 24 hours after birth *(26)*. Premature infants are most likely to have signs of infection within hours of delivery. Clinical evidence of septicemia, pneumonia, and meningitis are the most common manifestations of early-onset disease *(6)*. Meningitis occurs in 5–10% of infants but is much less common than bacteremia and pneumonia. The initial signs of infection are usually nonspecific and include tachypnea, cyanosis, grunting, tachycardia, lethargy, and poor feeding. For infants with pneumonia, the chest x-ray may have changes very similar to those associated with hyaline membrane disease.

An infant with signs of GBS infection beginning from 7 days to 3 months of age has late-onset GBS disease *(6)*. The median time of onset of late-onset disease is 3–4 weeks of age. Late-onset disease may present as bacteremia, meningitis, or focal infections, such as osteomyelitis, septic arthritis, or cellulitis. Intrapartum antibiotics have not been associated with a decline in the incidence of late-onset disease *(6)*.

Neonates with fever, hypothermia, or signs of bacteremia should have blood and urine obtained for cultures and, if there are respiratory symptoms, a chest x-ray. If the infant is stable, a lumbar puncture should also be done for evaluation of possible meningitis because meningitis can occur in 15% of neonates without positive blood cultures *(19)*. Infants with late-onset GBS disease may also have meningitis even when infection is diagnosed at another site *(6)*.

Because the risk of early-onset disease is high in infants born to mothers who have chorioamnionitis, cultures should be obtained from the newborn and antibiotics begun empirically as soon as possible after birth, even if the newborn is asymptomatic and screening for GBS colonization in the mother was negative *(19)*. Antibiotics that will treat GBS as well as other common pathogens in the newborn are recommended until the results of cultures are available.

Importantly, intrapartum antibiotic prophylaxis does not change the clinical spectrum of neonatal illness or the time of onset of early disease *(26)*. Intrapartum prophylaxis is effective in preventing early-onset GBS disease. Thus, asymptomatic newborns born to mothers who are colonized with GBS and receive 4 hours or more of intrapartum antibiotics according to the recommended dosing usually do not require evaluation *(19)*. Observation of the infant is generally recommended. Factors that indicate a full or limited evaluation of the newborn should be considered include maternal chorioamnionitis, evidence of neonatal sepsis or bacteremia, asymptomatic or symptomatic infants born preterm, or delivery less than 4 hours after antibiotic prophylaxis was provided *(19)*.

DIAGNOSTIC ASSAYS FOR GROUP B STREPTOCOCCUS

Cultures are the most common method at this time for diagnosis of GBS infection in neonates and for detection of colonization or infection in pregnant women. To improve the sensitivity of cultures for detection of colonization in pregnant women, the CDC has provided recommendations about the optimal time to obtain cultures during pregnancy, the optimum sites for obtaining cultures, and the processing of clinical specimens in the revised guidelines for prevention of perinatal GBS disease *(19)*. Important details for the clinician providing care to the pregnant woman are that (1) specimens should be obtained at 35–37 weeks of gestation; (2) the lower vagina, followed by the rectum, should be swabbed for culture (cervical cultures are not recommended); (3)

specimens can be collected in the outpatient setting by the health care provider or the patient if appropriate instructions have been provided; (4) swab(s) should be placed into a nonnutritive transport medium, in which GBS will be viable up to 4 days at room temperature or under refrigeration; and (5) labels on the specimens should identify that they are for GBS culture *(19)*.

The use of antenatal cultures to predict intrapartum colonization of women has several limitations. A significant factor is that colonization is not constant but may be intermittent or transient. Another variable is the method used by different practitioners to obtain specimens for culture may provide variation in the predictive value of the cultures. Studies have indicated that the predictive value of antenatal cultures is no greater than 87% and may be much lower *(27)*. Other limitations of antenatal cultures include the possibility that the results may not be available at the time of delivery or that the women did not receive prenatal care.

A final point about cultures in pregnant women that was previously mentioned is that a urine culture that grows any quantity of GBS, regardless of symptoms, is an indicator of heavy colonization, and the woman should receive intrapartum prophylaxis. Vaginal and rectal cultures are not needed *(19)*. To alert laboratories to the need to report any quantity of GBS, urine specimens for cultures require labeling that they are from pregnant women.

Rapid Assays

Rapid antigen assays utilizing the group-specific GBS carbohydrate have been developed for rapid diagnosis of infection. These antigens can be found in the body fluids of infected persons, including the cerebrospinal fluid (CSF), serum, and urine. This antigen is detected by hyperimmune polyclonal antisera or monoclonal antibodies using a number of different test formats, including countercurrent immunoelectrophoresis, enzyme immunoassay, and latex particle agglutination *(6)*. The assays vary in sensitivity, and false-positive assays using both serum and CSF have been reported *(6)*. Only CSF and serum are recommended fluids for testing in neonates and infants *(28)*. Antigen assays should not be used as a substitute for bacterial cultures for diagnosis of GBS because of their limitations but may be useful in addition to cultures for diagnosis.

Rapid assays that are sensitive and specific and can be adapted to a variety of clinical settings could be useful for identifying women with GBS colonization at the time of labor. Polymerase chain reaction-based rapid assays have been developed, and recent assays have been very sensitive and specific when compared with antenatal and intrapartum cultures *(29,30)*. Whether these assays will have a practical application in clinics and hospitals will require further experience with their use.

REFERENCES

1. McCracken GH. Group B streptococcus: the new challenge in neonatal infections. J Pediatr 1973;82:703–706.
2. Baker CJ, Barrett FF, Gordon RC, et al. Suppurative meningitis due to streptococci of Lancefield group B: a study of 33 infants. J Pediatr 1973;82:724–729
3. Zangwill KM, Schuchat A, Wenger JD. Group B streptococcal disease in the United States. 1990; report from a multistate active surveillance system. MMWR Morb Mortal Wkly Rep 1992;41(SS-6):25–32.

4. Schrag SJ, Zywicki S, Farley MM, et al. Group B streptococcal disease in the era of intra-partum antibiotic prophylaxis. N Engl J Med 2000;342:15–20.
5. Schrag SJ. The past and future of perinatal group B streptococcal disease prevention. CID 2004;39:1136–1138.
6. Edward MS, Baker CJ. Group B streptococcal infections. In Remington JS, Klein JO, eds. Infectious Diseases of the Fetus and Newborn Infant, 5th ed. Philadelphia: Saunders, 2001:1091–1156.
7. American Academy of Pediatrics. Group B streptococcal infections. In Pickering LK, ed. Red Book: 2003 Report of the Committee on Infectious Disease 26th ed. Elk Grove Village, IL: American Academy of Pediatrics, 2003: 584–591.
8. Baker CJ, Edwards MS. Group B streptococcal infections: perinatal impact and prevention methods. Ann NY Acad Sci 1988;549:193–202.
9. Easmon CSF, Hastings MJG, Clare AJ, et al. Nosocomial transmission of group B strepto-cocci. BMJ 1981;283:459–461.
10. Anthony BF, Okada DM, Habel CJ. Epidemiology of the group B streptococcus: maternal and nosocomial sources for infant acquisitions. J Pediatr 1979;95:435–436.
11. Boyer KM, Gadzala CA, Kelly PD, et al. Selective intrapartum chemoprophylaxis of neo-natal group B streptococcal early-onset disease: II. Predictive value of prenatal cultures. J Infect Dis 1983;148:802–809.
12. Pass MA, Gary BM, Khare S, et al. Prospective studies of group B streptococcal infections in infants. J Pediatr 1979;95:437–443.
13. Schuchat A, Deaver-Robinson K, Plikaytis BD, et al. Multistate case-control study of ma-ternal risk factors for neonatal group B streptococcal disease. Pediatr Infect Dis J 1994;13:623–629.
14. Baker CJ, Barrett FF. Transmission of group B streptococci among parturient women and their neonates. J Pediatr 1973;83:919–925.
15. Dillon HC, Khare S, Gray BM. Group B streptococcal carriage and disease: a 6-year pro-spective study. J Pediatr 1987;110:31–35.
16. Schrag SJ, Zywick S, Farley MM, et al. Group B streptococcal disease in the era of intra-partum antibiotic prophylaxis. N Engl J Med 2000;342:15–20.
17. Baker CJ, Edwards MS, Kasper DL. Role of antibody to native type III polysaccharide of group B streptococcus in infant infections. Pediatrics 1981;68:544–549.
18. Boyer KM, Gotoff SP. Strategies for chemoprophylaxis of GBS early-onset disease. J In-fect Disease 1983;148:802–802.
19. Centers for Disease Control and Prevention. Prevention of perinatal group B streptococcal disease. Revised guidelines from CDC. MMWR Morb Mortal Wkly Rep 2002;51(RR-11):1–22.
20. Mead PB. Infections of the female pelvis. In: Mandell GL, Bennett JE, Dolin R, eds. Prin-ciples and Practice of Infectious Diseases, 5th ed. Philadelphia: Churchill Livingstone, 2000:1235–1243.
21. American College of Obstetricians and Gynecologists, Committee on Obstetric Practice. Prevention of Early-Onset Group B Streptococcal Disease in Newborns (Opinion 173). Washington, DC: American College of Obstetricians and Gynecologists, 1996.
22. Centers for Disease Control and Prevention. Prevention of perinatal group B streptococcal disease: a public health perspective. MMWR Morb Mortal Wkly Rep 1996;45(RR-7):1–24.
23. American Academy of Pediatrics, Committee on Infectious Diseases/Committee on Fetus and Newborn. Revised guidelines for prevention of early-onset group B streptococcal (GBS) disease. Pediatrics 1997;99:489–496.
24. Schuchat A, Hilger T, Zell A, et al. Active Bacterial Core Surveillance of the Emerging Infections Program Network. Emerg Infect Dis 2001;7:92–99.
25. Schrag SJ, Zell ER, Lynfield R, et al. A population-based comparison of strategies to pre-vent early-onset group B streptococcal disease in neonates. N Engl J Med 2002;347:233–239.

26. Bromberger P, Lawrence JM, Braun D, et al. The influence of intrapartum antibiotics on the clinical spectrum of early-onset group B streptococcal infection in term infants. Pediatrics 2000;106:244–250.

27. Yancey MK, Schuchat A, Brown LK, et al. The accuracy of late antenatal screening cultures in predicting genital group B streptococcal colonization at delivery. Obstet Gynecol 1996;88:811–815.

28. FDA Alert. Safety alert re: risk of misdiagnosis of group B streptococcal infection. JAMA 1997;277:1343.

29. Davies HD, Miller MA, Faro S, et al. Multicenter study of a rapid molecular-based assay for the diagnosis of group B streptococcus colonization in pregnant women. Clin Infect Dis 2004;39:1129–1135.

30. Bergeron MG, Ke D, Menard C, et al. Rapid detection of group B streptococci in pregnant women at delivery. N Engl J Med 2000;343:175–179.

20

Listeria monocytogenes, Neisseria gonorrhoeae, and Other Bacteria

Katherine M. Knapp

LISTERIA MONOCYTOGENES

Introduction

Listeria monocytogenes is a motile Gram-positive bacterium that is a frequent cause of zoonotic infections, most often associated with abortion and meningoencephalitis in cattle and sheep. *L. monocytogenes* had been described as the etiologic agent of infectious mononucleosis soon after it was first isolated, but subsequent evidence revealed that the disease manifestations in humans are similar to those observed in animals. Human infections caused by this organism are not common. Neonates, pregnant women, and the elderly or immunocompromised are most at risk for infections caused by *L. monocytogenes*. Neonatal listeriosis is the most common form of the infection and is divided into early onset (manifesting in the first days of life) and late onset (after the first week of life) disease. The organism is widespread in the environment and is commonly found in soil and decayed matter. Almost all human cases are related to ingestion of contaminated food. Vegetable, meat, and dairy products have all been identified as source items in large outbreaks of listeriosis *(1–6)*.

The Organism

The microscopic appearance of the organism may vary greatly, depending on the age of the culture and laboratory techniques. Gram staining will typically reveal short Gram-positive rods. Younger cultures may have a more coccoid appearance. Older cultures tend to be Gram variable, and overdecolorization with Gram staining on direct examination may lead to the erroneous diagnosis of *Haemophilus influenzae* infection *(7)*. *L. monocytogenes* is typically described as having a characteristic "tumbling motility." *L. monocytogenes* will grow optimally on blood agar plates at 30–37°C. Colonies are surrounded by narrow zones of β-hemolysis.

Transmission

L. monocytogenes is a common organism in soil and decaying vegetation. Animals feeding on spoiled vegetation become infected and can subsequently reinfect the soil via fecal colonization. Humans can acquire the organism via direct transmission from

From: *Infectious Disease: Congenital and Perinatal Infections: A Concise Guide to Diagnosis*
Edited by: C. Hutto © Humana Press Inc., Totowa, NJ

animals: veterinarians and others have become infected while delivering infected animals. Farmers and abattoir workers have also been found to have higher rates of seropositivity and fecal carriage of *L. monocytogenes* than the general population *(7)*. However, the majority of human cases result from ingestion of contaminated food sources.

In the 1980s, there were several large outbreaks of food-borne listeriosis involving pregnant women and immunocompromised patients *(1–3,5)*. In the first such foodborne outbreak to be described, cabbage that had been fertilized with contaminated sheep manure was identified as the food source in a listeriosis outbreak in the Canadian Maritimes in 1980–1981 *(1)*.

Dairy products have long been identified as sources in outbreaks of *L. monocytogenes*. In one report from the 1980s, contaminated milk was the source, despite the fact that it had been properly pasteurized *(2)*. The mechanism by which this milk remained contaminated despite pasteurization remains unclear, although the authors speculated that this outbreak might have been caused by a large inoculum of *Listeria*.

In the 1990s, the Listeria Study Group of the Centers for Disease Control and Prevention published the results of microbiological, epidemiological, and risk factor studies conducted in the United States *(8,9)*. These studies definitively established the significant role of food items in transmission of *Listeria* during outbreaks and demonstrated that ingestion of soft cheeses and deli meats and, for immunosuppressed patients, ingestion of improperly cooked chicken are important risk factors for acquisition of infection. Reports of food-borne outbreaks in the late 1980s were well publicized and led to aggressive regulatory efforts to ensure proper food handling *(10)*. It appears that heightened awareness of listeriosis risks and improved regulatory control of food processing may have had some effect on the incidence of listeriosis in this country: The Listeriosis Study Group reported a 44% decrease in incidence of listeriosis (and a 48% decrease in death rate) from 1989 to 1993 *(10)*.

Perinatal infections are thought to comprise approx 30% of the total number of cases of listeriosis *(7)*. Maternal infection is transmitted to the infant transplacentally and perhaps via ascending infection as well. *L. monocytogenes* has been demonstrated to have a marked predilection for the fetoplacental unit.

Risk of Infection for the Mother and Child

Both fecal carriage of *L. monocytogenes* and cases of listeriosis are uncommon, although their exact incidences are difficult to determine. The majority of cases of listeriosis occur in immunocompromised adults. Gastrointestinal illness caused by *Listeria* is not considered a reportable incident, and many such self-limited infections may resolve without a microbiological diagnosis. In addition, in the absence of active surveillance systems, it is felt that cases of invasive listeriosis are more than likely underreported *(7)*.

Studies have suggested that the incidence of fecal or vaginal carriage of *Listeria* does not differ between pregnant and nonpregnant persons. Although pregnant women do not appear to have increased colonization rates over the general population, *Listeria* has a marked predilection for the placental unit. Pregnant women are advised to take precautionary measures to prevent food-borne listeriosis: they should avoid soft cheeses, thoroughly reheat leftovers and ready-to-eat items, and consider avoiding delicatessen meats. The Listeriosis Study Group reported a decrease in incidence of peri-natal disease from 17.4 to 8.6 cases per 100,000 births from 1989 to 1993 *(10)*. Asymp-tomatic fecal carriage that leads to vaginal colonization may explain the development of late-onset listeriosis in babies born to seemingly healthy mothers.

Although mother-to-child transmission is clearly the most likely mechanism by which infants become infected with *Listeria*, there have been several reports of nosocomially acquired listeriosis in neonates *(7,11)*. In these cases, poor infection con-trol measures have been implicated in the spread of infection from an infant with early-onset listeriosis to other infants, who subsequently develop manifestations of late-onset disease.

Prenatal Evaluation

Listeria monocytogenes has been demonstrated to have a predilection for the pla-centa and adjacent tissues. Gross examination of the infected placenta may reveal mul-tiple small whitish lesions. Histological evaluation of the placenta reveals microabscesses and acute villitis, usually accompanied by chorioamnionitis. *Listeria* may be transmitted from the mother to the fetus transplacentally or via ascending in-fection. Most identified cases of perinatal listeriosis occur in the third trimester or late second trimester. In the majority of these cases, infection is identified following a still-birth or preterm delivery of a septic infant. Maternal listeriosis occurring earlier in pregnancy is associated with septic abortion and is identified less commonly, although the incidence may be greater than is reported.

Although the mortality rate of perinatal listeriosis is quite high (40–50%), early treat-ment of the mother can decrease morbidity in the infant or even prevent transmission of disease. Maternal infection may be inapparent or nonspecific: Often, the mother will have a history of flu-like illness a few days to 2 weeks before delivery. Although these symptoms might be resolved by the time of delivery, it is common for infection and fever to precipitate delivery. Blood cultures from infected mothers are usually positive. Typically, infected mothers will deliver prematurely, more than two-thirds prior to 35 weeks estimated gestation.

Clinical Evaluation of the Neonate

Early-Onset Disease

Early-onset listeriosis typically manifests in the infant within the first 2 days of life, although symptoms may not be evident until later in the first week of life. The majority of infants will be symptomatic at birth. Meconium-stained amniotic fluid, cyanosis, and respiratory distress are common findings in the delivery room. Many infants will require ventilatory support. Pneumonia is a frequent finding and is usually nonspecific, although it may progress to a more nodular pattern. Severely infected infants may de-velop a granulomatous skin rash (granulomatosis infantisepticum) consisting of small raised lesions with an erythematous base. Biopsies of such rashes will reveal multiple bacteria along with a leukocytic infiltrate.

Laboratory evaluation of the infant with early-onset listeriosis is nonspecific. Leu-kocytosis with a "left shift" is common, as are findings of thrombocytopenia and ane-mia. Alternatively, the very sick infant may manifest neutropenia rather than leukocytosis. These laboratory values will not distinguish listeriosis from other perina-tal bacterial infections.

Late-Onset Disease

Late-onset disease is much less common than early-onset disease and usually affects term newborns 1–8 weeks after birth. Whereas meningitis is an uncommon presentation of early-onset disease, this finding characterizes more than 80% of cases of late-onset perinatal listeriosis. In most cases of late-onset disease, there is no maternal history of preceding illness. Most infants will have fever and irritability but may not appear severely ill, thus leading to delays in diagnosis. Other, much less common, manifestations of late-onset disease include colitis/diarrhea and sepsis in the absence of meningitis.

As with early-onset disease, laboratory findings are nonspecific. Cerebrospinal fluid (CSF) white cell counts are typically high, with a polymorphonuclear predominance. Elevated monocyte counts in the CSF may be seen rarely, in cases of prolonged disease. Gram stains of the CSF may be nondiagnostic because of low numbers of organisms or because of pleomorphic appearance of the organism, suggesting the presence of Gram-negative bacilli or Gram-positive cocci. Mortality from late-onset listeriosis is low when the disease is recognized promptly, and adverse sequelae are rare.

Diagnostic Assays

Isolation of the organism remains the only reliable means of diagnosing *L. monocytogenes* infection. Both maternal and infant blood cultures are often positive. Stool cultures should not be used to diagnose infection as 1–5% of healthy women will be culture-positive for *L. monocytogenes*. Serologic tests have historically been unreliable in diagnosing listeriosis. Agglutination reactions to whole-cell antigens are difficult to interpret because of the large degree of cross-reactivity with other Gram-positive organisms *(12)*. Complement fixation tests have shown low sensitivity and positive predictive value. Initial work in detection of anti-listeriolysin O antibodies has shown to be a promising area for future diagnostic testing *(13)*. Highly sensitive and specific polymerase chain reaction testing to detect *L. monocytogenes* deoxyribonucleic acid in CSF and tissue specimens is available through specialized laboratories *(12,14)*.

NEISSERIA GONORRHOEAE

Introduction

Neisseria gonorrhoeae is an aerobic, Gram-negative bacterium that was first observed in purulent urethral discharge and has since been well described as an etiologic agent of ophthalmia neonatorum. It has only been in the past few decades that other disease manifestations have been described in infants.

The Organism

N. gonorrhoeae is a Gram-negative diplococcus with adjacent sides flattened, also known as gonococcus. There are several other species of *Neisseria* known to colonize or cause disease in humans, including *Neisseria meningitidis* (meningococcus). *N. gonorrhoeae* is differentiated from these other species primarily by differences in sugar fermentation. Gonococci are usually cultured on chocolate blood agar in a carbon dioxide-enriched atmosphere during incubation. To avoid the overgrowth of normal flora from nonsterile sites, specimens may be inoculated onto a selective medium (e.g., modified Thayer-Martin medium).

There are four distinct colony types of *N. gonorrhoeae*. Types 1 and 2 are seen on primary isolation and are more virulent than types 3 and 4, which are only seen after repeated subculturing at 37°C. Types 1 and 2 have pili, which play a significant role in the initial attachment of the organism to host cells and inhibition of phagocytosis *(15)*. Colonies also differ in opacity: opaque colonies exhibit surface proteins that affect gonococcal interaction with cells, whereas transparent colonies lack these proteins. Pathogenic gonococcal isolates typically form opaque colonies on agar medium.

The *N. gonorrhoeae* strains may be distinguished from one another by different means of typing *(15)*. Auxotyping defines about 20 types of gonococci based on growth characteristics in the absence of certain amino acids and other substrates. Gonococci are also differentiated by typing methods based on the predominant outer membrane protein, protein I. There are three serogroups of gonococci (WI, WII, and WIII) encompassing nine antigenic types based on enzyme-linked immunosorbent assay of protein I. Typing using monoclonal antibodies to protein I offers the greatest discrimination among gonococcal strains; approx 50 serotypes belonging to two serogroups (1A and 1B) may be differentiated.

Transmission

There are an estimated 600,000 new gonococcal infections in the United States each year *(16)*. Rates of infection are highest in 15- to 24-year-olds and in non-white, urban populations. Infected males are usually symptomatic, with a purulent urethral discharge, and typically seek treatment before the occurrence of sequelae but often after sexual transmission to others. In contrast, gonococcal infection in women is often asymptomatic until complications (pelvic inflammatory disease) arise.

The majority of neonatal gonococcal infections follow vaginal delivery of the infant to an infected mother. Gonococcal infection has also been documented in infants born via cesarean section following rupture of membranes. Gonococcal infections in infants beyond the first month of life are almost always caused by sexual contact *(15)*.

Risk of Infection for the Mother and Child

Because of risks of neonatal infection and adverse outcome of pregnancy, it is recommended that pregnant women routinely be tested for gonorrhea at the first prenatal visit. Rates of gonorrhea are highest in young, non-white, urban women of low socioeconomic status. High-risk sexual behaviors and previous history of a sexually transmitted disease are additional risk factors for infection. Women at high risk of becoming infected with *N. gonorrhoeae* should have repeat testing later in pregnancy.

Pregnant women have a decreased risk of developing ascending gonococcal infection when compared with nonpregnant women. However, ascending infection during pregnancy may result in septic abortion or premature rupture of the membranes. Pregnant women with gonococcal infection are at a substantial risk of delivering prematurely. Infection during pregnancy has also been associated with chorioamnionitis and delayed delivery after membrane rupture. In addition to preterm birth, infants of untreated mothers are more at risk for perinatal distress (5–10%) and even death (2–11%).

Prenatal Evaluation

Mothers at high risk for gonococcal infection should have repeat testing late in pregnancy. Women diagnosed with gonorrhea during pregnancy should be retested closer to delivery, bearing in mind that reinfection is common. Endocervical cultures are recommended for women with premature rupture of membranes, septic abortion, or fever during labor and delivery. Infants born to mothers with untreated gonorrhea are at high risk of infection.

Clinical Evaluation of the Neonate

Ophthalmia neonatorum is the most widely recognized manifestation of gonococcal disease in the newborn infant. Soon after this entity was first described, Credé reported a decrease in the incidence of ophthalmia neonatorum following topical use of silver nitrate solution in the eyes of newborns *(15)*. *N. gonorrhoeae* is still a common cause of neonatal conjunctivitis and blindness in many parts of the world but is now rarely the etiologic agent of ophthalmia neonatorum in the United States and other developed countries. Infected infants develop an acute purulent conjunctivitis 2–5 days after birth. The exudates are typically thick and bilateral and may be hemorrhagic. Disease may manifest later in some infants, and some neonates may have only mild symptoms; therefore, gonococcal infection should be considered in *any* infant with conjunctivitis. If appropriate treatment is delayed, infection may spread to subconjunctival tissues and the cornea, where it may cause ulceration and perforation.

The differential diagnosis of ophthalmia neonatorum includes chemical conjunctivitis following prophylaxis, *Chlamydia trachomatis*, and herpes simplex virus infection. Eye irritation caused by silver nitrate prophylaxis is mild and usually develops by 6 hours after birth and resolves within the first day of life. *C. trachomatis* is the most common cause of neonatal conjunctivitis in developed countries and typically manifests within 5–14 days after birth. As with gonococcal infection, ophthalmic evidence of herpes simplex virus infection manifests within the first few days of life and may lead to corneal involvement. Fluorescein staining of the cornea is recommended in all cases of neonatal conjunctivitis.

Septic Arthritis

Arthritis is the most commonly recognized systemic manifestation of gonococcal disease in infants. Ophthalmia neonatorum is often not present in infants with gonococcal arthritis. Infants may have evidence of proctitis or vulvovaginitis. Arthritis typically develops after the first week of life and presents as refusal to move the limb. Multiple joint involvement is characteristic of gonococcal arthritis in the neonate. Infants have variable functional outcomes following arthritis, and those with hip involvement are at high risk for development of aseptic necrosis of the femoral head. Clinicians should be alert to the possibility of gonococcal arthritis in infants born to infected mothers and pay particular attention to the infant's limb movement throughout the neonatal course.

Other Neonatal Manifestations

In addition to the conjunctivas, infected maternal secretions may also directly inoculate the pharynx. Infants with pharyngeal involvement may develop a cough soon after birth. Other manifestations of local mucosal involvement, such as vaginitis and urethritis, typically present later in the neonatal period. There have been several reports of neonatal scalp abscesses following fetal electrode monitoring in infected pregnant women. Systemic manifestations of gonococcal infection other than arthritis are quite rare in neonates.

Diagnostic Assays

In cases of ophthalmia neonatorum, conjunctival specimens should be sent to the laboratory for Gram stain and culture on blood agar and Thayer-Martin agar. If gonococcal infection is suspected based on Gram stain or clinical history or is subsequently identified, rectal and pharyngeal specimens should also be obtained. Because of the increasing rates of antibiotic resistance in gonococcal infection, isolates should undergo susceptibility testing. Because patients with gonorrhea are often co-infected with *C. trachomatis*, infants with ophthalmia neonatorum should also be tested for chlamydia.

There is very little information about the use of the newer rapid methods of diagnosis in children. These nucleic acid probe and enzyme-linked immunosorbent assay tests have not been approved by the Food and Drug Administration for use in infants. Culture of the organism remains the only approved method by which to diagnose gonococcal infection definitively in children.

OTHER BACTERIA CAUSING PERINATAL DISEASE

Obviously, it is beyond the scope of this text to provide a detailed description of all other recognized bacterial pathogens in neonates. Of the many bacterial species that may be part of the normal flora of the infant or mother, there are certain ones that deserve further mention.

Staphylococcal Infections

Staphylococcus aureus has been described in nursery outbreaks for more than 100 years. It has only been recently that *Staphylococcus epidermidis* has received attention as an increasing cause of neonatal sepsis. *S. epidermidis* infections are especially common among infants who are premature or who otherwise require catheter placement, and this organism is the most frequent etiologic agent of sepsis in some neonatal intensive care units. Although positive blood cultures might be caused by contamination with skin flora during the specimen collection, the isolation of coagulase-negative staphylococci should not be readily dismissed.

Prevention of the spread of *S. aureus* colonization within the nursery is a challenging prospect. Neonatal staphylococcal skin infections include bullous impetigo, staphylococcal scalded skin syndrome, and toxic shock syndrome. Staphylococcal pneumonia is associated with significant mortality and is characterized by the formation of microabscesses, which may rupture and lead to empyema, and by the formation of pneumatocoeles because of obstruction of terminal bronchioles. Osteomyelitis is infrequent and manifests differently in neonates than in older children. In neonatal osteomyelitis, the membranous bones (scapula, maxilla) are affected as well as the long bones. In addition, neonates with osteomyelitis may not exhibit fever or laboratory abnormalities suggestive of infection. Staphylococcal endocarditis is rare in neonates.

Other Gram-Positive Bacteria

Infections caused by group A streptococci may be acquired intra- or postpartum. Infection may be acquired from an asymptomatic carrier or from someone with clinically apparent infection, such as pharyngitis. Disease manifestations in neonates include omphalitis, cellulitis, pneumonia, sepsis, meningitis, and osteomyelitis. Enterococcal infections have also been reported with increasing frequency in neonatal intensive care units. Pneumococcal infections are also seen more frequently in younger children and may mimic group B streptococcal infections in neonates.

Enterobacteriaceae

Infants may become colonized with maternal coliform bacteria during delivery. *Escherichia coli* is a frequent cause of neonatal urinary tract infections and may cause sepsis or meningitis. Citrobacter species (*Citrobacter diversus*) are associated with neonatal brain abscess. *Enterobacter sakazakii* and *Enterobacter cloacae* may cause severe necrotizing meningitis in neonates. Isolation of these Gram-negative organisms should prompt careful evaluation of the neonate; involvement of the central nervous system may at first be inapparent, and outcomes may be devastating if infection is not recognized and promptly treated. Infants with meningitis caused by these organisms should have follow-up lumbar punctures.

REFERENCES

1. Schlech WF III, Lavigne PM, Bortolussi R, et al. Epidemic listeriosis—evidence for transmission by food. N Engl J Med 1983;308:203.
2. Fleming DW, Cochi SL, MacDonald KL, et al. Pasteurized milk as a vehicle of infection in an outbreak of listeriosis. N Engl J Med 1985;312:404–407.
3. Linnan MJ, Mascola L, Lou XD, et al. Epidemic listeriosis associated with Mexican-style cheese. N Engl J Med 1988;319:823–828.
4. Aureli P, Fiorucci GC, Caroli D, et al. An outbreak of febrile gastroenteritis associated with corn contaminated by *Listeria monocytogenes*. N Engl J Med 2000;342:1236–1241.
5. Schlech WF III. Foodborne listeriosis. Clin Infect Dis 2000;31:770–775.
6. Centers for Disease Control and Prevention. Multistate outbreak of listeriosis—United States, 2000. MMWR Morb Mortal Wkly Rep 2000;49:1129–1130.
7. Bortolussi R, Schlech WF III. Listeriosis. In: Remington JS, Klein JO, ed. Infectious Diseases of the Fetus and Newborn Infant, 4th ed. Philadelphia: Saunders, 1995:1055–1073.
8. Schuchat A, Deaver KA, Wenger JD, et al. Role of foods in sporadic listeriosis. I. Case-control study of dietary risk factors. The Listeria Study Group. JAMA 1992;267:2041–2045.
9. Pinner RW, Schuchat A, Swaminathan B, et al. Role of foods in sporadic listeriosis. II. Microbiologic and epidemiologic investigation. The Listeria Study Group. JAMA 1992;267:2046–2050.
10. Tappero JW, Schuchat A, Deaver KA, et al. Reduction in the incidence of human listeriosis in the United States. Effectiveness of prevention efforts? The Listeriosis Study Group. JAMA 1995:273;1118–1122.
11. Schuchat A, Lizano C, Broome CV, et al. Outbreak of neonatal listeriosis associated with mineral oil. Pediatr Infect Dis J 1991;10:183–189.
12. Bille J, Rocourt J, Swaminathan B. Listeria, erysipelothrix, and kurthia. In: Murray PR, Baron EJ, Pfaller MA, et al., eds. Manual of Clinical Microbiology, 7th ed. Washington, DC: American Society for Microbiology, 1999:346–352.
13. Gholizadeh Y, Poyart C, Juvin M, et al. Serodiagnosis of listeriosis based upon detection of antibodies against recombinant truncated forms of listeriolysin O. J Clin Microbiol 1996:34;1391–1395.
14. Jaton K, Sahli R, Bille J. Development of polymerase chain reaction assays for detection of *Listeria monocytogenes* in clinical cerebrospinal fluid samples. J Clin Microbiol 1992:30;1931–1936.
15. Gutman LT. In: Remington JS, Klein JO, ed. Gonococcal Infection. Infectious Diseases of the Fetus and Newborn Infant, 4th ed. Philadelphia: Saunders, 1995:1087–1104.
16. Centers for Disease Control and Prevention. 1998 Guidelines for treatment of sexually transmitted diseases. MMWR Morb Mortal Wkly Rep 1998;47:59–70.

21

Mycobacterium tuberculosis

Kim Connelly Smith and Jeffrey R. Starke

DESCRIPTION OF ORGANISM

The genus, *Mycobacterium*, is classified in the order of Actinomycetales and the family Mycobacteriaceae. In general, species of mycobacteria that are pathogenic to humans are more acid fast, grow more slowly, form less pigment, and are more susceptible to chemotherapy than are saprophytic species.

Acid-fastness is the capacity to form stable mycolate complexes with certain arylmethane dyes such as carbol-fuchsin, crystal violet, and auramine and rhodamine, which are not readily removed even by rinsing with 95% ethanol plus hydrochloric acid. Acid-fastness is often regarded as the hallmark of mycobacteria, although other organisms such as *Nocardia* and *Cryptosporidium* display acid-fastness with modified stains. Mycobacteria appear red when stained with fuchsin (Ziehl-Neelsen or Kinyoun stains) and purple with crystal violet or exhibit yellow-green fluorescence under ultraviolet light when stained with auramine and rhodamine (Truant stain). Truant stain is the most sensitive, particularly important for use on specimens from children or extrapulmonary specimens from adults for whom the number of organisms is low.

Classic media for mycobacterial growth consisted of egg yolk and glycerin, with a malachite green dye to inhibit growth of other organisms. Mycobacterial also grow well in simple synthetic media, with an admixture of asparagines, glutamate, and amino acid mixtures (Middlebrook 7H9 medium). Isolation of *Mycobacterium tuberculosis* on solid media often takes 3–6 weeks. Traditional methods to determine drug susceptibility using solid media containing various antituberculosis drugs usually required an additional 2–3 weeks.

More rapid isolation, identification, and drug susceptibility testing can be carried out using liquid medium in an automated radiometric system known as BACTEC. A decontaminated, concentrated specimen is inoculated into a culture bottle containing carbon-14-labeled palmitic acid as the substrate. As mycobacteria metabolize the carbon-14 palmitic acid, carbon dioxide-14 accumulates in the headspace of the bottle, where the radioactivity can be measured. Cross contamination of bottles can occur, resulting in false-positive cultures, when the needle used to sample bottles on the automated system is not properly heated (and sterilized) between measurements. Using this and other similar liquid broth culture systems, the time for identification and drug susceptibility testing can be reduced to 1–3 weeks, depending on the size of the inoculum *(1)*.

From: *Infectious Disease: Congenital and Perinatal Infections: A Concise Guide to Diagnosis*
Edited by: C. Hutto © Humana Press Inc., Totowa, NJ

TIMING AND ROUTES OF TRANSMISSION

The pathogenesis of tuberculosis (TB) infection and disease during pregnancy is similar to that for nonpregnant individuals. The usual portal of entry of *M. tuberculosis* is the lung via inhalation of infected droplet nuclei discharged by an infectious individual. After several weeks of replication within the lungs, some organisms are carried within macrophages from the initial lung parenchymal focus to the regional lymph nodes. From there, organisms enter lymphatic and blood vessels and disseminate throughout the body; the genitalia, endometrium, and, if the woman is pregnant, the placenta may be seeded. Specific immunity develops in several more weeks in normal hosts, and both pulmonary and extrapulmonary infection are halted and walled off. If the host later becomes immunosuppressed, dormant organisms within these walled-off foci may become active, leading to so-called reactivation disease.

There are two major ways that TB infection in the mother can lead to infection of the fetus *in utero*. If dissemination of organisms through the blood and lymphatic channels occurs during pregnancy, the placenta may be infected directly. This can occur as part of an asymptomatic dissemination that accompanies the mother's initial infection or can be a complication of pulmonary or disseminated TB disease in the mother. Infection with *M. tuberculosis* that occurs during pregnancy, as opposed to dormant infection that occurred prior to pregnancy, poses a greater risk to the fetus. The second mechanism by which a fetus can be infected with *M. tuberculosis* is directly from established genitourinary TB in the mother. Genital TB is most likely to start around menarche and can have a long and relatively asymptomatic course. The fallopian tubes are most often affected, followed by the uterus, ovaries, and cervix *(2)*. Sterility is a common complaint with genitourinary TB, explaining one reason why congenital TB is a rare disease. Tuberculosis in the mother as a complication of in vitro fertilization has been described *(3)*.

Congenital (acquired *in utero*) TB can be acquired in one of three ways: (1) from the infected placenta via the umbilical vein; (2) by inhalation of infected amniotic fluid; and (3) by ingestion of infected amniotic fluid. Neonatal (acquired after birth) TB can be acquired in four different ways: (1) by inhalation of infected droplets; (2) by ingestion of infected droplets; (3) by ingestion of infected milk (theoretical only); and (4) by contamination of traumatized skin or mucous membranes *(4)*. It is often not possible to elucidate the route of infection in a particular neonate. However, it is important to try to identify the source of infection so the person infecting the infant can be treated and transmission stopped.

Infection of the fetus through the umbilical cord with *M. tuberculosis* is rare, with fewer than 300 cases reported in the English language literature. These infants' mothers frequently suffer from TB disease during pregnancy or soon after. The intensity of lymphohematogenous spread during pregnancy is one of the factors that determine if congenital TB will occur. *M. tuberculosis* has been demonstrated in the deciduas, amnion, and chorionic villi of a hematogenously infected placenta. Organisms also can reach the placenta by direct extension from a tuberculous salpingeal tube. However, even massive involvement of the placenta does not necessarily give rise to congenital infection. It is not clear if the fetus can be infected directly from the mother's bloodstream without a caseous lesion forming first in the placenta, but this route of transmission has been demonstrated in experimental animal models.

Congenital infection of the infant also can occur through aspiration or ingestion of infected amniotic fluid. If the caseous lesion in the placenta ruptures directly into the amniotic cavity, the fetus can inhale or ingest the bacilli. This route of transmission is likely if the infant has multiple primary foci in the lung, gut, or middle ear.

Postnatal acquisition of *M. tuberculosis* through airborne inoculation is the most common route of transmission to the neonate. Any adult in the neonate's environment, including health care workers, can be a source of airborne transmission. Historical studies suggest that 40% of infants with untreated, postnatally acquired TB infection develop disease within 1 year. In one study of 48 infants exposed during the pretreatment era to their mothers with pulmonary TB, 21 became infected; of the infants who developed TB disease, signs such as fever, tachypnea, weight loss, and hepatosplenomegaly developed in 4–8 weeks *(5)*. Because newborn infants infected with *M. tuberculosis* are at a very high risk of developing serious forms of disease, public health investigation of an adult with TB whose close contacts include a pregnant woman or newborn should be undertaken emergently.

RISK OF MATERNAL INFECTION

Between 1985 and 1992, there was a 20% increase in the total number of TB cases in the United States and a 40% increase among children *(6)*. Factors contributing to the resurgence included increased immigration, the human immunodeficiency virus (HIV) epidemic, a decline in public health services, and a rise in homeless and incarcerated populations. Rates among young adults of childbearing age increased dramatically and contributed to increased rates in children. At the same time, the emergence of multidrug-resistant TB was recognized as a new threat because it is very difficult to cure, with high mortality rates even with therapy. National and international efforts, as well as increased funding to combat the problem, stopped the rise of TB in the United States in 1993. Since the 1992 peak, the rate of TB has dropped 50%, from 10.5 cases per 100,000 people in 1992 to 5.2 cases per 100,000 in 2002 *(7)*. Still, an estimated 4–6% of the US population or about 15 million people are infected with TB. Without treatment for latent infection, this group represents a large reservoir from which future cases of active disease will emerge. Worldwide, TB remains one of the leading causes of death from an infectious agent, with one-third of the world's population infected, 8 million new cases and approx 2 million deaths reported each year *(8)*. Tuberculosis is a significant public health problem, especially in our global community.

Assessing the risk for maternal infection depends on epidemiologic and individual risk factors. Geographically, in the United States TB is most common in areas with ethnically diverse populations, large urban areas, coastal states, and states bordering Mexico. An estimated 30–50% of recent immigrants have latent TB infection, and many will develop active TB within 5 years of moving to the United States. Between 1992 and 2002, the percentage of cases in the United States from foreign-born individuals increased from 27 to 51% *(7)*. For all other populations, the rate of TB cases has decreased since 1993. In foreign-born and poor minority populations, almost 40% of the cases in women occur before 35 years of age, during the childbearing years. Other risk factors, such as HIV infection, incarceration, and recent immigration, are more common in young adults, who are more likely to have contact with children. Higher rates among young minority women, especially in lower socioeconomic groups, account for

Table 1
High-Risk Groups for Tuberculosis (TB) Infection and Disease

Groups at high-risk of exposure or infection
    Close contacts of person with TB
    Foreign-born persons from high-risk countries (Asia, Africa, Latin America, Russia,
        eastern Europe)
    Residents and employees of high-risk congregate settings (correctional institutions,
        nursing homes, homeless shelters, hospitals serving high-risk populations, drug
        treatment centers)
    Medically underserved, low-income populations
    High-risk racial or ethnic minority populations
    Injection drug users
    Children exposed to adults in high-risk categories

Groups at higher risk of developing disease once infected
    Immunosuppressed patients, including HIV infected
    Recent TB infection (within past 2 years)
    Persons with certain medical conditions (diabetes mellitus, silicosis, cancer, end-stage
        renal disease, gastrectomy, low body weight $\leq 10\%$ ideal)
    Injection drug users
    History of inadequately treated TB
    Children ≤ 4 years of age, especially infants

the fact that 87% of TB cases in children in the United States occurred in minority populations in 2002 *(7)*.

Pregnancy is a time when young women access health care on a regular basis and presents an opportunity to screen for and prevent disease. Physicians should be aware of and ask questions regarding symptoms of active TB as well as screen for risk factors for latent TB infection. Any patient with risk factors or symptoms should have a tuberculin skin test. If the skin test is positive, a complete physical examination looking for active disease and a chest radiograph should be obtained. High-risk groups for TB infection and disease are listed in Table 1 *(9)*. The most significant risk factor for TB infection is a history of exposure to someone with contagious TB. Some providers use questionnaires as a screening tool for risk factors.

Opinions about the effects of pregnancy on TB have varied over time. Most studies since the 1950s have shown no significant difference in active TB rates in pregnant women compared to nonpregnant women or the general population *(10)*. Based on the most recent data, pregnancy does not appear to increase the risk of progression to active TB in women with latent TB infection *(11)*. The risk in pregnant women is comparable to the general population, with about 5% of those with latent infection progressing to active disease within 2 years after infection, and an additional 5% developing active TB disease later in life.

RISK OF FETAL OR PERINATAL INFECTION

Tuberculosis in the neonate may be acquired congenitally or postnatally following contact with a contagious adult. Congenital TB is extremely rare. The most common route of infection for young infants is after birth, via respiratory exposure to an adult in the home with active pulmonary TB. Any infectious adult, including the mother, family members, frequent visitors to the home, hospital or day care staff, could be a source of postnatal infection.

Infants and young children are particularly vulnerable to TB if infected, and they have a much higher risk of progression to active disease than adults. Infected infants are more likely to have extrapulmonary and disseminated TB, which can progress early and rapidly, as soon as 1 month following infection (12). TB meningitis and miliary TB are usually fatal if unrecognized and untreated. Sometimes, the infant will become seriously ill with TB so quickly that the adult source case may not be recognized until after the investigation of household and family contacts is initiated. Because infants may quickly progress to more serious forms of TB following infection, they should be evaluated and placed on prophylactic therapy as soon as possible following exposure whether the source case is the mother or another adult in the home (13).

The key to assessing the risk of exposure or infection for infants is determining the infectiousness of adults in the home. For an adult to be contagious, he or she must aerosolize mycobacteria by coughing. In most cases, contagious adults with TB have pulmonary disease with abnormal findings on chest x-ray and symptoms of chronic cough, fever, and weight loss. Sputum smears usually show acid-fast bacilli (AFB) on microscopic examination, and cultures are positive for TB.

The presentation of TB is the same in pregnant and nonpregnant women. One study in 27 pregnant women with culture-confirmed TB reported the following symptoms: 74% had cough; 41% had weight loss; 30% had fever, malaise, or fatigue; 19% had hemoptysis; and 20% were asymptomatic; all had abnormal radiographs (14). Pulmonary disease is most common in pregnant women, with extrapulmonary TB seen in about 5–10% of cases, the same as in the general adult population (15). Any patient with symptoms of TB should be evaluated carefully, especially if she belongs to a high-risk group. Treatment is universally recommended for women diagnosed or suspected to have active TB during pregnancy. Untreated progressive disease may pose increased risks of mortality to the mother and the fetus, especially if diagnosed late in pregnancy (16).

Transmission of TB to the fetus during pregnancy is rare but is more likely to occur if the mother has disseminated TB, such as miliary disease or TB meningitis, or in rare cases when the genitourinary tract is involved. In hematogenous congenital TB, the primary focus of infection in the infant is usually the liver, although it is possible for the bacilli to pass the liver, to go through the foramen ovale to the main circulation and into the lungs, and to establish a primary pulmonary focus.

Pulmonary disease during pregnancy is unlikely to spread to the fetus, especially if appropriate treatment is given to the mother. However, untreated pulmonary disease in the mother or any household contact has a high likelihood of transmission to the infant once the baby is born. Adults on appropriate treatment usually become asymptomatic and AFB smears become negative within 2–4 weeks. Patients with at least three consecutive AFB smear- and culture-negative sputum samples are no longer considered contagious. As long as the patient remains on therapy and is monitored for symptoms and sputum conversion, there is no longer need for isolation after the sputum smears become negative. Adherence to therapy is essential for the treatment and cure of TB. Most health departments, including the Centers for Disease Control and Prevention,

Table 2
Classification of the Tuberculin Skin Test Reaction by Measurement of Induration

≥5 mm	≥10 mm	≥15 mm
Recent contacts with infectious TB case	Children ≤ 4 years of age	Persons with no known risk factors for TB
Immunosuppressed patients	Children in contact with high-risk adults	
Patients with fibrotic changes on chest radiograph (old healed TB)	Foreign-born people from high-prevalence countries	
	Residents and employees of high-risk congregate settings (nursing homes, correctional facilities, homeless shelters)	
	Injection drug users	
	Health care workers in high-risk settings	
	Certain medical conditions (e.g., diabetes mellitus, silicosis)	

recommend directly observed therapy for patients with active disease. Directly observed therapy requires a third party, usually a nurse or outreach worker, to observe the patient taking every dose of medication. Women and children living in an environment with ongoing exposure are at continued risk of infection with TB as well as the possibility of exposure to multidrug-resistant TB, which is more likely to develop in nonadherent patients.

PRENATAL EVALUATION

During pregnancy, women should be screened routinely for risk factors for TB. Women identified with risk factors, either from travel, employment, medical conditions, or exposure, should have a Mantoux tuberculin skin test. If the skin test is positive, measuring 5, 10, or 15 mm of induration or greater, depending on individual risk factors (Table 2), a chest radiograph should be done to evaluate for pulmonary disease. Of course, standard precautions should be taken to protect the fetus when x-rays are obtained. A careful physical examination, looking for extrapulmonary disease, is important as well because 15–20% of cases of TB in adults may involve sites other than the lungs, the most common are lymph nodes, pleura, and bones or joints *(7)*.

Unless the patient has tuberculin skin testing on a regular basis, such as health care workers, it may be difficult to know when the infection occurred. It is still important to ask about household or other close contacts with symptoms of active TB, which may have infected the mother, especially because untreated pulmonary TB in the home would be a serious threat to a newborn infant. More than 90% of adults with active pulmonary TB have symptoms of chronic cough. Any contacts with suspicious symptoms should be referred for tuberculin skin testing and chest radiography before the infant is exposed to the environment.

Patients with documented recent skin test conversion, from negative to positive, are at increased risk of developing active disease within 2 years of infection. Of healthy adults with untreated latent TB infection, 5–10% will develop active TB, half within 2 years of skin test conversion. Whether to treat women during pregnancy for latent TB infection when there is no evidence of active disease has been controversial. Some experts recommend delaying isoniazid therapy until 3 months postpartum because of reports of increased risk of hepatotoxicity; others advocate treating during the pregnancy.

Women with evidence of active TB disease should have specimens collected for culture. Results of the AFB smears are usually available within 24 hours but are not specific for *M. tuberculosis*. Rapid nucleic acid techniques, such as the polymerase chain reaction, are sometimes helpful. In women with suspected extrapulmonary TB, specimens should be collected from appropriate sites. Pathologic evaluation of tissue may be helpful in cases of lymph node or other organ involvement. In cases of suspected disseminated TB, such as miliary or TB meningitis, appropriate specimens should be collected from the mother, including cerebral spinal fluid, and the placenta should be examined for evidence of granulomatous lesions or AFB after delivery. Suspected genitourinary TB usually requires biopsy, pathologic evaluation, and culture of the tissue. Cultures are often negative in cases of extrapulmonary TB, and the diagnosis may be based on clinical or pathological evidence alone.

POSTNATAL EVALUATION OF THE INFANT

Distinguishing between congenital and postnatally acquired TB is often difficult; although this distinction may be clinically insignificant as it does not alter treatment of the infant. In congenital TB, which is extremely rare, the infant must be infected prior to or at the time of birth. Congenital transmission should be considered if the mother has untreated active disease at the time of delivery or soon after. The risk to the fetus is greater in cases of disseminated disease in the mother, such as meningitis or miliary TB, or in cases involving the genitourinary tract, when organisms may infect the amniotic fluid or placenta. Guidelines for diagnosing congenital TB based on previously published criteria by Beitzke *(17)* were revised and updated in 1994 by Cantwell and coworkers *(18)* and suggest the following criteria for diagnosing congenital TB: (1) lesions in the first week of life; (2) a primary hepatic complex or caseating hepatic granulomas; (3) TB infection of the placenta, maternal genital tract, or both; or (4) exclusion of postnatal transmission by a thorough contact investigation. Congenital TB is rare, with only about 300 cases ever reported in the English-language literature *(18)*. Postnatally acquired TB remains the most common route of transmission for infants with TB.

The clinical presentation of infants and newborns with TB will vary by the site of involvement and the age of onset. With congenitally acquired TB, symptoms may be present at birth but more commonly present within the first 2–3 weeks of life. The most frequent presenting findings for congenital TB reported by Cantwell et al. are shown in Table 3 *(18)*. In contrast, infants with postnatally acquired TB usually present after 1 month of age, the shortest incubation time for *M. tuberculosis* to progress to active disease following infection.

The symptoms of TB disease in infants are often nonspecific and may resemble more common generalized infections. Cough, fever or fever of unknown origin, as well as decreased appetite are the most common presenting symptoms reported in infants with postnatally acquired TB *(19)*. Respiratory distress or respiratory failure may be seen in advanced pulmonary disease. Infants with meningitis may have classic find-

Table 3
Most Common Presenting Signs and Symptoms in Infants With Congenital TB

Signs and symptoms	Percentage
Hepatosplenomegaly	76
Respiratory distress	72
Fever	48
Lymphadenopathy	38
Abdominal distention	24
Lethargy or irritability	21
Ear discharge	17
Papular skin lesions	14
Vomiting, apnea, cyanosis, jaundice, seizures, and petechiae	each <10

Adapted from ref. *18.*

ings, such as vomiting, lethargy, meningismus, seizures, or irritability. As many as 20% of infants and 50% of older children with active TB may have no symptoms or physical findings at the time of diagnosis, and these are discovered during the epidemiologic investigation of the household contacts of an adult with active disease. Therefore, it is important to examine carefully any child exposed to contagious TB, even if there are no symptoms at the time of the evaluation.

Infants born to mothers with TB and infants with TB generally are not considered contagious. There is no need for isolation of the baby except in rare cases of severe pulmonary involvement if the infant has positive AFB smears. Standard precautions should be taken when handling pulmonary or gastric secretions, especially in intubated infants. In cases of suspected maternal pulmonary TB, some experts recommend separating the infant from the mother until contagious disease in the mother can be excluded *(13)*. Others allow limited contact of the mother and infant for breast-feeding and bonding but suggest no rooming-in to reduce exposure time and prophylaxis with isoniazid to protect the infant *(13,20)*.

Evaluation of infants suspected to have TB can be difficult because the history and physical findings are often nonspecific, and AFB smears and cultures may be negative. There is no contraindication to tuberculin skin testing in infants, but a negative test is considered unreliable in infants less than 3–6 months of age. Following infection, 4–12 weeks is usually required for the skin test to become reactive; however, TB disease may develop as soon as 1 month after infection. Because of the delay in skin test conversion, an infant or child may develop active TB before the skin test becomes positive. The risk in infants of progression to active disease after infection may be as high as 45% in the first year of life, whereas the lifetime risk of disease in healthy untreated adults is between 5 and 10%. Because infants and children younger than 4 years of age are at increased risk of developing active TB if they are not treated, a chest radiograph, physical examination and isoniazid prophylaxis (for at least 3 months) are recommended following exposure in this age group regardless of the initial tuberculin skin test or chest radiograph results *(13)*. At 3–6 months after exposure, if the repeat tuberculin skin test is negative, infection is excluded, and isoniazid prophylaxis may be discontinued. In cases of ongoing exposure in the household because of nonadherence or failure of therapy, isoniazid should be continued until the tuberculin skin test is negative 3 months after the exposure has been broken either by separation or effective treatment of the adult source case.

The diagnostic evaluation of infants and children with suspected TB disease generally should be initiated in the hospital for the proper collection of specimens and cultures. Children are generally unable to provide sputum specimens because of poor tussive force and a lack of sputum production. Early morning gastric fluids collected by aspiration prior to eating or awakening represent pulmonary secretions brought up by the respiratory cilia and swallowed during the night. If at least three specimens are collected properly on consecutive mornings, the yield on mycobacterial culture has been shown to be as sensitive as bronchoaveolar lavage. In cases of clinically proven disease, cultures from infants younger than 12 months of age are more often positive (70%) than cultures from older children (40%) *(19)*. AFB smears are usually negative in children because of the low bacterial load, but infants with extensive pulmonary disease may have positive smears.

Children with clinical findings consistent with extrapulmonary TB should have specimens collected from the site of involvement. Fine-needle or excisional biopsy sent for pathology and culture may be diagnostic for TB lymphadenitis. Urine specimens for mycobacterial culture may be positive in patients with renal involvement or miliary TB. Middle ear fluid, bone marrow aspirate, and liver or pulmonary biopsy have been successful in identifying *M. tuberculosis* in some cases of congenital disease *(21,22)*.

Because of the generally poor yield of specimens from children with TB, negative AFB smears, TB cultures, or polymerase chain reaction do not exclude the diagnosis of TB. In culture-negative cases, the diagnosis is usually made using clinical criteria. Any infant with a positive tuberculin skin test and physical or radiographic findings consistent with TB disease meets the clinical criteria for diagnosis. In cases with negative tuberculin skin tests, the diagnosis is made when clinical findings are consistent with TB and an adult contact with contagious TB has been identified. Clinical response to TB therapy may also support the diagnosis in culture-negative or unclear cases *(12)*.

Direct Diagnostic Assays and Interpretation

The timely diagnosis of congenital TB is often difficult. Suspecting or confirming that the mother has disseminated or genitourinary TB is usually required to make a premortem diagnosis. The majority of reported cases have been diagnosed postmortem.

AFB Stain

In developing countries, the AFB stain is often the only available diagnostic test for TB. The fluorescent stain (auramine and rhodamine or Truant stain) is more sensitive than the traditional Kinyoun or Ziehl-Neelsen stains. Approximately 70% of adults with pulmonary TB have a positive AFB stain of sputum. An AFB stain of genitourinary excretions or the uterine endothelium is rarely positive in women with genitourinary TB. An AFB stain of the placenta may be positive, but finding organisms in the placenta does not prove congenital TB. However, by the time an infant with congenital TB becomes symptomatic with pulmonary disease, an AFB stain of tracheal secretions or a gastric aspirate is often markedly positive. Congenital TB has been diagnosed by AFB stain of liver tissue, bone marrow, and cerebrospinal fluid. Although other mycobacteria are indistinguishable from *M. tuberculosis* in an AFB stain, finding a positive AFB stain from a neonate with an illness consistent with congenital TB is almost diagnostic of the disease.

Mycobacteria Culture

Absolute confirmation of congenital TB requires isolating the organism from a body fluid or tissue. Growth using traditional culture media often requires 3–6 weeks of incubation. However, techniques employing radiometric systems using liquid media allow for isolation of the organism in 10–14 days in most cases. These automated systems also have antimicrobial agent-containing bottles; full identification and drug susceptibility testing of organisms usually can be accomplished within 3 weeks.

About 90% of adults with pulmonary TB have positive sputum cultures when multiple specimens are obtained. However, TB can be culture confirmed from only 20–40% of children with TB using either tracheal secretions or gastric aspirates as the source for culture. Extrapulmonary TB also can be difficult to confirm with culture. Only 25–50% of adults with disseminated or genitourinary TB have positive cultures. When evaluating a neonate for congenital TB, the placenta should always be examined and cultured. Because of overwhelming dissemination, confirmation of congenital TB by culture is often possible and should be attempted more often. In one review of congenital TB cases, positive cultures for *M. tuberculosis* were found in 10 of 12 gastric aspirates, 3 of 4 liver biopsies, 3 of 3 lymph node biopsies, and 2 of 4 bone marrow aspirations *(21)*. Open lung biopsy with culture also has been used to establish the diagnosis *(23)*.

Nucleic Acid Amplifications

Numerous published studies have shown that various nucleic acid amplification (NAA) techniques, most detecting the mycobacterial insertion element IS6110, have sensitivity and specificity greater than 90% for detecting pulmonary TB in adults when they are applied to sputum. However, the Food and Drug Administration has approved the use of these tests only for AFB stain-positive sputum specimens because the somewhat low specificity means that, when the tests are applied to AFB stain-negative specimens, the majority of positive results in the NAA tests will be falsely positive. The NAA tests have been applied to other body fluids and tissues, but false-negative results are common, and false-positive results can be misleading if careful patient selection (high index of suspicion) has not occurred.

Several published studies have evaluated NAA tests for diagnosis of pulmonary TB in children *(22)*. When compared with the clinical diagnosis of TB in children, the average sensitivity has been 40–60%, and the specificity has been 80–95%. A negative NAA test does not eliminate TB as a diagnostic possibility, and a positive test is not absolute confirmation of TB. There are no published studies examining the use of NAA in the mother, placenta, or neonate to establish the diagnosis of congenital TB.

Serology and Antigen Detection

Despite dozens of studies published over the past few decades, serology and antigen detection have found little place in the diagnosis of TB in adults or children. However, in 2001 a new test, the QuantiFERON-TB (Cellestis Limited, Carnegie, Victoria, Australia) was approved by the Food and Drug Administration for the diagnosis for latent

TB infection in adults *(24)*. The test measures the release of interferon-γ in whole blood in response to stimulation by purified protein derivative. This test has not been approved for use in children yet.

CONCLUSION

In the United States, TB continues to be a problem, especially among recent immigrants from high-risk countries and persons who have been in contact with adults with contagious disease. Congenital TB, tuberculosis acquired prior to birth, is quite rare. Transmission to infants after birth, either from the mother or other contagious household contacts, is more common. The diagnosis may be difficult, and a high index of suspicion as well as awareness of the risk factors and presenting symptoms are important. The presentation of TB in infants may be similar to other more common infections, and currently available diagnostic tests have low sensitivity in children. Diagnosis is often based on the clinical presentation of the infant coupled with finding TB disease in the mother or other close contacts. Tuberculosis may be rapidly progressive and life threatening to infants and young children. Therefore, when contagious pulmonary disease is diagnosed in an adult who has contact with children, it should be considered a public health emergency.

REFERENCES

1. Cantanzaro A, Davidson BL, Fujiwara PI, et al. Rapid diagnostic tests for tuberculosis—progress but no gold standard. Am J Respir Crit Care Med 1997;155:1804–1814.
2. Schaefer G, Zervondakis IA, Fuchs FF, et al. Pregnancy and pulmonary tuberculosis. Obstet Gynecol 1995;46:706–715.
3. Addis GM, Anthony GS, Semple P, et al. Miliary tuberculosis in an in-vitro fertilization pregnancy: a case report. Eur J Obstet Gynecol Reprod Biol 1988;27:351–353.
4. Starke JR. Tuberculosis: an old disease but a new threat to the mother, fetus and neonate. Clin Perinatol 1997;24:107–127.
5. Kendig EL Jr, Rodgers WL. Tuberculosis in the neonatal period. Am Rev Tuberc Pulm Dis 1958;77:418–422.
6. Cantwell MF, Snider DE Jr, Cauthen GM, Onorato IM. Epidemiology of tuberculosis in the United States, 1985 through 1992. JAMA 1994;272:535–539.
7. Centers for Disease Control and Prevention, Division of Tuberculosis Elimination. Surveillance reports: reported tuberculosis in the United States, 2000. August 2001. Available at: www.cdc.gov/nchstp/tb/surv/surv2000.htm. Accessed August 2001.
8. Dye C, Scheele S, Dolin P, Pathania V, Raviglione MC. Consensus statement: global burden of tuberculosis: estimated incidence, prevalence, and mortality by country: WHO Global Surveillance and Monitoring Project. JAMA 1999;282:677–686.
9. Centers for Disease Control and Prevention. Core Curriculum on Tuberculosis: What a Clinician Should Know, 4th ed. Atlanta, GA: US Department of Health and Human Services, 2000.
10. Espinal MA, Reingold AL, Lavendra M. The effects of pregnancy on the risk of developing active tuberculosis. J Infect Dis 1996;173:488–491.
11. Ormerod P. Tuberculosis in pregnancy and the puerperium. Thorax 2001;56:494–499.
12. Smith KC. Tuberculosis in children. Curr Probl Pediatr 2001;31:1–34.
13. American Academy of Pediatrics. Tuberculosis. In: Pickering LK, ed. 2000 Red Book: Report of the Committee on Infectious Diseases, 25th ed. Elk Grove Village, IL: American Academy of Pediatrics, 2000; pp. 593–613.

14. Good JT, Iseman MD, Davidson PT, et al. Tuberculosis in association with pregnancy. Am J Obstet Gynecol 1981;140:492–498.
15. Wilson EA, Thelin TJ, Dilts PV. Tuberculosis complicated by pregnancy. Am J Obstet Gynecol 1972;115:526–529.
16. Figueroa-Damien R, Arredondo-Garcia JL. Pregnancy and tuberculosis: influence of treatment on perinatal outcome. Am J Perinatol 1998;15:303–306.
17. Beitzke H. Ueber die angeborene tuberkuloese Infektion. Ergeb Gesamte Tuberkuloseforsch 1935;7:1–30.
18. Cantwell MF, Shehab ZM, Costello AM, et al. Brief report: congenital tuberculosis. N Engl J Med 1994;330:1051–1054.
19. Vallejo JG, Ong LT, Starke JR. Clinical features, diagnosis, and treatment of tuberculosis in infants. Pediatrics 1994;94:1–7.
20. Denby M, Banks J, Coody D, Smith K, Yetman R. Infant born to a mother with a positive tuberculin skin test—practice guidelines. J Pediatr Health Care 1996;10:31–34.
21. Hageman J, Shulman S, Schreiber M, et al. Congenital tuberculosis: critical reappraisal of clinical findings and diagnostic procedures. Pediatrics 1980;66:980–984.
22. Khan EA, Starke JR. Diagnosis of tuberculosis in children: increased need for better methods. Emerg Infect Dis 1995;1:115–123.
23. Stallworth JR, Brasfield DM, Tiller RE. Congenital miliary tuberculosis proved by open lung biopsy specimen and successfully treated. Am J Dis Child 1980;14:320–321.
24. Mazurek GH, Villarino ME, Centers for Disease Control and Prevention. Guidelines for using QuantiFERON-TB test for diagnosing latent *Mycobacterium tuberculosis* infection. MMWR Recomm Rep 2003;52:15–18.

22

Toxoplasma gondii

Aida Chaparro and Charles D. Mitchell

INTRODUCTION

The ability to diagnose congenital toxoplasmosis has been hampered by both the lack of a readily available means of isolating the causative organism *Toxoplasma gondii* and the apparent inability of many commercially available serological assays to detect *Toxoplasma*-specific immunoglobulin (Ig) M or IgA in congenitally infected infants because of inadequate sensitivity. This chapter concisely reviews the current state of the art of diagnosing congenital *Toxoplasma* infection and reviews present guidelines for making this diagnosis both pre- and postnatally.

MICROBIOLOGY

Of the six known species of *Toxoplasma*, only one, *T. gondii*, has commonly been recognized as a human pathogen. *T. gondii* is an obligate, intracellular protozoan parasite that phylogenetically is classified within the same subclass Coccidia as *Cryptosporidium*, another protozoan pathogen associated with acquired immunodeficiency syndrome. *T. gondii* has a diverse range of hosts, including most species of mammals, birds, and some reptiles.

The life cycle is composed of a sexual phase that occurs only within the gut epithelium of members of the cat family (its only known definitive host) and an asexual phase. Although the latter may occur within the definitive host, it usually takes place following infection of an intermediate host (humans, other mammals, birds, and reptiles). Two morphological stages of the life cycle are found in the intermediate host: the motile, proliferating tachyzoite, which is present during acute infection, and the tissue cyst *(1)*. The tissue cyst develops in brain and muscle tissue following acute infection as the host's immune response contains the infection, and is the hallmark of chronic infection. The size of the tissue cyst may vary considerably relative to the number of bradyzoites or slowly replicating organisms contained within the cyst. Although tissue cysts have usually been thought of as "dormant," certain reports have suggested a slow turnover of bradyzoites within the cyst and periodic cyst rupture. The released bradyzoites may revert to tachyzoites and give rise to clinical disease if the host's immunity is severely impaired. Hence, effective immunological control of acute and chronic *Toxoplasma* infection most likely results from intact humoral and cellular im-

From: *Infectious Disease: Congenital and Perinatal Infections: A Concise Guide to Diagnosis*
Edited by: C. Hutto © Humana Press Inc., Totowa, NJ

mune responses against a diversity of antigens associated with both forms of this organism *(1,2)*.

EPIDEMIOLOGY

Acquired toxoplasmosis commonly occurs as a result of the (1) ingestion of food contaminated with sporulated oocysts, (2) ingestion of undercooked meat containing tissue cysts, or (3) contact with soil or other material (i.e., cat litter) contaminated by cat feces containing viable oocysts. Very few cases have been reported as a result of transfusion, transplant of a contaminated organ, or laboratory accident.

Toxoplasma gondii has a ubiquitous global distribution, with serological evidence of human infection found on at least five different continents *(1)*. In general, the seroprevalence of *Toxoplasma* increases with increasing age as a result of horizontal acquisition, but it has been noted to vary considerably among different geographical areas *(3)*. The seroprevalences of *Toxoplasma* in the United States have previously been noted to vary between 3% in Denver and 35% in Miami, with Boston and Palo Alto, California, having intermediate rates of 10 and 14%, respectively. The seroprevalences of *Toxoplasma* in Africa, Europe, and Latin America, however, are considerably higher, with rates that vary between 21 (London) and 72% (Paris), 23 (Zambia) and 81% (Central African Republic), and 59 (Santiago, Chile) and 65% (Belo Horizonte, Brazil) *(3)*. The overwhelming majority of cases of congenital transmission result from the acquisition of primary maternal *Toxoplasma* infection during pregnancy. Most cases of primary infection in immunocompetent hosts are asymptomatic or nonspecific and as such are not investigated. Some cases, however, may present as a syndrome-like "infectious mononucleosis." The development of a "mono"-like illness in a pregnant woman, especially if it is associated with lymphadenopathy and fatigue without fever, should prompt an investigation for acute acquired toxoplasmosis *(4)*. In geographical regions where the seroprevalence is higher (i.e., France, certain Central American countries), the threshold for testing for primary infection is usually lower. Serological tests for *Toxoplasma* IgM and IgG are the most common laboratory methods used to diagnose primary infection and are described in Table 1.

The risk of acquiring primary infection is increased among patients who ingest undercooked meat or have contact with oocysts in soil or cat feces. Given the right soil conditions, the oocysts may remain viable for several months. The risk of transplacental transmission is highest when the mother is infected late during gestation. In contrast, the frequency of symptomatic neonatal infection is lowest among these infants. Although the risk of congenital infection among infants born to mothers initially infected early during gestation is considerably lower, the frequency of symptomatic neonatal disease is much higher *(1,2)*. Previous data have suggested that the prevalence of congenital infection in the United States may range between 2 per 1000 (reported during the 1970s) and 1 per 12,000 births (data derived from a prospective study published during 1994). Of note, a relatively few cases have been reported in chronically infected pregnant women with impaired cell-mediated immunity (usually as a result of profound immunosuppression induced by human immunodeficiency virus [HIV] coinfection) *(3)*.

Table 1
Guidelines for the Prenatal Diagnosis of Congenital Toxoplasmosis

I. Diagnosis of maternal infection

    Initial screening for primary maternal infection can be done by requesting a *T. gondii*-specific ELISA for *Toxoplasma* IgG and IgM (available in most clinical laboratories)

    Confirmation (if indicated) of the diagnosis of primary maternal infection may be done by submitting maternal serum to a reference laboratory for

    Sabin-Feldman dye test for *T. gondii* IgG, also IgM, IgA, and IgE ISAGA/DS-ELISA and IgG agglutination AC/HS assay (*see* text for more information)

II. Diagnosis of congenital infection

Following confirmation of primary maternal infection

    1. Initial nonspecific screening for fetal infection can be performed by

      a. Serial obstetrical ultrasounds looking for an increase in the ventricular-hemisphere ratio suggestive of ventricular dilations secondary to hydrocephalus

      b. White blood cell count, eosinophil count, platelets, liver function tests, and total IgM on fetal blood

    2. Specific testing for fetal infection can be performed by one of the following methods:

      a. Amniocentesis to screen amniotic fluid for *T. gondii* by gene amplification (PCR)

      b. Amniocentesis to obtain fluid for mouse inoculation

      c. Cordocentesis to obtain fetal blood for isolation by mouse inoculation and serological testing for *T. gondii* IgM

DIAGNOSIS OF PRIMARY *TOXOPLASMA* INFECTION IN THE PREGNANT WOMAN

Most cases of acquired *T. gondii* infection in the immunocompetent pregnant woman are mild or inapparent *(1,5)*. When symptomatic infection does occur, it most commonly presents with lymphadenopathy, malaise, and fatigue without fever *(1,5–9)*. Symptomatic disease presenting as encephalitis or chorioretinitis most commonly occurs among severely immunocompromised patients *(5)*.

Although acute toxoplasmosis has been rarely diagnosed by detecting the parasite in body fluids, tissues, or secretions; serological testing remains the most common and useful method of diagnosing acute infection *(5,10–12)*. High levels of *Toxoplasma*-specific IgG antibodies suggest acute infection, but they cannot reliably distinguish between recently acquired infection and infection acquired prior to conception or in the distant past *(5,13)*. The key question is whether the acute infection occurred during gestation or prior to conception. If the latter is true, then the presence of a pre-existing maternal immune response should protect the fetus from infection.

In acute infection, IgG and IgM antibodies generally rise within 1–2 weeks. IgM antibodies usually persist for 1 year postinfection but have been reported to persist for up to 18 months postinfection *(5,14)*. IgM-positive results should be confirmed by a *Toxoplasma* reference laboratory *(15)*. Confirmatory testing with serologic profile (including the Sabin-Feldman dye test; IgM, IgA, and IgE enzyme-linked immunosorbent assay [ELISA] and/or immunosorbent agglutination assay [ISAGA]; and the differential agglutination test) has also been useful in distinguishing recently acquired infections *(10–12,16)*.

Prenatal serological screening to detect maternal infection is routinely used in many European countries *(5)*. French guidelines recommend that nonimmune pregnant women be tested every month throughout pregnancy to detect seroconversion *(17–20)*. In the United States, targeted screening is recommended only if there are suspicious prenatal ultrasound findings, such as hydrocephalus, intracranial calcifications, microcephaly, fetal growth restriction, ascites, or hepatosplenomegaly *(5)*. All HIV-1-infected women should be screened for latent *Toxoplasma* infection. If seropositive, then the mother should be followed for the occurrence of clinical disease secondary to reactivation *(5,21)* and their infants screened for congenital infection, especially if they are profoundly immunosuppressed.

PRENATAL DIAGNOSIS OF CONGENITAL TOXOPLASMOSIS

The occurrence of primary maternal infection postconception must be confirmed before any attempt is made at diagnosing infection *in utero*. Although many clinical laboratories are capable of making a preliminary diagnosis of primary infection based on the acquisition of *Toxoplasma* IgG antibodies and a reactive *Toxoplasma* IgM assay, these results should be confirmed in a reference laboratory before any invasive procedures are performed. Table 1 describes the guidelines for making the prenatal diagnosis of congenital infection. Given its utility and the relative safety of amniocentesis, polymerase chain reaction (PCR) testing of amniotic fluid for *T. gondii* has been labeled as the method of choice for diagnosing *in utero* infection. Cordocentesis (aspiration of fetal blood following transabdominal insertion of a sterile needle into the umbilical vein) has also been used successfully to document infection *in utero* and may be used as an alternative method of diagnosis if necessary *(1,22,23)*. The reported rate of fetal loss associated with this procedure is 0.3 per 1000 *(1)*. It should be remembered that even if the fetus is found to not be infected, the at-risk infant should be reevaluated during the neonatal period as transplacental infection may not have occurred until very late in pregnancy.

CONGENITAL TOXOPLASMOSIS AND CLINICAL DISEASE

Although there are certain clinical signs that may be present in the infant with symptomatic congenital toxoplasmosis, the ability to diagnose this condition on clinical grounds is often problematic. The spectrum of disease manifestations may vary widely and mimic other transplacentally or perinatally acquired infections. Also, the majority of congenitally infected infants (approx 70–90%) are asymptomatic at birth *(1,3,4,24–27)*. Many of these infants will not have any signs or symptoms until months to years later, when they present with significant clinical sequelae, most frequently affecting the eye or the brain *(27–32)*. In many cases, this may not be caused as much by delayed onset of disease as late recognition of the condition *(1)*.

Some 20% of asymptomatic neonates have been noted previously to have clinically silent ocular or neurological disease *(1,31)*. Disease with delayed onset occurs most often among premature infants, usually during the first 3 months of life. Ocular disease can reactivate months or even years later among immunocompetent as well as immunocompromised patients. There is, however, as yet no reliable method of predicting which infants will develop subsequent complications *(27)*. Thus, it is important to diagnose congenital toxoplasmosis early and start specific therapy to lessen the possibility of such complications. Unless the primary care provider has a high index of suspicion for congenital toxoplasmosis, the diagnosis may be missed and the infant not treated appropriately until after blindness, mental retardation, or even death has occurred. A small percentage of congenitally infected infants may continue to have subclinical infection that may not be detected unless the condition is suspected.

A neonate presenting with overt symptomatic disease may have the classic triad of hydrocephalus (secondary to periaqueductal stenosis), intracranial calcifications, and chorioretinitis (typically bilateral, focal, necrotizing retinitis). This triad, however, occurs in only a minority of symptomatic patients *(27,33)*. The clinical manifestations are usually protean and include one or more of the following manifestations, which occur in more than 50% of affected infants: diffuse maculopapular rash, generalized lymphadenopathy, hepatosplenomegaly, jaundice, ocular disease (cataracts, microphthalmia, optic atrophy, and chorioretinitis), abnormal spinal fluid, convulsions, fever, and anemia *(1,27,34)*.

Congenitally infected infants born to mothers dually infected with both *Toxoplasma* and HIV-1 are also at high risk for having HIV-1 infection *(35–38)*. Although these infants may be asymptomatic during the neonatal period, they may subsequently develop rapidly progressive HIV-1 disease complicated by clinically apparent congenital toxoplasmosis.

GUIDELINES FOR THE DIAGNOSIS OF CONGENITAL TOXOPLASMOSIS IN A NEONATE OR YOUNG INFANT

Table 2 describes the diagnostic workup of an infant suspected of having congenital toxoplasmosis. The practitioner should have a high index of clinical suspicion for congenital infection when confronted with the following scenarios: (1) symptomatic neonatal disease consistent with congenital toxoplasmosis, (2) a history of documented primary maternal *T. gondii* infection during pregnancy, or (3) a history of HIV1 coinfection when the mother has had either reactivated clinical toxoplasmosis (cerebritis or chorioretinitis) during pregnancy or is profoundly immunosuppressed. Infants born to chronically infected mothers who are similarly immunosuppressed for another reason may also be at risk for congenital infection. All at-risk infants should be evaluated to document or rule out congenital infection and assess the degree of involvement.

At-risk infants who present during the neonatal period should have a complete diagnostic workup as the chances of isolating the organism are best during the first several days of life. Congenital infection is highly likely if the organism is detected and the assays for *Toxoplasma* IgM, IgA, or IgE are positive. Repeat testing of all infants with reactive *Toxoplasma* IgM, IgA, or IgE should be done to confirm the presence of congenital infection. Follow-up serological testing of all infants who are strongly suspected of having a congenital infection and are nonreactive in these assays should also be done in case the synthesis of *Toxoplasma*-specific antibodies is delayed until 3–4 months of age. This delay may occur as a result of late transplacental transmission, the presence of circulating maternal antibody, or concomitant anti-*Toxoplasma* therapy. Congenitally infected infants with perinatally acquired HIV-1 infection may not be able to synthesize any *Toxoplasma*-specific antibodies if they have rapidly progressive HIV-1 disease. In these last cases, the diagnosis may have to rely on the detection of the organisms or the presence of the typical clinical and radiologic findings.

Table 2
Guidelines for the Diagnosis of Congenital Toxoplasmosis in a Neonate or Young Infant

I. Clinical evaluation

  History and physical examination including a neurological and ophthalmologic examina
  tion, which must include fundoscopy

  Auditory testing (brain stem response to 20 dB)

II. Non-specific laboratory evaluation

  Laboratory: Complete blood cell count with differential and platelet count; serum quanti
  tative immunoglobulins; liver function tests, including γGTP and bilirubin; urinalysis,
  serum creatinine; CSF cell count; protein; and glucose

  Radiologic: Brain computed tomographic scan with and without contrast; chest x-ray

III. *Toxoplasma*-specific laboratory evaluation

  1. Serologic: *Toxoplasma*-specific IgG and IgM: IgM ISAGA or DS-ELISA are preferred
     IgM assays because of superior sensitivity (~80 and 75%, respectively)[a]; Sabin-Feldman
     dye test ideally is used for IgG (although most laboratories use ELISA assays)

  2. Other serologic assays: IgA DS-ELISA, IgE ISAGA/ELISA may also be useful for
     diagnosis[b]

  3. CSF serology: Obtain *T. gondii*-specific IgG and IgM antibodies

  4. Isolation/detection of the organism:

     a. Inoculate into mice or tissue culture samples from placenta, umbilical cord, or infant
        blood

     b. Test amniotic fluid (if available), infant blood, and CSF for *T. gondii* deoxyribo-
        nucleic acid using PCR

Modified with permission from ref. *1*.

[a]Commercially available EIA assays for *T. gondii* IgG and IgM are useful for detecting acquired infection; they are less sensitive for detection of congenital infection. If an IgM EIA is equivocal or negative and there is a high index of suspicion for congenital infection, serum should be sent to a reference laboratory for serum IgG testing or other antibody testing.

[b]The same test should be performed using maternal serum and the IgM ELISA can be substituted for the ISAGA; on maternal serum, the IgG agglutination AC/HS assay should also be obtained.

The diagnosis of congenital infection among infants who present beyond the neonatal period rests primarily on the demonstration of a repeatedly positive *Toxoplasma* IgM, IgA, or IgE and a persistently positive or rising *Toxoplasma* IgG titer.

LABORATORY DIAGNOSIS OF CONGENITAL TOXOPLASMOSIS

All neonates suspected of having a congenital infection should have a complete blood cell count *(20)*, including a platelet count to screen for thrombocytopenia *(40,41)* and eosinophilia *(42)* (although the latter has not been a common finding in many infected infants), and liver function tests. A lumbar puncture should be done to determine if there is a disproportional increase in cerebrospinal fluid (CSF) protein relative to the degree of pleocytosis *(25,43,44)* and a computed axial tomographic scan of the brain with contrast to detect diffuse cerebral calcifications *(27)*. Every infant suspected to be congenitally infected (especially those who are asymptomatic) should have a thorough ophthalmologic examination to detect any ocular complications (i.e., chorioretinitis) (Table 1) *(1)*.

Serological Diagnosis of Congenital Toxoplasma Infection

Although there are a number of direct and indirect assays available to detect infection with *Toxoplasma*, serological testing remains the most common means of diagnosing toxoplasmosis *(1,3,4,24–26)*. The results of such testing, however, must be interpreted carefully. The diagnosis of acute acquired infection can be made by finding the simultaneous presence of *Toxoplasma* IgM and IgG antibodies or the demonstration of a fourfold rise in IgG titers *(1)*. The sensitivity of the commonly employed Diagnostic Clinical Laboratory techniques for these antibodies is adequate for many cases of acquired infection but not all, especially when it involves the confirmation of primary infection during pregnancy. These same assays are usually inadequate in cases of congenital infection.

In both of these scenarios, the appropriate clinical specimens should be submitted to a reference laboratory with expertise in the serological diagnosis of toxoplasmosis to either confirm or refute the presence of infection. Table 3 contains a brief description of the various methods that have been developed to detect *Toxoplasma*-specific antibodies. That numerous assays employing different methodologies have had to be developed hints at the difficulties previously encountered with serological testing. The antigenic structure of *T. gondii* is extremely complex, composed of several proteins (both membrane and cytoplasmic) from different phases of the life cycle. This may partially explain the discrepancy in the ability of different assays to detect *Toxoplasma*-specific antibodies. Certain antigens cross-react with normal human proteins, as evidenced by the presence of "natural" anti-*Toxoplasma* IgM antibodies in the sera of uninfected patients.

Furthermore, methodologic difficulties and lack of standardization have prevented a single assay from being widely adopted. The continuing improvements in various ELISA assays (i.e., double-sandwich [DS] ELISAs for *Toxoplasma*-specific IgM and IgA) and the further development of immunosorbent agglutination assays for IgM, IgA, and IgE, with their greater sensitivity and specificity, should lend impetus to the need to standardize these tests. Once standardized, it is hoped they will then become more widely available in many diagnostic laboratories in the United States.

Toxoplasma-specific IgG antibodies typically achieve a peak concentration 1–2 months following acute infection and remain positive for life following both acute and congenital infection. Although the Sabin-Feldman dye test is the standard *(45,46)* against which all other assays should be judged, many clinical laboratories have adopted various commercially available *Toxoplasma* IgG ELISA assays. The IgG indirect immunofluorescence assay (IFA) measures the same antibody as the dye test and is easier to perform, but it is highly laboratory dependent. False-negative results may occur in sera with low titers, and sera that contain antinuclear antibodies may yield false-positive results. The results from IgG ELISA assays correlates well with the dye test and the IFA, but these have not been standardized as yet *(47)*.

Toxoplasma-specific IgG declines continuously (approximate half-life 30 days) in the uninfected infant as the transplacentally acquired maternal antibody is catabolized. It usually becomes undetectable sometime between 6 and 12 months of age *(48,49)*. Among congenitally infected infants, depending on the timing of *in utero* infection, the *Toxoplasma* IgG may decline initially and not begin to rise until 3–4 months of

Table 3
Serological Assays for *Toxoplasma gondii*-Specific Antibodies and the Diagnosis of Congenital Infection

Sabin Feldman Dye Test: The dye test is the gold standard for the detection of *Toxoplasma*-specific IgG but requires the availability of a mouse facility to generate the fresh tachyzoites used in this assay. It is available only in reference laboratories. Following incubation in normal saline and methylene blue, the parasite swells and stains deep blue. Pretreatment of the parasites with antibody containing sera and complement produces lysis. Lysed organisms appear thin and distorted and fail to stain with the dye. The IgG titer reported is that dilution of serum at which half of the organisms are not killed (appear stained). The titers are determined by comparison to a reference serum and expressed in international units (IU) per milliliter of serum.

Indirect Hemagglutination Test: Red cells tagged with *T. gondii* agglutinate when sera containing specific antibodies are added. It is not recommended for the diagnosis of primary infection during pregnancy because of the delay in the rise in *T. gondii* IgG titers. It is also not recommended for the diagnosis of congenital toxoplasmosis as false-negative reactions have been observed in cases with high dye test titers.

Complement Fixation Test: Complement-fixing IgG antibodies appear later than those demonstrable by the dye test. The antigen preparations used in this test have not been standardized; therefore, this test cannot be recommended for routine use for infants.

Agglutination Test: This method is very sensitive in detecting specific IgM and is routinely used as part of the mouse inoculation assay. It has primarily been used in Europe to screen for *T. gondii* IgM and IgG but is not widely available in the United States. The differential agglutination method (HS/AC) has been demonstrated to be capable of differentiating between acute vs chronic infection.

IFA Test: Slide preparations of killed *T. gondii* are incubated with serial dilutions of the patient's serum. A positive reaction is detected by the fluorescence of the organisms when examined under the microscope. Correlation with the dye test in detecting IgG antibodies is excellent, but reliable and reproducible titers are difficult to obtain. False-positive results occur with sera that contain antinuclear antibodies. The IFA test has been adapted for the demonstration of IgM antibodies to *T. gondii*, but the sensitivity and specificity of this assay when used to diagnose congenital infection is poor. The sensitivity is only 25%; the specificity is marred by the occurrence of false-positive reactions. Thus, although IFA may detect *Toxoplasma*-specific IgM, it should not be used as the only means of diagnosing congenital infection.

Conventional ELISA: This method has largely replaced other tests in the routine clinical laboratory because of its availability, rapid turnaround time, simplicity, reliability in most clinical situations, and capability of performing tests on multiple clinical specimens at the same time. It has been used successfully to detect *Toxoplasma*-specific IgG, IgM, IgA, and IgE in the pregnant woman, fetus, and neonate. IgG ELISA titers correlate well with the results of the dye test, but the conventional IgM ELISA (IgM-EIA) detects IgM in only 50% of congenitally infected infants. False-positive reactions have also been a problem. Commercial kits are presently available to detect *Toxoplasma* IgG and IgM.

(continued)

Table 3 *(Continued)*
Serological Assays for *Toxoplasma gondii*-Specific Antibodies and the Diagnosis of Congenital Infection

Double-Sandwich or Capture Enzyme-Linked Immunosorbent Assay(DS-ELISA or DS-EIA):
These assays differ from the conventional ELISA in that they employ plates with wells that are coated with antihuman IgM or IgA antibodies (rather than antigen) to bind these specific antibodies. The IgM DS-EIA has become the most widely used method for the demonstration of *T. gondii* IgM. It avoids false-positive results (related to rheumatoid factor) and false-negative results (secondary to competition from maternal IgG) previously seen with the IFA. The sensitivity of the IgM DS-EIA among congenitally infected infants approaches 73% during the neonatal period and 81% during the first month of life. The DS-ELISA for the detection of *T. gondii*-specific IgA is more sensitive than either the IgM-EIA or the IgM ISAGA for the diagnosis of congenital infection when the commercial assay is appropriately standardized.

Enzyme-Linked Immunofiltration Assay: Preliminary data suggest that this assay may hold great promise as a means of detecting IgA and IgE in congenitally infected infants, although it is not available commercially. It employs a Millipore filter as a solid-phase, immunoprecipitation to determine antibody specificity, and immunofiltration to determine antibody isotypes. Pinon et al. *(64)* were able to diagnose 94% of congenitally infected infants by 3 months of age using a combination of IgA enzyme-linked immunofiltration and IgM ISAGA.

ISAGA: The ISAGA combines the sensitivity and specificity of the direct agglutination and the DS-ELISA for *T. gondii* IgM, IgA, and IgE. The sensitivity and specificity of the ISAGA for IgM is superior to both the IgM IFA and the IgM ELISA and detects *T. gondii* IgM both earlier and later than other assays. The ISAGA has also been used to detect *T. gondii* IgA and IgE. The IgM ISAGA has been widely used by several investigators. A commercial assay is available from Bio-Meriux (Lyon, France).

Immunoblot: Although a modification of the Western blot assay has been useful in identifying some congenitally infected infants (based on the presence of select antigen-antibody bands not found in maternal sera), it is primarily a research tool.

IgG Avidity Testing: Based on the increasing avidity of IgG antibodies during the transition from acute to chronic infection, this assay (which correlates well with the HS/AC agglutination assay) has proven to be useful in excluding acute infection during the earlier part of pregnancy. However, because of a lack of consensus on a standard procedure and the lack of availability, it cannot be recommended presently for routine use in the diagnosis of congenital infection.

---

age. If the mother and her infant are infected close to birth, the infant's *Toxoplasma* IgG may not be detectable until a few months of age. Consequently, the diagnosis may be missed. This phenomena may also explain why the most sensitive serological assays for *Toxoplasma* IgM (i.e., IgM immunosorbent agglutination [ISAGA], etc.) only have a sensitivity of 75–80% for detecting congenital infection.

Two additional clinical scenarios in which the *Toxoplasma*-specific antibody may be impaired relate to congenitally infected infants who are also perinatally infected with HIV or whose anti-*Toxoplasma* therapy is begun perinatally or soon after birth. Such treatment, if it is begun early in infection, reduces antigenic challenge by killing tachyzoites, thus blunting antibody synthesis. Serological rebound occurs in a majority of such infants 2–6 months following cessation of therapy *(49–53)*. Typically, once established the *Toxoplasma* IgG titer will remain positive for life. Congenitally infected infants who have rapidly progressive HIV-1 disease may not be able to synthesize *Toxoplasma*-specific antibodies *(38)*.

Typically, IgM antibodies can be detected 1–2 weeks following acute infection, peak in 1 month, and decline thereafter. In many cases, they may become undetectable within 6–9 months. The IgM antibody, however, may persist for several more months. Although the IgM IFA and the conventional IgM ELISA can usually detect *Toxoplasma*-specific IgM following acute infection *(54–56)*, the IgM DS-ELISA and IgM ISAGA are both more sensitive and specific and should be used to screen for *Toxoplasma* IgM associated with congenital infection *(47,57–60)*. Antinuclear antibodies *(61)* and rheumatoid factor *(62)* may cause false-positive results with the IgM IFA. The sensitivity of the IgM double-sandwich enzyme immunoassay (DS-EIA) among congenitally infected infants is 73% during the neonatal period and 81% during the first months of life. The sensitivity of the IgM ISAGA approaches 75–80% among congenitally infected infants and usually detects *Toxoplasma* IgM both earlier and later than many other assays *(63)*.

Toxoplasma-specific IgA and IgE usually decline to undetectable levels sooner than IgM and are helpful in determining the timing of acute infection during pregnancy (especially when the initial infection pre-dated conception and the *Toxoplasma* IgM is still positive). IgA production parallels IgM production, with peak levels occurring approx 2 months following initial infection and then declining quickly *(48,52)*. *Toxoplasma*-specific IgE as detected by the IgE ISAGA has a similar pattern of development but decreases more rapidly than do IgA antibodies *(64)*.

As with *Toxoplasma* IgM, the documentation of *Toxoplasma* IgA or IgE in neonatal sera is diagnostic of congenital infection (unless a materno-fetal transfusion has occurred). Follow-up testing for these antibodies should probably be performed at more than 2 weeks of age to confirm their presence if the initial assays are reactive. Prior reports have suggested that the sensitivity of the *Toxoplasma* IgA and IgE assays for detecting congenital infection may in fact be superior to that previously noted with IgM testing *(52,64)*, and although the development of commercial kits for *Toxoplasma* IgA is encouraging, they are as yet not reliable *(65,66)*. There are as yet no commercial kits to test for *Toxoplasma* IgE *(64)*.

Direct Isolation of Toxoplasma

Isolation of this obligate intracellular parasite from amniotic fluid or neonatal blood provides unequivocal proof of infection *(67–69)* but requires the availability of a clinical laboratory that is proficient in these procedures. Furthermore, the results may not be available for a period of weeks. An attempt to isolate the parasite from cord or peripheral blood of the newborn should, however, be made as a definitive serological diagnosis may not be possible during the first weeks or months of infection. Blood (in a serum tube) should ideally be drawn from the infant within the first week of life as the frequency of detectable parasitemia decreases after this point. Specimens of CSF and other bodily fluids as indicated (i.e., peritoneal fluid, amniotic fluid in the case of pre-natal diagnosis, etc.) should also be submitted for testing. Although the specimen should be processed and inoculated as soon as possible to prevent the death of the organism, specimens should be kept at 4°C if short-term storage or shipping is re-quired. Freezing should be avoided (1).

Because the organism is most likely to reside within the white blood cells in patients with parasitemia, the buffy coat layer should be separated from the plasma and pro-cessed for subsequent inoculation. The separation of the buffy coat from the plasma should also lessen the chance of T. gondii-specific antibodies interfering with the de-tection of the organism (1). If the blood clot from a serum tube is used, the clot should be triturated in a small amount of normal saline and drawn into a syringe. Placental tissue from all infants suspected of congenital infection (stored at 4°C without fixative) should also be processed by trypsin digestion and inoculated into mice (1,24). Positive results have previously been found to correlate well with congenital infection.

Isolation of T. gondii by Tissue Culture Inoculation

Although isolation by tissue culture inoculation has been used by certain investiga-tors with some success, the consensus seems to be that this method is a less-sensitive method than mouse inoculation (67,70). Inoculated cultures of human embryonic fi-broblasts grown on coverslips are incubated for 72–96 hours, fixed, and processed for indirect immunofluorescence using anti-T. gondii-specific antibody. Although this method would be most useful when an early diagnosis is needed (positive results may be obtained in 4–5 days), its relative insensitivity and lack of availability have lessened its importance as a diagnostic tool.

Isolation by Mouse Inoculation

Mouse intraperitoneal inoculation has been considered the gold standard for demon-stration of this organism (1). At 5–10 days after injection, peritoneal fluid should be examined for the presence of tachyzoites. Demonstration of the organism is proof of infection (67–69). If no organisms are recovered, mouse serum should be tested for T. gondii antibodies 6 weeks postinjection (the preferred method of testing is agglutina-tion as this requires only a small amount of serum). Confirmation of infection once antibodies are found should be performed by examination of the brain for the presence of cysts (1). Although earlier serological testing of the mice may detect antibodies sooner, definitive results from this assay are usually not available for at least 3–6 weeks.

Detection of T. gondii by PCR

The development of a PCR assay capable of detecting T. gondii has significantly enhanced the ability to detect congenital infection. Grover (71) demonstrated the util-ity of a PCR assay (employing primers for the repetitive B1 gene) as a means of mak-ing a rapid prenatal diagnosis. In this study, PCR correctly identified T. gondii in amniotic fluid samples from 7 of 9 congenitally infected infants studied. No false posi-tives were reported.

Subsequent reports (72) have documented that PCR testing of amniotic fluid have equivalent sensitivity, specificity, and positive and negative predictive valves as con-ventional assays (i.e., mouse inoculation and serological assays) (44,73–77). PCR test-ing will most likely become the preferred method of testing because of its rapid turnaround time, reliability, safety, simplicity, and low cost. PCR has also been shown to be capable of detecting *T. gondii* in CSF, ascitic fluid, blood, urine, and placental tissue *(78,79)*. There is as yet insufficient data about the utility of these sources compared to amniotic fluid. The use of PCR on amniotic fluid without having to use fetal blood samples represents perhaps the greatest advancement in prenatal diagnosis of *T. gondii* infection in the fetus.

PCR will most likely replace the other two methods of isolation of the parasite described above, although there are disadvantages. These include the following: (1) PCR's primary utility as a means of making the diagnosis prenatally, (2) limited availability of PCR at this time; (3) occasional false-negative assays (false-positive assays appear to be rare), and (4) like any of the other conventional assays, failure to detect materno-fetal transmission occurring after amniocentesis close to partuition.

Detection of T. gondii-*Specific Antigens and Cell-Mediated Immunity*

Serological detection of *T. gondii* antigens by ELISA and demonstration of a specific cell-mediated immune response as assessed by antigen-specific lymphocyte transformation have both been used previously to detect congenital infection. There is as yet insufficient data regarding their respective sensitivity and specificity to warrant their inclusion as part of the standard diagnostic workup.

FINAL COMMENTS

Although the focus of this chapter is diagnosis, treatment for congenital toxoplasmosis is available. For information, refer to the comprehensive discussion of treatment in the chapter, "Toxoplasmosis" by Remington et al. in the fifth edition of Remington and Klein's classic text, *Infectious Diseases of the Fetus and Newborn (1)*. Unlike congenital rubella, there is a therapeutic regimen (pyrimethamine and sulfadiazine with folinic acid supplementation) that is beneficial. As is the case with neonatal herpes, this regimen is most effective when started early, before overt clinical disease has developed.

REFERENCES

1. Remington JS, McLeod R, Thulliez, P, Desmonts G. Toxoplasmosis. In: Remington JS, Klein JO, eds. Infectious Diseases of the Fetus and Newborn Infant, 5th ed. Philadelphia: Saunders, 2001:205–346.
2. Smith J, McNeil G, Zhang Y, et al. Serological recognition of *Toxoplasma gondii* cyst antigens. In: Gross U, ed. *Toxoplasma gondii*. Berlin: Springer, 1996:67–75.
3. Mitchell C. Toxoplasmosis. In: Pizzo P, Wilfert C, eds. Pediatric AIDS, 2nd ed. Baltimore, MD: Williams and Wilkins, 1994:419–431.
4. Boyer K, Remington J, McLeod R. Toxoplasmosis. In: Feigin R, Cherry J, Demmler G, Kaplan S, eds. Textbook of Pediatric Infectious Diseases, 5th ed. Philadelphia: Saunders, 2004:2755–2770.
5. Gross U, Roggenkamp A, Janitschke K, et al. Improved sensitivity of the polymerase chain reaction for the detection of *Toxoplasma gondii* in biological and human clinical specimens. Eur J Clin Microbiol 1992;11:33–39.
6. Jones JL, Lopez A, Wilson M, Schulkin J, Gibbs R. Congenital toxoplasmosis: a review. Obstet Gynecol Survey 2001;56:296–305.
7. Remington JS, Gentry LO. Acquired toxoplasmosis: infection vs disease. Ann N Y Acad Sci 1970;174:1006–1017.

8. Siim JC. Clinical and diagnostic aspects of human acquired toxoplasmosis. Human Toxoplasmosis 1960;53–79.

9. Remington JS. Toxoplasmosis in the adult. Bull N Y Acad Med 1974;50:211–227.

10. Jones TC, Kean BH, Kimbal AC. Acquired toxoplasmosis. N Y State J Med 1969;69:2237–2242.

11. Wallon M, Dunn D, Slimani D, et al. Diagnosis of congenital toxoplasmosis at birth: what is the value of testing for IgM and IgA? Eur J Pediatr 1999;158:645–649.

12. Villena I, Aubert D, Brodard V, et al. Detection of specific immunoglobulin E during maternal, fetal and congenital toxoplasmosis. J Clin Microbiol 1999;37:3487–3490.

13. Dunn D, Wallon M, Peyron F, et al. Mother to child transmission of toxoplasmosis: risk estimates for clinical counseling. Lancet 1999;353:1899–1900.

14. Montoya JG, Remington JS. *Toxoplasma gondii*. In: Mandel GL, Bennett JE, Dolin R, eds. Mandel, Douglas, and Bennetts' Principles and Practice of Infectious Diseases, 5th ed. Philadelphia: Churchill Livingstone, 2000:2858–2888.

15. Wilson M, McAuley JM. *Toxoplasma*. In: Murray PR, Baron ES, Pfaller MA, et al., eds. Manual of Clinical Microbiology, 7th Ed. Washington, DC: ASM Press, 1999:1374–1382.

16. Wilson M, Remington JS, Clavet C, et al. Evaluation of six commercial kits for detection of human immunoglobulin M antibodies to *Toxoplasma gondii*. J Clin Microbiol 1997;35:3112–3115.

17. Liesenfield O, Montoya JG, Tathineni NJ, et al. Confirmatory serologic testing for acute toxoplasmosis among women reported to have positive *Toxoplasma* immunoglobulin M antibody titers. Am J Obstet Gynecol 2001;184:140–145.

18. Romand S, Wallon M, Franck J, et al. Prenatal diagnosis using polymerase chain reaction on amniotic fluid for congenital toxoplasmosis. Obstet Gynecol 2001;97:296–300.

19. Robert-Gangneux F, Gavinet MF, Ancelle T, et al. Value of prenatal diagnosis and early postnatal diagnosis of congenital toxoplasmosis: retrospective study of 110. J Clin Microbiol 1999;37:2893–2898.

20. Foulon W, Pinon JM, Stray-Pedersen B, et al. Prenatal diagnosis of congenital toxoplasmosis: a multicenter evaluation of different diagnostic parameters. Am J Obstet Gynecol 1999;181:843–847.

21. Bader TJ, Macones GA, Asch DA. Prenatal screening for toxoplasmosis. Obstet Gynecol 1997;90:457–464.

22. American College of Obstetricians and Gynecologists. Perinatal Viral and Parasitic Infections. Washington, DC: American College of Obstetricians and Gynecologists, 2000. ACOG Practice Bulletin 20.

23. Robert-Gangneux F, Commerce V, Tourte-Schaefer C, et al. Performance of Western blot assay to compare mother and newborn anti-*Toxoplasma* antibodies for the early neonatal diagnosis of congenital toxoplasmosis. Eur J Clin Microbiol Infect Dis 1999;18:648–654.

24. Glasser L, Delta BG. Congenital toxoplasmosis with placental infection in monozygotic twins. Pediatrics 1965;35:276–283.

25. Desmonts G, Couvreur J. toxoplasmosis in pregnancy and its transmission to the fetus. Bull N Y Acad Med 1974;50:146–159.

26. Alford CA, Stagno S, Reynolds DW. Congenital toxoplasmosis: clinical laboratory and therapeutic considerations with special reference to sub clinical disease. Bull N Y Acad Med 1974;50:160–181.

27. Alford CA, Foft JW, Blankenship WJ, et al. Subclinical central nervous system disease of neonates: a prospective study of infants born with increased levels of IgM. J Pediatr 1969;75:1167–1178.

28. Eichenwald HF. A study of congenital toxoplasmosis with emphasis on clinical manifestations, sequelae and therapy. In: Siim JC, ed. Human Toxoplasmosis. Copenhagen: Munksgaard, 1960:41.

29. Wilson CB, Remington JS, Stagno S, et al. Development of adverse sequelae in children born with sub clinical congenital *Toxoplasma* infection. Pediatrics 1980;66:767–774.
30. Koppe JG, Loewer-Sieger DH, de Roever-Bonnet H. Results of 20-year follow-up of congenital toxoplasmosis. Lancet 1986;1:254–256.
31. Saxon SA, Knight W, Reynolds DW, et al. Intellectual deficits in children born with subclinical congenital toxoplasmosis: a preliminary report. J Pediatr 1973;8:2792.
32. Guerina NG, Hsu HW, Meissner HC, et al. Neonatal serologic screening and early treatment for congenital *Toxoplasma gondii* infection. The New England Regional *Toxoplasma* Working Group. N Engl J Med 1994;330:1858–1863.
33. Lebech M, Andersen O, Christensen NC, et al. Feasibility of neonatal screening for *Toxoplasma* infection in the absence of prenatal treatment. Danish Congenital Toxoplasmosis Study Group. Lancet 1999;353:1834–1837.
34. Foulon W, Naessens A, Ho-Yen D. Prevention of congenital toxoplasmosis. J Perinat Med 2000;28;337–345.
35. Feldman HA. Toxoplasmosis. Pediatrics 1958;22:559–574.
36. Mitchell CD, Erlich SS, Mastrucci MT, et al. Congenital toxoplasmosis occurring in infants perinatally infected with human immunodeficiency virus I. Pediatr Infect Dis J 1990;9:512–518.
37. Cohen-Addad NE, Joshi VV, Sharer LR, et al. Congenital toxoplasmosis: pathologic support for a chronology of events. J Perinatol 1988;8:328–331.
38. O'Donohoe JM, Brueton MJ, Holliman RE. Concurrent congenital human immunodeficiency virus infection and toxoplasmosis. Pediatr Infect Dis J 1991;10:627–628.
39. Miller MJ, Remington JS. Toxoplasmosis in infants and children with HIV infection or AIDS. In: Pizzo PA, Wilfert CM, eds. Pediatric AIDS: The Challenge of HIV Infection in Infants, Children and Adolescents. Baltimore, MD: Williams and Wilkins, 1990:299–307.
40. Roberts F, McLeod R, Boyer K. Toxoplasmosis. In: Katz S, Gershon A, Hotez P, eds. Krugman's Infectious Diseases of Children, 10th ed. St. Louis, MO: Mosby, 1998:538–570.
41. Miller MJ, Seaman E, Remington JS. The clinical spectrum of congenital toxoplasmosis: problems in recognition. J Pediatr 1967;70:714–723.
42. Hendenstrom G, Huldt G, Langercrantz R. Toxoplasmosis in children. A study of 83 Swedish cases. Acta Pediatr 1961;50:304–312.
43. Couvreur J, Desmonts G, Girre JY. Congenital toxoplasmosis in twins. A series of 14 pairs of twins: absence of infection in one twin in two pairs. J Pediatr 1976;89:235–240.
44. Callahan WP, Russell WO, Smith MG. Human toxoplasmosis: a clinicopathologic study with presentation of five cases and review of the literature. Medicine 1946;25:343–397.
45. Pelloux H, Guy E, Angelici MC, et al. A second European collaborative study on polymerase chain reaction for *Toxoplasma gondii*, involving 15 teams. FEMS Microbiol Lett 1998;165:231–237.
46. Sabin AB, Feldman HA. Dyes as micro chemical indicators of a new immunity phenomenon affecting a protozoon parasite (*Toxoplasma*). Science 1948;108:660–663.
47. WHO Expert Committee on Biological Standardization. Twentieth report. WHO Tech Rep Ser 1968;384:1–100.
48. Balsari A, Poli G, Molina V, et al. ELISA for *Toxoplasma* antibody detection: a comparison with other serodiagnostic tests. J Clin Pathol 1980;33:640–643.
49. Gross U, Luder CG, Hendgen V, et al. Comparative immunoglobulin G antibody profiles between mother and child (CGMC test) for early diagnosis of congenital toxoplasmosis. J Clin Microbiol 2000;38:3619–3622.
50. Zufferey J, Hohlfeld P, Bille J, et al. Value of the comparative enzyme-linked immunofiltration assay for early neonatal diagnosis of congenital *Toxoplasma* infection. Pediatr Infect Dis J 1999;18:971–975.
51. McAuley J, Roizen N, Patel D, et al. Early and longitudinal evaluations of treated infants and children and untreated historical controls with congenital toxoplasmosis. Clin Infect Dis 1994;18:38–72.

52. Djurkovic-Djakovic O, Romand S, Nobre R, et al. Serologic rebounds after 1-year-long treatment for congenital toxoplasmosis. Pediatr Infect Dis J 2000;19:81–83.

53. Bessieres MH, Berrebi A, Rolland M, et al. Neonatal screening for congenital toxoplasmosis in a cohort of 165 women infected during pregnancy and influence of in utero treatment on the results of neonatal tests. Eur J Obstet Gynecol Reprod Biol 2001;94:37–45.

54. Villena I, Aubert D, Leroux B, et al. Pyrimethamine-sulfadoxine treatment of congenital toxoplasmosis; follow-up of 78 cases between 1980 and 1997. Reims Toxoplasmosis Group. Scan J Infect Dis 1998;30:295–300.

55. Remington JS. The present status of the IgM fluorescent antibody technique in the diagnosis of congenital toxoplasmosis. J Pediatr 1969;75:1116–1124.

56. Stagno S, Thiermann E. Valor de la immunofluorescencia indirecta en el diagnostico serologico de la toxoplasmosis aguda. Bol Chil Parasit 1970;25:915.

57. Aparicio Garrido A, Cour Boveda I. Aplicacion de la immunofluorescencia al estudio de las fracciones immunoglobulinicas en el diagnostico de la toxoplasmosis adquirida y congenita. Rev Clin Esp 1972;125:37–42.

58. Siegel JP, Remington JS. Comparison of methods for quantitating antigen-specific immunoglobulin m antibody with a reverse enzyme-linked immunosorbent assay. J Clin Microbiol 1983;19:63–70.

59. Naot Y, Remington JS. An enzyme-linked immunosorbent assay for detection of IgM antibodies of *Toxoplasma gondii*: use for diagnosis of acute acquired toxoplasmosis. J Infect Dis 1980;142:757–766.

60. Naot Y, Desmonts G, Remington JS. IgM enzyme-linked immunosorbent assay test for the diagnosis of congenital *Toxoplasma* infection. J Pediatr 1981;98:32–36.

61. Paul M, Petersen E, Pawlowski ZS, et al. Neonatal screening for congenital toxoplasmosis in the Poznan region of Poland by analysis of *Toxoplasma gondii*-specific IgM antibodies eluted from filter paper blood spots. Pediatr Infect Dis J 2000;19:30–36.

62. Araujo FG, Barnett EV, Gentry LO, et al. False-positive anti-*Toxoplasma* fluorescent-antibody tests in patients with antinuclear antibodies. Appl Microbiol 1971;22:270–275.

63. Hyde B, Barnett EV, Remington JS. Method for differentiation of nonspecific from specific *Toxoplasma* IgM fluorescent antibodies in patients with rheumatoid factor. Proc Soc Exp Biol Med 1975;148:1184–1189.

64. Pinon J, Puygauthier-Toubas D, Marx-Chemla C, et al. Detection of specific immunoglobulin E in patients with toxoplasmosis. J Clin Microbiol 1990;28:1739–1743.

65. Wallon M, Dunn D, Slimani D, et al. Diagnosis of congenital toxoplasmosis at birth: what is the value of testing for IgM and IgA? Eur J Pediatr 1999;158:645–649.

66. Naessens A, Jenum PA, Pollak A, et al. Diagnosis of congenital toxoplasmosis in the neonatal period: a multicenter evaluation. J Pediatr 1999;135:714–719.

67. Wallon M, Claudie C, Rubio S, et al. Value of cerebrospinal fluid cytochemical examination for the diagnosis of congenital toxoplasmosis at birth in France. Pediatr Infect Dis J 1998;17:705–710.

68. Hayes K, Billson FA, Jack I, et al. Cell culture isolation of *Toxoplasma gondii* from an infant with unusual ocular features. Med J Aust 1973;1:1297–1299.

69. Harvas JA, Fiol M, Caimari M, et al. Central nervous system congenital toxoplasmosis mimicking brain abscesses. Pediatr Infect Dis J 1987;6:491–492.

70. Coffey JD Jr. Congenital toxoplasmosis 38 years ago [letter to the editor]. Pediatr Infect Dis 1985;4:214.

71. Abbas AMA. Comparative study of methods used for the isolation of *Toxoplasma gondii*. Bull WHO 1967;36:344–346.

72. Grover CM, Thulliez P, Remington JS, et al. Rapid prenatal diagnosis of congenital *Toxoplasma* infection by using polymerase chain reaction in amniotic fluid. J Clin Microbiol 1990;28:2297–2301.

73. Hohlfeld P, Daffos F, Costa J, et al. Prenatal diagnosis of congenital toxoplasmosis with a polymerase chain reaction test on amniotic fluid. N Engl J Med 1994;331:695–699.

74. Van de Ven E, Melchers W, Galama J, et al. Identification of *Toxoplasma gondii* infections by B1 gene amplification. J Clin Microbiol 1991;19:2120–2124.

75. Dupouy-Camet J, Bougnoux ME, Lavreda de Souza S, et al. Comparative value of polymerase chain reaction and conventional biological tests for the prenatal diagnosis of congenital toxoplasmosis. Ann Biol Clin 1992;50:315–319.

76. Frisker-Hidalgo H, Pullout H, Racine C, et al. Detection of *Toxoplasma gondii* in 94 placentae from infected women by polymerase chain reaction, in vivo, and in vitro cultures. Placenta 1998;19:545–549.

77. Jenum PA, Holberg-Petersen M, Melby KK, et al. Diagnosis of congenital *Toxoplasma gondii* infection by polymerase chain reaction (PCR) on amniotic fluid samples. The Norwegian experience. APMIS 1998;106:680–686.

78. Bergstrom T, Ricksten A, Nenonen N, et al. Congenital *Toxoplasma gondii* infection diagnosed by PCR amplification of peripheral mononuclear blood cells from a child and mother. Scand J Infect Dis 1998;30:202–204.

79. Gratzl R, Hayde M, Kohlhauser C, et al. Follow-up of infants with congenital toxoplasmosis detected by polymerase chain reaction analysis of amniotic fluid. Eur J Clin Microbiol Infect Dis 1998;17:853–858.

80. Cazenovia J, Forester F, Besieges M, et al. Contribution of a new PCR assay to the prenatal diagnosis of congenital toxoplasmosis. Prenat Diagn 1992;12:119–127.

23

Chlamydia trachomatis

Margaret R. Hammerschlag

THE ORGANISM

Chlamydiae are obligate intracellular pathogens that have established a unique niche within the host cell. Until recently, the order Chlamydiales contained one family, Chlamydiaceae, which contained one genus, *Chlamydia*, with four recognized species: *Chlamydia trachomatis, Chlamydia psittaci, Chlamydia pneumoniae*, and *Chlamydia pecorum*. The species most important in human disease are *C. trachomatis* and *C. pneumoniae. C. trachomatis* infection is the most prevalent sexually transmitted pathogen and infectious disease in the United States today *(1)*. The Centers for Disease Control and Prevention estimates that the number of new *C. trachomatis* infections exceeds 4 million annually *(1,2)*. *C. pneumoniae* is now recognized as an important respiratory pathogen, and *C. psittaci* is primarily a zoonosis.

Taxonomic analysis using the 16S and 23S ribosomal ribonucleic acid (RNA) genes have suggested that the order Chlamydiales contains at least four distinct groups at the family level, and that within the family Chlamydiaceae there are two distinct lineages *(3)*. Under this analysis, the family Chlamydiaceae would be split into two genera: *Chlamydia*, which would contain *C. trachomatis* and two new species, *Chlamydia muridarum* and *Chlamydia suis*, and *Chlamydophila*, which would contain *C. pecorum*, *C. pneumoniae*, and *C. psittaci* and three new species split off from *C. psittaci*. The *Chlamydia* genus is also distinguished from species of the new genus *Chlamydophila* by the presence of the glycogenlike amorphous substance in the inclusions and susceptibility to sulfonamides.

Chlamydiae are characterized by a unique developmental cycle with morphologically distinct infectious and reproductive forms: elementary body (EB) and reticulate body (RB). Chlamydiae have a Gram-negative envelope without detectable peptidoglycan, although genomic analysis has revealed that both *C. trachomatis* and *C. pneumoniae* encode for proteins forming a nearly complete pathway for synthesis of peptidogylcan, including penicillin-binding proteins *(3)*. This is the basis for the so-called chlamydial peptidoglycan paradox, as it has been known for decades that chlamydia development is sensitive to β-lactam antibiotics.

Chlamydiae also share a group-specific lipopolysaccharide antigen and utilize host adenosine triphosphate for the synthesis of chlamydial protein. Although chlamydiae are auxotrophic for three of four nucleoside triphosphates, they do encode functional

From: *Infectious Disease: Congenital and Perinatal Infections: A Concise Guide to Diagnosis*
Edited by: C. Hutto © Humana Press Inc., Totowa, NJ

glucose-catabolizing enzymes, which can be used for generation of adenosine triphosphate *(3)*. As with peptidoglycan synthesis, for some reason these genes are turned off. All chlamydiae also encode an abundant protein called the major outer membrane protein (MOMP or OmpA), which is surface exposed in *C. trachomatis* and *C. psittaci* but apparently not in *C. pneumoniae*. The major outer membrane protein is the major determinant of the serologic classification of *C. trachomatis* and *C. psittaci* isolates.

Following infection, the infectious EBs, which are 200–400 µm in diameter, attach to the host cell by a process of electrostatic binding and are taken into the cell by endocytosis, which does not depend on the microtubule system. Within the host cell, the EB remains within a membrane-lined phagosome. The phagosome does not fuse with the host cell lysosome. The inclusion membrane is devoid of host cell markers, but lipid markers traffic to the inclusion, which suggests a functional interaction with the Golgi apparatus. The EBs then differentiate into RBs that undergo binary fission. After approx 36 hours, the RBs differentiate into EBs. At about 48 hours, release may occur by cytolysis or by a process of exocytosis or extrusion of the whole inclusion, leaving the host cell intact. Chlamydiae may also enter a persistent state after treatment with certain cytokines, such as γ-interferon, treatment with antibiotics, or restriction of certain nutrients, although in the persistent state metabolic activity is reduced. The ability to cause prolonged, often subclinical, infection is one of the major characteristics of Chlamydiae.

TIMING AND ROUTES OF INFECTION

Epidemiological evidence strongly suggests that the infant acquires chlamydial infection from the mother during vaginal delivery. Ascending infection through intact membranes during pregnancy can occur, but is very rare. Depending on the population examined, cervical infection with *C. trachomatis* has been reported in 2–30% of pregnant women attending prenatal clinics *(4–8)*. In most studies, chlamydial infection was far more prevalent than gonococcal infection. The prevalence of chlamydial infection is associated more weakly with socioeconomic status, urban or rural residence, and race or ethnicity than are gonorrhea and syphilis. The prevalence of *C. trachomatis* infection is consistently higher than 5% among sexually active adolescent and young adult women attending outpatient clinics, regardless of the region of the country, location of the clinic (urban or rural), and the race or ethnicity of the population. Among sexually active adolescents, prevalences commonly exceed 10% and may exceed 20% *(9)*. Decreasing age at first intercourse and increasing age at marriage have contributed importantly to the higher prevalence of *C. trachomatis* infection. Infection with *C. trachomatis* tends to be asymptomatic and of long duration.

RISK OF MATERNAL INFECTION DURING PREGNANCY

The majority of women, including pregnant women, with chlamydial infection are asymptomatic. Results from a National Institutes of Health-sponsored multicenter study of 8000 pregnant women (Vaginal Infection and Prematurity Study Group) found that cervical polymorphonuclear (PMN) leukocytes were poor predictors of the existence of chlamydial infection *(8)*. The predictive values of cervical mucopus and cervical PMNs were lower than those reported in nonpregnant women. Cervical friability was also an insensitive indicator.

Infection with *C. trachomatis* in pregnancy has been inconsistently linked to preterm delivery, low birth weight, and premature rupture of the membranes. A major problem with several of these studies has been the confounding presence of other infections, especially the genital mycoplasmas (*Mycoplasma hominis* and *Ureaplasma urealyticum*) and the organisms involved with bacterial vaginosis, which also may have adverse effects on the pregnancy and fetus *(5,10)*. Results from the Vaginal Infection and Prematurity study found an increase in risk of low birth weight among children of women who were colonized with genital mycoplasmas and *Trichomonas*. Chlamydial infection was associated with a nonsignificant increase in risk for low birth weight infants following adjustment for these other risk factors *(8)*. Women with mucopurulent cervicitis, defined as 30 or more PMN cells per 1000× field, were twice as likely to deliver a low birth weight infant. However, mucopurulent cervicitis had very poor sensitivity, specificity, and positive predictive value as an indicator of chlamydial infection in pregnant women. A later study of more than 10,000 pregnant women from the same group found a very strong association of preterm delivery of a low birth weight infant and bacterial vaginosis *(10)*. General opinion today is that evidence for adverse effects of *C. trachomatis* infection during pregnancy is minimal. Infection with *C. trachomatis* has definitively been linked to postpartum endometritis and salpingitis.

RISK OF FETAL OR NEONATAL INFECTION WHEN INFECTION IN THE MOTHER IS DIAGNOSED OR SUSPECTED

An infant born to a woman with active cervical infection with *C. trachomatis* is at risk of acquiring the infection during passage through the infected birth canal. Approximately 50–75% of infants born to infected women become infected at one or more anatomic sites, including the conjunctiva, nasopharynx, rectum, and vagina (Table 1). Overall, the nasopharynx is the most frequently infected site in the infant. Approximately 30–50% of infants born to *Chlamydia*-positive mothers will develop conjunctivitis *(11–14)*. Studies in the 1980s identified *C. trachomatis* in 14–46% of infants younger than 1 month of age presenting with conjunctivitis. Chlamydia ophthalmia appears to occur much less frequently now secondary to systematic screening and treatment of pregnant women. The incubation period is 5–14 days after delivery. *C. trachomatis* is usually not detectable in the eye or nasopharynx immediately after birth unless there has been prolonged rupture of membranes. At least 50% of infants with chlamydial conjunctivitis also have nasopharyngeal infection. The presentation varies extremely, ranging from mild conjunctival injection with scant mucoid discharge to severe conjunctivitis with copious purulent discharge, chemosis, and pseudomembrane formation. The conjunctiva can be friable and may bleed when stroked with a swab. Chlamydial conjunctivitis needs to be differentiated from gonococcal ophthalmia in some infants, especially those born to mothers who did not receive any prenatal care, had gonorrhea during pregnancy, or abused drugs. Overlap in both incubation periods and presentation is possible.

The majority of nasopharyngeal infections in infants are asymptomatic and may persist for 3 years or more. *C. trachomatis* pneumonia develops in only about 30% of infants with nasopharyngeal infection. In those who develop pneumonia, the presentation and clinical findings are characteristic. Infants with *C. trachomatis* pneumonia usually present between 4 and 12 weeks of age. A few cases have been reported presenting as early as 2

Table 1
Selected Studies of Perinatal Chlamydial Infection

Author (reference), year, city	Prevalence of maternal genital infection		Proportion of infants born to infected mother who developed chlamydial infection			
	Total	No. infected (%)	Total	Conjunctivitis	Pneumonia	NP	Rectum/vagina
Frommell et al. *(11)*, 1979, Denver	340	30 (8.8)	67	39%	11%	6%	NS
Schachter et al. *(14)*, 1986, San Francisco	5531	262 (4.7)	131	17.6%	16%	11.5%	14%
Hammerschlag et al. *(13)*, 1989, Brooklyn	4357	341 (8)	45	15%	1%	4%	NS

NP, nasopharynx; NS, not studied.

weeks of age, but no cases have been seen beyond 4 months of age. The infants frequently have a history of cough and congestion with an absence of fever *(15,16)*.

On physical examination the infant is tachypneic, and rales are heard on auscultation of the chest; wheezing is distinctly uncommon. There are no specific radiographic findings except hyperinflation. A review of chest films of 125 infants with chlamydial pneumonia revealed bilateral hyperinflation; diffuse infiltrates with a variety of radiographic patterns, including interstitial and reticulonodular; atelectasis; and bronchopneumonia. Lobar consolidation and pleural effusions were not seen. Significant laboratory findings include peripheral eosinophilia (>300 cells/cm^3) and elevated serum immunoglobulins *(15,16)*.

Infants born to *Chlamydia*-positive mothers also may become infected in the rectum and vagina *(14)*. Although infection at these sites appears to be totally asymptomatic, the infection may cause confusion if detected later, especially in the setting of suspected child sexual abuse. Subclinical rectal and vaginal infection may occur in as many as 14% of infants born to *Chlamydia*-positive women; some of these infants still were culture-positive at 18 months of age *(17)*.

PRENATAL EVALUATION OF MOTHER

The Centers for Disease Control and Prevention 2002 Guidelines for the Treatment of Sexually Transmitted Diseases recommend that screening for *C. trachomatis* be performed at the first prenatal visit and in the third trimester for women at increased risk (i.e., women <25 years of age and women who have had a new or more than one sexual partner or whose partner has other partners *[1]*). If screening is performed only during the first trimester, a longer period exists for acquiring infection before delivery. The major purpose of screening is to prevent postnatal maternal complications (i.e., endometritis) and chlamydial infection in the infant. As stated, evidence for adverse effects during pregnancy is minimal. Anecdotal evidence suggests that systematic screening for *C. trachomatis* infection and treatment of pregnant women has resulted in a significant reduction in perinatally acquired infection in infants *(18)*. However, infection in the infant may still occur if the mother was missed on screening or, more frequently, was reinfected later in pregnancy because of failure to treat the sexual partner or new sexual partner.

DIAGNOSTIC TESTS FOR EVALUATION OF CHLAMYDIA INFECTION IN THE MOTHER AND INFANT

As *C. trachomatis* is an obligate intracellular parasite, isolation of the organism must be performed in tissue culture, with culture confirmation by staining with species-specific fluorescent monoclonal antibodies and identification of the characteristic intracytoplasmic inclusions with microscopy. Until recently, the gold standard of diagnosis of *C. trachomatis* infection in women was isolation by culture from the cervix *(2)*. Culture requires careful specimen collection and stringent transport conditions with maintenance of the cold chain and requires 48–72 hours to perform. In addition, culture methods for *C. trachomatis* are not standardized; therefore, there can be significant variation in performance from laboratory to laboratory. Serology, using either the microimmunofluorescence test or enzyme immunoassays (EIAs), is not suitable for the diagnosis of genital *C. trachomatis* infection *(19)*.

Several types of nonculture tests for detection of *C. trachomatis* in clinical speci-mens have been available in the past. These include EIAs, specifically Chlamydiazyme (Abbott Diagnostics, Chicago, IL) and MicroTrak EIA (Genetic Systems, Seattle, WA) and direct fluorescent antibody (DFA) tests, including Syva MicroTrak (Genetic Sys-tems, Seattle, WA) and Pathfinder (Sanofi-Pasteur, Chaska, MN) and a deoxyribo-nucleic acid (DNA) hybridization assay, GenProbe Pace II (GenProbe, San Diego, CA), were introduced in the 1980s *(20)*.

The DFA test was less sensitive than culture (70–90% depending on the site and clinical status) but highly specific (≥95%). The DFA was best suited for high-preva-lence populations when culture was not available; however, the very nature of the test made it difficult to use for screening large numbers of specimens.

Unlike the DFA, EIAs were semiautomated and suitable for processing large num-bers of specimens. EIAs use either a polyclonal or a monoclonal antibody directed against the *Chlamydia* genus-specific lipopolysaccharide antigen. These tests will de-tect other chlamydia species, specifically *C. pneumoniae*, if used for respiratory speci-mens.

The direct nucleic acid probe was until recently the most commonly used nonculture test for detection of *C. trachomatis* in many hospital and public health laboratories in the United States. Using chemiluminescence, the probe hybridizes to a species-specific sequence of chlamydial 16S ribosomal RNA. The performance of the probe assay has been similar to available EIAs, with sensitivities of 75–80% and specificities greater than 99%. This assay is not a nucleic acid amplification test. Neither EIAs nor DNA probe are sensitive enough to detect *C. trachomatis* in urine from women.

A major advance in the diagnosis of *C. trachomatis* infection during the past decade has been the introduction of nucleic acid amplification tests (NAATs *[20,21]*). These tests have high sensitivity, perhaps even detecting 10–20% greater than culture, while retaining high specificity (>98–99%). There are currently three commercially avail-able NAATs approved by the Food and Drug Administration (FDA): polymerase chain reaction (PCR; Amplicor, Roche Molecular Diagnostics, Nutley, NJ), transcription-mediated amplification (TMA; GenProbe), and strand displacement amplification (SDA; ProbeTec, Becton Dickson, Sparks, MD). A fourth assay, ligase chain reaction (LCR)-LCx *Chlamydia trachomatis* Assay (Abbott Diagnostics), was withdrawn from the market by Abbott in June 2002 because of performance problems. PCR and SDA are DNA amplification tests; all use primers that target gene sequences on the cryptic *C. trachomatis* plasmid, which has approx 10 copies per cell. TMA is an RNA amplifi-cation assay that uses reverse transcriptase and a T7 polymerase to produce anywhere from 1 million to 1 billion copies of an RNA target. Unlike the DNA amplification assays, TMA is isothermal; that is, it does not require the use of a thermocycler, which is necessary for PCR or LCR. As shown in Table 2, EIAs can detect a minimum of 10^4–10^5 organisms; culture can detect 10–100 organisms, and NAATs can detect 1–10 organisms.

Amplification tests are more sensitive than currently available EIAs and nonamplification DNA probe assays. One such study found PCR to be 37% more sen-sitive than the DNA probe. However, these tests are not all equivalent. False-negatives caused by inhibitors of DNA polymerase are more of a problem than false-positives caused by amplicon carryover. Inhibitor appears to be more frequent in cervical speci-mens and urine. Inhibitory substances in urine from pregnant women include β-human

Table 2
Relative Limits of Detection of Different Technologies
Used to Diagnose *C. trachomatis*

	Number of organisms/sample[a]
Amplified DNA/RNA	$1–10^1$
Culture	$10^1–10^2$
DFA	$10^1–10^3$
EIA	$10^3–10^5$
DNA probe	$10^3–10^4$

[a]Log number of chlamydial elementary bodies.

chorionic gonadatropin, crystals, nitrites, and hemoglobin. Of note, there are no inhibition controls included with any of the currently available kits. Also, there are rare strains of *C. trachomatis* that lack the cryptic plasmid and thus would not be detected by PCR.

Currently available commercial NAATs have FDA approval for cervical swabs from women, urethral swabs from men, and urine from men and women. However, the sensitivity for detection of *C. trachomatis* in urine from women is less than for the cervix (78–96%). The use of noninvasive specimens such as urine is especially useful in high-prevalence populations such as sexually active adolescents *(9)*. A second-generation TMA was just recently approved for vaginal specimens from women.

Urine specimens for NAATs should be collected as directed by the test manufacturer. The patient should not have urinated within the previous hour, and women should be instructed not to clean the perineum prior to voiding. The first catch of 10–20 mL urine should be collected in a clean collection cup and refrigerated immediately at 2–8°C. However, a midstream catch urine has been reported to be effective for testing with LCR. Longer times (>3 hours) since the last void appeared to reduce the sensitivity of antigen tests for urine from women. This appears to be less of an issue with the amplification tests. The time the urine specimen is left at room temperature should be minimized because the low pH and high urea content can rapidly denature DNA present in the specimen, especially at temperatures greater than 25°C. Although PCR is currently not approved for use with frozen urine specimens, freezing and thawing may actually improve the sensitivity of PCR by eliminating transient inhibitory factors that are present in some specimens.

NAATs should probably not be used as a test of cure within 3 weeks of treatment. More than 40% of follow-up urine specimens from female patients who were initially positive by PCR and 73.3% of those initially positive by LCR were still positive 1–3 days after treatment with single-dose azithromycin. Only at 15 days posttherapy did all specimens test negative *(10)*.

Isolation by culture remains the preferred method for detection of *C. trachomatis* from the conjunctiva, nasopharynx, vagina, or rectum of infants. Several nonculture methods have FDA approval for diagnosis of chlamydial conjunctivitis. They include EIAs, specifically Chlamydiazyme and MicroTrak, and DFAs, including Syva MicroTrak and Pathfinder. These tests appear to perform well with conjunctival specimens with sensitivities greater than or equal to 90% and specificities greater than or equal to 95% compared with culture *(22,23)*. The performance with nasopharyngeal specimens has not been as good, with sensitivities ranging from 33 to 90%. The DNA probe does not have approval for any site in children. Data on use of NAATs in children are limited. Preliminary data suggest that PCR (Amplicor) is equivalent to culture for detection of *C. trachomatis* in the conjunctiva and nasopharynx of infants with conjunctivitis *(18)*. However, no NAATs are currently approved by the FDA for this indication.

REFERENCES

1. Centers for Disease Control and Prevention. Sexually transmitted diseases treatment guidelines 2002. MMWR Morb Mortal Wkly Rep 2002;51:1–78.
2. Centers for Disease Control and Prevention. Screening tests to detect *Chlamydia trachomatis* and *Neisseria gonorrhoeae* infections—2002. MMWR Morb Mortal Wkly Rep 2002;51:1–38.
3. Rockey DD, Lenart J, Stephens RS. Genome sequencing and our understanding of chlamydiae. Infect Immunol 2000;68:5473–5479.
4. Bell TA, Stamm WE, Kuo CC, Wang SP, Holmes KK, Grayston JT. Risk of perinatal transmission of *Chlamydia trachomatis* by mode of delivery. J Infect 1994;29:165–169.
5. Berman SM, Harrison HR, Boyce WT, Haffner WJJ, Lewis M, Arthur JB. Low birth weight, prematurity, and postpartum endometritis. Association with prenatal cervical *Mycoplasma hominis* and *Chlamydia trachomatis* infection. JAMA 1987;257:1189–1194.
6. McGregor JA, French JI. *Chlamydia trachomatis* infection during pregnancy. Am J Obstet Gynecol 1991;164:1782–1789.
7. Miller JM, Martin DH. Treatment of *Chlamydia trachomatis* infections in pregnant women. Drugs 2000;60:597–605.
8. Nugent RP, Hillier SL. Mucopurulent cervicitis as a predictor of chlamydia infection and adverse pregnancy outcome. Sex Transm Dis 1992;19:198–202.
9. Gaydos CA, Crotchfelt KA, Howell MR, Kralian S, Hauptman P, Quinn TC. Molecular amplification assays to detect chlamydial infections from high school female students and to monitor the persistence of chlamydia DNA after therapy. J Infect Dis 1998;177:417–424.
10. Hillier SL, Nugent RP, Eschenbach DA, et al. Association between bacterial vaginosis and preterm delivery of a low-birth-weight infant. The Vaginal Infections and Prematurity Study Group. N Engl J Med 1995;333:1737–1742.
11. Frommell GT, Rothenberg R, Wang SP, McIntosh K. Chlamydial infection of mothers and their infants. J Pediatr 1979;95:28–32.
12. Hammerschlag MR, Chandler JW, Alexander ER, English M, Koustky L. Longitudinal studies on chlamydial infections in the first year of life. Pediatr Infect Dis J 1982;1:395–401.
13. Hammerschlag MR, Cummings C, Roblin PM, Williams TH, Delke I. Efficacy of neonatal ocular prophylaxis for the prevention of chlamydial and gonococcal conjunctivitis. N Engl J Med 1989;320:769–772.
14. Schachter J, Grossman M, Sweet RL, Holt J, Jordan C, Bishop E. Prospective study of perinatal transmission of *Chlamydia trachomatis*. JAMA 1986;255:3374–3377.
15. Beem MO, Saxon EM. Respiratory-tract colonization and a distinctive pneumonia syndrome in infants infected with *Chlamydia trachomatis*. N Engl J Med 1997;296:306–310.
16. Harrison HR, English MG, Lee CK, Alexander ER. *Chlamydia trachomatis* infant pneumonitis: comparison with matched controls and other infant pneumonitis. N Engl J Med 1978;298:702–708.
17. Bell TA, Stamm WE, Wang SP, Kuo CC, Holmes KK, Grayston JT. Chronic *Chlamydia trachomatis* infections in infants. JAMA 1992;267:400–402.
18. Hammerschlag MR, Roblin PM, Gelling, M, Tsumura N, Jules J, Kutlin A. Use of polymerase chain reaction for the detection of *Chlamydia trachomatis* in ocular and nasopharyngeal specimens from infants with conjunctivitis. Pediatr Infect Dis J 1997;16:293–297.

19. Moss TR, Darougar S, Woodland RM, Nathan M, Dines RJ, Cathrine V. Antibodies to chlamydia species in patients attending a genitourinary clinic and the impact of antibodies to *Chlamydia pneumoniae* and *Chlamydia psittaci* on the sensitivity and the specificity of *Chlamydia trachomatis* serology tests. Sex Transm Dis 1993;20:61–65.
20. Black CM. Current methods of laboratory diagnosis of *Chlamydia trachomatis* infection. Clin Microbiol Rev 1997;10:160–184.
21. Chernesky MA. Nucleic acid tests for the diagnosis of sexually transmitted diseases. FEMS Immunol Med Microbiol 1999;24:437–446.
22. Hammerschlag MR, Roblin PM, Cummings C, Williams TH, Worku M, Howard LV. Comparison of enzyme immunoassay to culture for the diagnosis of chlamydial conjunctivitis and respiratory infection in infants. J Clin Microbiol 1987;25:2306–2308.
23. Roblin PM, Hammerschlag MR, Cummings C, Williams TH, Worku M. Comparison of two rapid microscopic methods and culture for detection of *Chlamydia trachomatis* in ocular and nasopharyngeal specimens from infants. J Clin Microbiol 1989;27:968–970.

24
Mycoplasma and Ureaplasma

Ken B. Waites

INTRODUCTION

The concept that *Mycoplasma hominis* and *Ureaplasma* spp could be important pathogens that may affect pregnancy outcomes and the health of neonates was first given serious consideration in the 1960s and early 1970s when reports of postpartum endometritis with septicemia, chorioamnionitis, and low birth weight caused by these organisms began to appear and a treatment trial of pregnant women given tetracycline showed a significant beneficial effect on birth weight for their infants *(1–4)*. Since those days, a great many more case reports have been described, and numerous clinical studies have been performed in an attempt to clarify what roles, if any, these organisms play as agents responsible for invasive infections in neonates, premature labor, spontaneous abortion, stillbirth, and chronic lung disease of prematurity.

Despite more than 30 years of study, many aspects of the biology and clinical importance of genital mycoplasmas and ureaplasmas are still incompletely understood for a variety of reasons. These include (1) the high prevalence of these organisms in healthy persons; (2) poor design of many of the earlier research studies, which attempted to relate the mere presence of mycoplasmas or ureaplasmas in the lower urogenital tract to pathology in the upper tract or in offspring; (3) failure to consider multifactorial aspects of some maternal conditions and potential confounders (e.g., bacterial vaginosis); (4) unfamiliarity of clinicians and microbiologists with the complex and fastidious nutritional requirements for mycoplasmas and ureaplasmas and the methods for their proper detection; and (5) considering these organisms only as a last resort in conditions thought more likely to be caused by other micro-organisms.

An extensive review of the published literature on perinatal and neonatal aspects of mycoplasmal and ureaplasmal infections is beyond the scope of this chapter. Therefore, commentary focuses on the latest information pertinent for clinicians who need to understand the basic biology of these fascinating micro-organisms, when to consider them as possible etiologies of perinatal or neonatal conditions, and how to approach diagnosis from both clinical and laboratory standpoints. Reference texts are available for more detailed analyses of evidence for and against a pathogenic role for mycoplasmas and ureaplasmas in the conditions mentioned briefly in subsequent sections of this publication *(5,6)*.

From: *Infectious Disease: Congenital and Perinatal Infections: A Concise Guide to Diagnosis*
Edited by: C. Hutto © Humana Press Inc., Totowa, NJ

MOLLICUTES AS AGENTS OF HUMAN DISEASE

Classification and Cell Biology

Mycoplasmas and ureaplasmas are eubacteria classified in the class Mollicutes, which evolved from clostridium-like ancestors through the process of gene deletion. There are more than 150 species currently named in the class Mollicutes, 16 of which are known to have humans as their primary host. Mollicutes represent the smallest self-replicating organisms, both in cellular dimensions and genome, that are capable of cell-free existence. The extremely small genome, less than 600 kbp for the smallest mollicute *Mycoplasma genitalium*, and drastically limited biosynthetic capabilities explain the parasitic or saprophytic existence of these organisms, their sensitivity to environmental conditions, and their fastidious growth requirements. Mollicutes associated with humans range from coccoid cells of about 0.2–0.3 μm diameter (e.g., ureaplasmas and *Mycoplasma hominis*) to tapered rods 1–2 μm in length and 0.1–0.2 μm in width in the case of *Mycoplasma pneumoniae*. All mollicutes totally lack a cell wall barrier, making them unique among prokaryotes. Lack of a cell wall also renders these organisms insensitive to the activity of β-lactam antimicrobials, prevents them from staining by Gram stain, and is largely responsible for their pleomorphic form.

The small cellular mass also means that mollicutes cannot be detected by light microscopy, and they do not produce visible turbidity in liquid growth media. Typical colonies require examination under a stereomicroscope to visualize their morphologic features. Mollicutes have never been found as freely living organisms in nature because they depend on a host cell to supply them with the things they need for their parasitic existence. Another characteristic of most members of the class Mollicutes is the requirement for sterols in artificial growth media, supplied by the addition of serum, to provide necessary components of the triple-layer cell membrane that gives structural support to the osmotically fragile organism. Maintenance of osmotic stability is especially important in these bacteria because of the lack of a rigid cell wall. Although mycoplasmas and ureaplasmas can flourish within an osmotically stable environment in their chosen eukaryotic host, they are extremely susceptible to desiccation, a fact that greatly impacts the need for proper handling of clinical specimens in which cultural isolation is to be attempted and the need for close contact for transmission of infection from person to person. The small size, complex and fastidious nutritional requirements of mollicutes makes them challenging for detection and characterization by the microbiologist and historically has greatly hampered the ability of diagnostic laboratories to provide reliable services for their detection and identification.

Mollicute Species Pathogenic in Humans

Most research in perinatal and neonatal pathology has focused on two organisms, *M. hominis* and the bacterium formerly known as *Ureaplasma urealyticum,* because they are clearly the most significant in terms of disease-producing potential in pregnant women and neonates. However, it is relevant to mention briefly three other pathogenic mycoplasmal species that may contribute to perinatal and neonatal conditions to a lesser extent.

M. pneumoniae is well known as a major respiratory tract pathogen in older children and adults and has been detected many times in infants younger than 1 year, but it is rarely considered to be of much importance in the perinatal or neonatal period and is believed to be uncommon. It was not detected by culture in an evaluation of more than 1500 neonates *(5)*. Nonetheless, this mycoplasma is a common cause of respiratory infections in women of childbearing age; it has been transmitted transplacentally with subsequent detection in the nasopharynx from a neonate with congenital pneumonia *(7)* and is therefore worthy of further study as a potential pathogen in this setting. More sensitive diagnostic tests such as the polymerase chain reaction (PCR) assay might yield different results if the culture-based study mentioned above was repeated.

M. genitalium was first detected in men with urethritis, and it has since been estimated to occur in 9–20% of men with urethritis and in up to 20% of women with urethritis or cervicitis *(8)*. This organism has the smallest genome known for any free-living micro-organism, grows very slowly, and cannot be readily detected by culture. The PCR assay has facilitated clinical studies of *M. genitalium* as evidence mounts for its role in male urethritis, pelvic inflammatory disease, and possibly cervicitis *(8)*.

Blanchard et al. *(9)* did not detect *M. genitalium* by PCR or culture in 232 amniotic fluids. Three studies have found *M. genitalium* in a very small percentage of pregnant women (3.9–6.2%) but were unable to relate the presence of this mycoplasma to preterm birth or other adverse pregnancy outcomes *(10–12)*. Vertical transmission of *M. genitalium* from mother to neonate has also been reported *(13)*, but its significance in neonates is unknown. Thus far, compelling evidence for an important role in pregnancy outcome or neonatal disease for this mycoplasma is lacking, but studies addressing this topic have been somewhat limited, and it is inappropriate to completely discount its significance based on information available at the present time.

Mycoplasma fermentans may also be pathogenic for humans in some settings, with most recent attention given to its role as an opportunist in persons with human immunodeficiency virus infection and acquired immunodeficiency syndrome and to a possible association with chronic arthritic conditions. *M. fermentans* is known to inhabit the lower and upper urogenital tracts of some adults. Furthermore, this mycoplasma has been detected by culture in placental tissue and in amniotic fluid in the presence of inflammation, but no studies have been performed to evaluate its occurrence and significance in neonates *(14)*.

Soon after ureaplasmas were first identified in the 1950s and were subsequently characterized, it became apparent that these organisms could be subclassified into several serotypes. Data obtained from 16S ribosomal ribonucleic acid sequencing has led to the further breakdown of the 14 serotypes into two biovars or clusters. The two biovars were designated as distinct species. Biovar 1 (parvo) became *Ureaplasma parvum*, whereas biovar 2 (T960) became *U. urealyticum*. Biovar 1 is the more common of the two biovars isolated in clinical specimens, especially pregnant women, but both species may occur simultaneously in the same person.

There has long been speculation that there may be differential pathogenicity of the various serotypes, biovars, and species. There was no conclusive evidence for this difference in pathogenicity for several years, and this was related to some degree to inefficient and imprecise methods for their accurate differentiation and the fact that many persons may harbor more than one serotype in their urogenital tract. The availability of the PCR assay has enabled a more rigorous assessment of whether one biovar or species is more pathogenic than the other. Kim et al. *(15)* found no difference in pregnancy outcome and magnitude of intra-amniotic inflammatory response, chorioamnionitis, birth weight, or gestational age at delivery or neonatal morbidity in 77 women whose amniotic fluid contained ureaplasmas detected by PCR according to biovar. Zheng *(16)* suggested that the property of invasiveness for ureaplasmas is likely not limited to one or a few particular serotypes, and that perhaps antigen variability and host factors may be more important determinants for *Ureaplasma* infections than different serotypes *per se*.

However, a few limited studies have identified some differences regarding pathogenicity between the two biovars. Abele-Horn et al. *(17)* found biovar 2 to be dominant in patients with pelvic inflammatory disease as well as in women who had had miscarriages, and it seemed to have more adverse effects on pregnancy outcome regarding birth weight, gestational age, and preterm delivery than biovar 1. Others have shown that biovar 2 can be isolated more frequently from patients with a history of recurrent miscarriages than from normal pregnant women *(18)*.

Martinez *(19)* found no differences in antimicrobial susceptibilities or occurrence of the two ureaplasmal species in amniotic fluids of women with adverse pregnancy outcomes vs isolates from the lower urogenital tract of healthy pregnant women. In contrast, two other studies found more tetracycline resistance in biovar 2 than in biovar 1 *(17,20)*. The apparent contradictory results of some of these studies suggest that differencenos in antimicrobial susceptibilities, when they are observed, may reflect the history of antimicrobial exposure, the population studied, and other local environmental and host factors rather than a different capacity of the organism to acquire the *tet* (M) transposon in some instances. Based on the modest, and somewhat contentious evidence for differential pathogenicity for the two ureaplasmal species available at the present time and limitations of widely available technology for organism identification, it is neither practical nor necessary to distinguish between the two *Ureaplasma* species for clinical purposes. Therefore, diagnostic laboratories should appropriately designate cultures as positive for *Ureaplasma* spp and leave it at that.

Table 1 summarizes the major conditions of adults and infants that have been purported to be associated with or caused by *M. hominis, M. genitalium,* and *Ureaplasma* spp and the relative strengths, based on published evidence, for their roles in these conditions. The discussion of the clinical importance of these organisms has been divided into two major categories: maternal aspects and neonatal aspects.

Routes of Transmission and Maternal Considerations

Following puberty, colonization of the male and female lower urogenital tract by *M. hominis* and *Ureaplasma* spp usually occurs as a result of sexual activity. Up to 80% of women may harbor ureaplasmas and more than 50% may harbor *M. hominis*. These organisms are also commonly found in the lower urogenital tract of pregnant women, and they usually persist throughout pregnancy, providing a reservoir for transmission to the developing fetus and neonate *(5)*. In most healthy adults, mycoplasmas and ureaplasmas exist primarily as commensals, associated with the mucosal surfaces, and rarely cause serious invasive disease. However, in persons who are immunocompromised, especially if hypogammaglobulinemic, invasion of extragenital sites can occur. If one considers pregnant women and preterm infants to have an altered immune status, it is not surprising that these organisms can cause invasive and destructive disease when given the right circumstances.

Ureaplasma spp can be transmitted from a colonized woman to her newborn infant *in utero* either transplacentally from the mother's blood or by an ascending route sec-

Table 1
Conditions Known To Be Associated With or Caused by *Mycoplasmas* **and** *Ureaplasmas*

Disease	*Ureaplasma* spp	*M. hominis*	*M. genitalium*
Adults			
Male urethritis	+	–	+
Chronic prostatitis	±	–	±
Epididymitis	±	–	–
Urinary calculi	+	–	–
Pyelonephritis	±	+	–
Bacterial vaginosis	±	±	–
Cervicitis	–	–	±
Pelvic inflammatory disease	–	+	+
Infertility	±	–	–
Chorioamnionitis	+	–	–
Spontaneous abortion	±	±	–
Extragenital disease (including arthritis)	+	+	+
Infants			
Prematurity/low birth weight	+	–	–
Intrauterine growth retardation	±	–	–
Postpartum/postabortal fever	+	+	–
Congenital pneumonia	+	+	–
Chronic lung disease	±	–	–
Meningitis	+	+	–
Abscesses	+	+	–

–, no association or causal role demonstrated. In some conditions for *M. genitalium*, this may reflect the fact that no studies using appropriate techniques to detect this organism have been performed.
+, causal role.
±, significant association and/or strong suggestive evidence, but causal role not proven. (Modified from ref. *29*.)

ondary to colonization of the mother's urogenital tract, or at delivery by passage through a colonized birth canal. The rate of vertical transmission has been reported to range from 18 to 55% among full-term infants and from 29 to 55% among preterm infants *(21)*. *Ureaplasma* spp and *M. hominis* can be isolated from neonates born to mothers with intact membranes and delivered by cesarean section and from amniotic fluid during early pregnancy *(5,21)*. The rate of vertical transmission is not affected by method of delivery but is significantly increased when chorioamnionitis is present. The rate of colonization also appears to be higher in very low birth weight infants *(21)*.

The first studies attempting to make a correlation of mycoplasmas and ureaplasmas with postpartum endometritis were based on cervicovaginal cultures and caused much confusion with their inconclusive results *(5)*. However, both *M. hominis* and *Ureaplasma* spp can be detected in the bloodstream of some women with postpartum or postabortal fever, with *M. hominis* being the more common. This condition is usually self-limited, but some cases of dissemination to joints resulting in arthritis may occur.

Isolation of *Ureaplasma* spp, but not *M. hominis,* from the chorioamnion has been consistently associated with histologic chorioamnionitis and is inversely related to birth weight, even when adjusting for duration of labor, rupture of fetal membranes, and presence of other bacteria. These organisms can invade the amniotic cavity and persist for several weeks when fetal membranes are intact and initiate an intense inflammatory reaction in the absence of labor *(22–24)*. Even though these conditions may be clinically silent, these findings are strongly supportive of a causal role for *Ureaplasma* spp in chorioamnionitis. *M. hominis* seems rarely to invade the chorioamnion and amniotic fluid in the absence of other micro-organisms, and data to support an independent role for this mycoplasma in either histologic or clinical amnionitis are modest at best. Chorioamnion colonization with *Ureaplasma* spp was associated with a threefold increased risk of post-cesarean delivery endometritis, an association that increased to eightfold in women in whom onset of labor was spontaneous *(25)*. The extent to which genital mycoplasmas may produce clinical amnionitis is unclear because some women whose placentas show significant evidence of inflammation and from whom genital mycoplasmas can be isolated from chorioamnion or amniotic fluid may not have evidence of clinical amnionitis.

Intrauterine infection is believed to be a major cause of preterm labor and can be documented in approximately one-fourth of all preterm births. The earlier the gestation age at delivery, the higher the frequency of intra-amniotic infection *(26)*. This relationship is believed to be related to the concept that uterine contractions may be induced by cytokines, prostaglandins, and phospholipases produced by micro-organisms *(27)*. *M. hominis* and *Ureaplasma* spp can be isolated from endometrial tissue of healthy, nonpregnant women, indicating they may be present at the time of implantation and might therefore be involved in early pregnancy losses *(5)*.

Studies of women from whom ureaplasmas and *M. hominis* were isolated from endometrium or placenta have shown a consistent association with spontaneous abortion, but this has not proven true for studies limited to sampling the lower genital tract *(28)*. Isolation of *Ureaplasma* spp in pure culture from amniotic fluid obtained from women with intact fetal membranes who experienced subsequent fetal loss in the presence of histological chorioamnionitis has been documented by multiple investigators, indicating that in some cases the role of this organism is causal *(22–24)*.

Other circumstantial evidence linking ureaplasmas to spontaneous abortion, low birth weight, intrauterine growth retardation, and preterm labor includes reports of successful pregnancies following antimicrobial treatment and serological studies *(5)*. Underlying problems that complicate complete understanding of any potential role for genital mycoplasmas in low birth weight are that *M. hominis* and, to a lesser extent, *Ureaplasma* spp can be components of the varied flora that occur with bacterial vaginosis, and this condition is itself associated with low birth weight *(28–31)*, problems in experimental study designs that failed to consider potential roles for organisms other than genital mycoplasmas, or use of control groups of uncertain comparability.

Neonatal Infections

M. hominis and *Ureaplasma* spp can be isolated from organs of aborted fetuses and stillborn infants in pure culture and in the presence of an inflammatory response *(5)*. Ureaplasmas are more commonly detected in products of early abortions and midtrimester pregnancy losses than from induced abortions, and they are more commonly detected in endometrium of habitual aborters and from placentas of aborted fetuses than from controls *(5)*. Several studies have reported an association between isolation of *Ureaplasma* spp from the chorioamnion and perinatal morbidity and mortality *(5,32,33)*. Because these studies did not attempt to detect the organisms directly in the infants, it is uncertain whether the problems experienced by the infants were caused by infection or complications of prematurity. However, when investigations were designed to culture directly the lower respiratory tract, blood, and cerebrospinal fluid (CSF), it became evident that both *Ureaplasma* spp and *M. hominis* can cause a variety of clinically significant infections in neonates.

Retrospective as well as prospective studies and well-documented case reports indicated *Ureaplasma* spp can cause congenital pneumonia *(5)*. Proof for causality includes isolation of the organism in pure culture from affected lungs of neonates and from the chorioamnion, demonstration of a specific immunoglobulin M response, presence of histologic pneumonia and chorioamnionitis, clinical manifestations of respiratory distress, and demonstration of the organisms in lung tissue by immunofluorescence and electron microscopy. In some instances, ureaplasmas have been detected from multiple sites in neonates before and after death. Although individual case reports suggested *M. hominis* may cause pneumonia in newborns, it has not been implicated as a common cause in prospective studies *(5)*. No convincing evidence exists to support a significant role for *Ureaplasma* spp or *M. hominis* as common independent causes of pneumonia in otherwise healthy infants beyond the neonatal period.

In the late 1980s, bacteremia and progression to chronic lung disease of prematurity and death were described in very low birth weight infants who were infected with *Ureaplasma* spp in the lower respiratory tract *(34–37)*. Presence of ureaplasmas in the lower respiratory tract has also been significantly associated with radiographic evidence of pneumonia when compared with uninfected infants, and precocious dysplastic changes were also significantly associated with the presence of these organisms *(38)*. Further studies have shown that infants from whom ureaplasmas were isolated from endotracheal secretions had significantly more neutrophils in endotracheal secretions, attesting to their inflammatory potential *(39)*.

An explanation for the association of perinatal infections caused by *Ureaplasma* spp and development of chronic lung disease relates to intrauterine exposure to proinflammatory cytokines that are released in response to infection, which persists because antimicrobials commonly used are not active against this organism. Chronic inflammation then increases the requirement for supplementary oxygen, which can lead to dysplastic changes in the airways as a result of oxygen toxicity or a synergistic effect between the ureaplasmas and hyperoxia. It is also speculated that this cytokine cascade may induce both preterm labor and inflammation in the airways, which triggers the lung injury sequence before birth.

Several additional studies performed during the 1990s confirmed that there was a significant association between chronic lung disease of prematurity and the presence of *Ureaplasma* spp in the lower respiratory tract of preterm neonates *(40)*. This association was also detected in studies performed after introduction of exogenous surfactant *(39)*. This relationship has not been shown consistently in all investigations performed to date *(41–44)*, but two studies from Europe supported a role for *Ureaplasma* spp in chronic lung disease of prematurity even as technological advances in neonatology continue to improve survival of very low birth weight infants *(45,46)*. A summary and review of all published studies on the role of ureaplasmas in neonatal lung disease through 2004 was published by Waites *(47)*.

There are also data to suggest that infants with perinatal ureaplasmal infections have a significantly greater need for hospital care during the first year of postnatal life *(48)*. Further evidence of the inflammatory potential for this organism comes from animal models that indicate *Ureaplasma* spp can induce pneumonia and chronic inflammation *(49–51)*.

Despite numerous studies and considerable data supporting an association, demonstration of a cause-and-effect relationship between *Ureaplasma* spp and chronic lung disease or prematurity has not been conclusively proven. Even though treatment with intravenous erythromycin may eradicate ureaplasmas from the lower respiratory tract of neonates, at least temporarily *(52)*, small randomized trials of erythromycin treatment initiated early in the neonatal period have failed to show a benefit in reducing chronic lung disease *(47)*. A larger treatment trial would provide greater insights regarding whether targeted antimicrobial therapy can reduce the incidence of morbidity and mortality associated with chronic lung disease.

Both *M. hominis* and *Ureaplasma* spp have been isolated from maternal and umbilical cord blood and the blood of neonates. Both species can also invade the CSF *(53,54)*, resulting in either mild, subclinical meningitis without sequelae or neurological damage with permanent handicaps. Mononuclear or polymorphonuclear pleocytosis and elevated protein have been reported, but in some cases inflammation is minimal or absent. CSF glucose concentrations are usually normal. Most reported cases have involved preterm infants; full-term infants with neurological defects, including meningomyelocele; or older children with ventriculoperitoneal shunts, but infections in otherwise normal full-term infants have also been described.

Cases of *M. hominis* CSF infection in infants are more numerous than those that can be attributed to *Ureaplasma* spp because the former is much more readily detected without specialized methods. There appears to be an association with hydrocephalus and intraventricular hemorrhage in preterm infants with *Ureaplasma* CSF infections *(54,55)*. A report of a brain abscess in a neonate in which both *M. hominis* and *Ureaplasma* spp were isolated concomitantly proved these organisms can cause focal central nervous system infection as well as meningitis *(56)*. Relatively little is known about the long-term prognosis and neurodevelopmental outcomes for infections of the central nervous system caused by *M. hominis* or *Ureaplasma* spp because most available information comes from individual case reports, many of which provided scant information beyond the immediate period following infection and short-term prospective studies.

In addition to the above examples, occasional cases have appeared in the literature describing other conditions that bear consideration by clinicians. These include infections of pericardial fluid causing cardiac tamponade *(57)* and subcutaneous abscesses associated with forceps delivery *(58)* or an internal heart monitor *(59)*. Two studies have described isolation of *Ureaplasma* spp from the respiratory tract and blood in infants with persistent pulmonary hypertension of the newborn and suggested there may be a possible association or interaction between the ureaplasmas and the vascular events that characterize this syndrome *(60,61)*. Other isolations of these organisms from urine and conjunctiva are more difficult to evaluate because of the uncertain contribution of these bacteria to illness in these cases.

DIAGNOSTIC APPROACH

Because of the frequency with which genital mycoplasmas inhabit the lower urogenital tract of healthy adult women, there is no justification for performance of screening cultures. However, because they can produce invasive infections in a subpopulation of those who are colonized in the lower urogenital tract, cultures using methods that circumvent cervical contamination may be useful in some cases to confirm a microbiological diagnosis in conditions such as pelvic inflammatory disease.

Formulating recommendations for performing diagnostic evaluations for genital mycoplasmas in pregnant women is both complex and problematic. Many women who have significant histologic evidence of chorioamnionitis do not have clinical manifestations of infection, and only half of those who have a culture-positive chorioamnion will have positive amniotic fluids that may be readily obtainable for culture prior to delivery. Blood and amnionitic fluid cultures for mycoplasmas can be useful in women who have clinical evidence of amnionitis. Cultures may also be obtained in women with postpartum fever and endometritis if a microbiological diagnosis is desired. However, because most cases of postpartum fever caused by genital mycoplasmas resolve without sequelae, often without specific treatment, and the fact that chemotherapy with broad-spectrum antimicrobials to cover a wide array of possible micro-organisms is usually successful, the cost of mycoplasmal cultures may not always be justified.

Routine screening of neonates is not clinically justified based on the available evidence that many healthy neonates may be colonized without consequence. However, if there is clinical, radiologic, or laboratory evidence of pneumonia, meningitis, or overall instability suggestive of sepsis, particularly in preterm neonates in whom there are no obvious alternative etiologies, infection with *M. hominis* or *Ureaplasma* spp should be considered, and appropriate diagnostic studies should be obtained. It may also be useful to assess preterm neonates whose birth weight is less than 1250 g for the presence of ureaplasmas if they have respiratory distress that lasts more than a few hours after birth. Obtaining mycoplasmal cultures is particularly important if routine bacteriological studies fail to yield an etiologic agent within 2–3 days.

There are no specific clinical features that will provide clues to the clinician that these organisms may be involved in a particular condition. Thus, continued vigilance and an awareness of the possible contribution of genital mycoplasmas should always be considered earlier rather than later in ill neonates, particularly those born preterm. It should be noted that many serious, invasive, neonatal infections caused by the genital mycoplasmas have been detected after several days have passed without identification of a microbial etiology using conventional means or if the neonate fails to improve after institution of antimicrobial therapy with β-lactams and aminoglycosides. Unless specific diagnostic tests are requested, it is very unlikely that a mycoplasmal etiology will be identified. Possible exceptions may occasionally occur because *M. hominis* will sometimes grow after 3 or more days on routine bacteriological media, but this should not be assumed. Treatment of mycoplasmal infections and the value of antimicrobial susceptibility testing are discussed in reference texts and reviews *(14,47)*.

DIAGNOSTIC TESTING

Stains and Culture-Based Tests

Culture is still the most widely used means for detection and identification of genital mycoplasmas in clinical specimens, and it remains the accepted reference standard *(14,62)*. The relative rapidity of their growth will allow cultural detection and presumptive identification of these organisms within 2–5 days with an analytical sensitivity comparable to that of the PCR assay. The main challenges that may be encountered by clinicians are finding an experienced laboratory capable of performing and interpreting the results of mycoplasmal cultures and the careful attention required for proper specimen collection and transport to ensure that viable organisms are obtained and preserved until received in the diagnostic laboratory.

Stains

Mycoplasmal and ureaplasmal cells are too small to be visualized in Gram-stained preparations of clinical specimens or cultures, and the lack of a cell wall precludes uptake of crystal violet or safranin. However, the Gram stain may prove useful to exclude contaminating bacteria. Giemsa stains may be used, but the results can be difficult to interpret because of debris and artifacts in clinical specimens that can be confused with mycoplasmas because of their small size. Deoxyribonucleic acid (DNA) fluorochrome stains may be useful to determine whether micro-organisms are present in a clinical specimen or culture, but they do not distinguish mycoplasmas from other bacteria *(62)*.

Specimen Collection and Transport

Cultures of nasopharyngeal, throat, and endotracheal secretions of neonates are appropriate to evaluate respiratory infection. Gastric aspirates and throat and nasal swabs are less desirable because they may not always accurately reflect the microbiology of the lower respiratory tract because some infants may be colonized in other locations without ill effects. If urogenital specimens from adults are of interest, urethral swabs, urine, and cervical or vaginal swabs are acceptable. Urine samples from females are most meaningful when obtained by catheter or suprapubic aspiration and if numbers of organisms are quantitated. Endometrial tissue, tubal samples, or pouch of Douglas fluid can be obtained to confirm mycoplasmal etiology of postpartum fever. For women with clinical amnionitis, amniotic fluid, blood, and placenta should be cultured. Other sterile fluids from neonates, such as CSF and blood, are suitable for culture, as are wound aspirates, abscess fluid, and tissue collected by biopsy or autopsy.

Mollicutes are extremely sensitive to adverse environmental conditions, particularly to drying and heat, so great care must be taken to ensure proper specimen collection and transport. Clinical specimens from neonates will usually be of very small volumes or quantities. Therefore, they should always be collected and placed in appropriate transport medium immediately to prevent desiccation and loss of organism viability. If larger samples, such as lung tissue collected at autopsy or placenta, can be placed in a sterile screw-capped container and sent to the laboratory immediately, no additional transport medium is necessary. However, if there is any delay anticipated or if specimens have to be shipped to a laboratory off site, addition of transport medium is essential.

Transport medium such as Shepard's 10B broth is acceptable for transport of *M. hominis* as well as *Ureaplasma* spp. This medium is available commercially (Remel

Laboratories, Lenexa, KS) or can be prepared locally *(62)*. 2 SP (10% v/v heat-inactivated fetal calf serum with 0.2*M* sucrose in 0.02*M* phosphate buffer, pH 7.2), which is also used for transport of specimens for chlamydial cultures, is also acceptable. Other media available commercially for transport and storage of specimens include Stuart's medium, A3B, and arginine broth. From a practical standpoint, transport media can be kept frozen in small volumes in a freezer located in a clinical unit so that it can be rapidly thawed and used to inoculate specimens at bedside.

When swabs are obtained, care must be taken to sample the desired site vigorously to obtain as many cells as possible because mycoplasmas are cell associated. Calcium alginate, Dacron, or polyester swabs with aluminum or plastic shafts are preferred. Wooden shaft cotton swabs should be avoided because of potential inhibitory effects. Swabs should be vigorously swirled in the appropriate transport broth, pressed against the side of the tube to express as much fluid as possible, and discarded.

Endotracheal secretions from neonates who are intubated can be collected using a small-bore suction catheter connected to a vacuum outlet. The catheter is passed through the endotracheal tube, and suction is applied. The tip of the suction catheter is cut with a sterile scalpel blade. Then, 1 mL of 10B broth is drawn into a 3-mL syringe to which a 21-gage needle is attached. The tip of the suction catheter is placed into the tube from which the broth was drawn, and the needle is used to flush the catheter with broth, forcing the respiratory secretions into the tube, which is then transported to the laboratory.

Fluids such as CSF or urine should be obtained according to standard clinical procedures and inoculated immediately into transport media in an approx 1:10 ratio. Mycoplasmas and ureaplasmas are inhibited by sodium polyanethol sulfonate present in most commercial blood culture media, so this is not an acceptable means for detection. Commercial blood culture media designed for use in automated instruments may support growth of *M. hominis*, but the instruments usually do not flag the bottles containing this organism as positive *(63)*. Successful isolation of *M. hominis* and *Ureaplasma* spp from blood can be achieved by inoculating blood directly into liquid mycoplasmal growth media such as 10 B broth in at least a 1:10 ratio.

Specimens should be refrigerated if immediate transportation to the laboratory is not possible. If specimens must be shipped or if the storage time is likely to exceed 24 hours prior to processing, the specimen in transport medium should be frozen to prevent loss of viability. Specimens can be stored for long periods in appropriate growth or transport media at −70°C or in liquid nitrogen. Storage at −20°C for even short periods will result in loss of viability. Frozen specimens may be shipped with dry ice to a reference laboratory if necessary.

Growth Media

There are a variety of commercial and nonproprietary culture medium formulations that have been used to detect *M. hominis* and *Ureaplasma* spp. Their merits and relative disadvantages have been reviewed *(62)*. Shepard's 10B broth is an ideal choice for general use because it can be used for cultivation of both *M. hominis* and *Ureaplasma* spp with A8 agar *(62)* as the corresponding solid medium. In the event that other mycoplasmal species are to be sought, alternative methods such as the PCR assay should be utilized because culture techniques are not well established for other species. Even though 10B broth and A8 agar are available commercially, the comparability of the commercially prepared products to nonproprietary formulations in their ability to support the growth of these fastidious organisms has not been documented, so internal quality control should be practiced *(62)*. There are a number of complete diagnostic kits for detection and identification of *M. hominis* and *Ureaplasma* spp; these are sold commercially in several European countries, but none is available in the United States. A comprehensive discussion and description of these products is available elsewhere *(64)*.

Specimen Processing and Interpretation

It is beyond the scope of this chapter to describe in depth the procedures that must be undertaken in a diagnostic laboratory to recover mycoplasmas and ureaplasmas from clinical specimens. Refer to reference microbiology texts *(14,62,64)* that deal with this topic for specific information, and only general comments are provided here.

Specimens should be mixed, and fluids should be centrifuged and the pellet serially diluted to at least 10^{-3} and inoculated into liquid and solid medium. Tissues should be minced in broth prior to diluting. Subculture of each dilution onto agar is an extremely important step in the cultivation process because it will help overcome possible interference by antibiotics, antibodies, and other inhibitors, including bacteria that may be present in clinical specimens. Omission of this critical dilution step can be one reason why some laboratories have difficulty in recovering the organisms. Dilution also helps to overcome the problem of rapid decline in culture viability, which is particularly common with ureaplasmas, and it also provides information about the number of organisms present in the specimen. Colonies develop best when agar plates are incubated in an atmosphere of 95% N_2 plus 5% CO_2 *(14)*, but successful isolation is also possible using an atmosphere of room air plus 5% CO_2 or in a candle jar.

Growth in 10B broth is suggested by an alkaline shift and change in color of the medium from yellow to pink because of urea hydrolysis by *Ureaplasma* spp or arginine hydrolysis by *M. hominis*. Such changes may be evident in 24 hours or less in the case of *Ureaplasma* spp and in 24–28 hours for *M. hominis*. Turbidity in broth cultures indicates bacterial contamination. Positive broths should always be subcultured to agar immediately because the primary inoculum does not always grow. Subcultures must be performed soon after the color change occurs, particularly if the organism is *Ureaplasma,* because the culture can lose viability within hours. Occurrence of pinpoint colonies on bacteriological media such as Columbia agar that do not produce a recognizable Gram reaction warrants subculture to mycoplasma media because of the possibility they may be *M. hominis*.

Colonies of *Ureaplasma* spp and *M. hominis* growing on A8 agar are shown in Figs. 1 and 2. Except for hydrolysis of urea and development of characteristic colonies on A8 agar that are unique for ureaplasmas, biochemical and colonial features are insufficient for definitive species distinction. However, colony morphology in conjunction with the biochemical profile, body site of origin, and rate of growth will often allow presumptive identification of the most common clinically significant species of large colony mycoplasmas. An arginine-hydrolyzing, urease-negative organism that produces fried egg colonies within 3–4 days of incubation may be presumptively identified as *M. hominis*, and in most instances no further work-up is required. Mycoplasmas that require more definitive identification can be submitted to a reference laboratory for characterization by PCR or other immunologic procedures in the event that this is

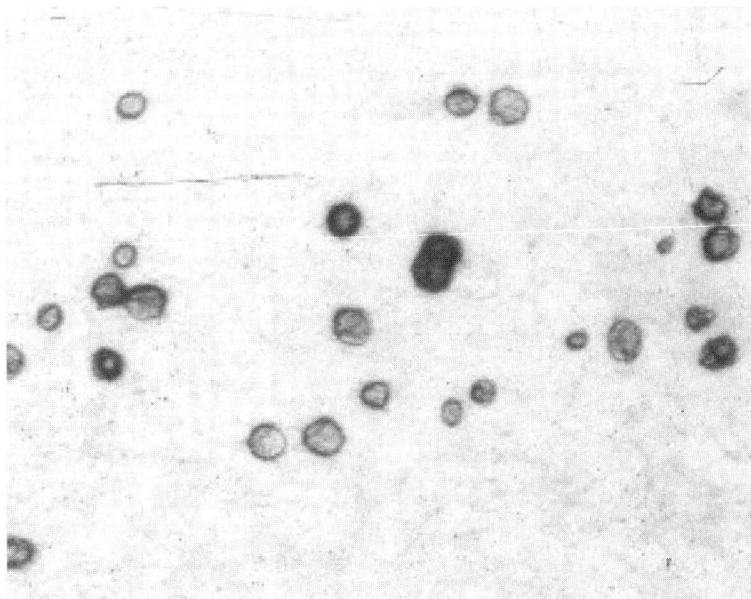

Fig. 1. Colonies of *Ureaplasma* spp growing on A8 agar after 48 hours of incubation as they appear under 126× magnification using a stereomicroscope. Colonies are typically 15–30 μm in diameter and have a brownish granular appearance caused by urease activity in the presence of the $CaCl_2$ indicator contained in the agar.

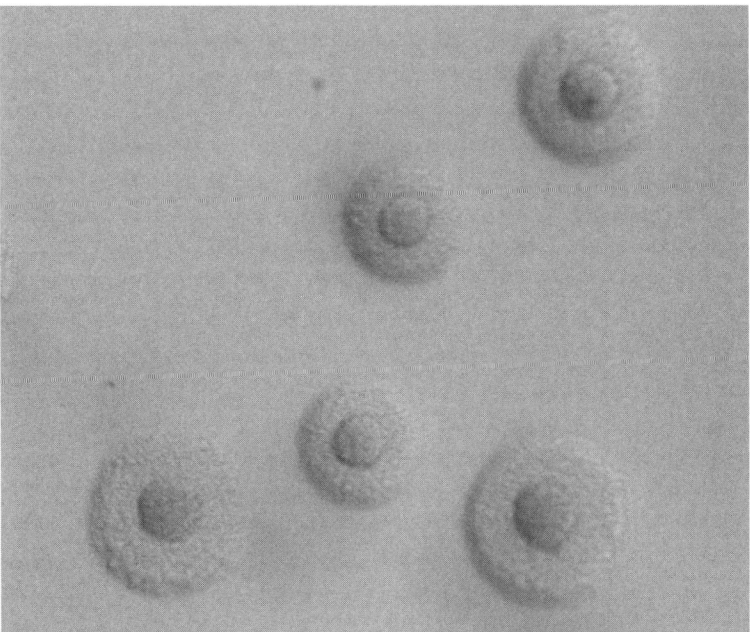

Fig. 2. Colonies of *Mycoplasma hominis* growing on A8 agar after 72 hours of incubation as they appear under 126× magnification using a stereomicroscope. Colonies are typically 200–300 μm in diameter and demonstrate the fried egg appearance characteristic of this organism.

clinically indicated. This may be relevant when the organism is present in a clinically significant infection of a normally sterile site.

Nonamplified Probes and Antigen Detection Systems

In the early 1980s, there was some interest in development of DNA probes and antigen detection systems for *M. pneumoniae*, but this technology was largely abandoned because of the low sensitivity of these assays and the more widespread development of nucleic acid amplification assays that were superior in many aspects. In view of the rapidity and relative ease for detection of *M. hominis* and *Ureaplasma* spp by culture, alternative methods based on nonamplified probes or antigen detection systems have never generated much interest.

Nucleic Acid Amplification

Nucleic acid amplification assays, particularly PCR, have been described for all mycoplasmas and ureaplasmas that are known to be significant pathogens for humans. Theoretically, PCR can detect a single organism or a single copy of the targeted gene when purified DNA is used, greatly exceeding the detection threshold of culture, which is approx 100–1000 cells under optimum conditions. PCR is also a very good tool for identification of an unknown mycoplasma previously obtained by culture, and it can be used for characterization of strains within a species.

Practically, PCR technology is less valuable for routine diagnostic purposes in the case of the more rapidly growing and relatively easily cultivable organisms, such as *M. hominis* and *Ureaplasma* spp, except in specific cases when isolation by culture could be difficult, such as fixed tissue samples. For slow-growing organisms, such as *M. pneumoniae*, and especially for extremely fastidious species for which optimum cultivation techniques are not established, such as *M. genitalium*, the use of PCR assays may be the only practical means of detecting their presence *(14)*.

Presently, PCR detection for mycoplasmas is still too labor intensive, expensive, and complex to be carried out routinely in most diagnostic laboratories and is not offered. Some drawbacks must still be corrected, such as the presence of inhibitors in the specimens and laboratory contamination. The possible development of commercial PCR kits in the future should bring about better standardization of the technique, and if available at a reasonable cost, PCR could become a major method for the diagnosis of mycoplasmal and ureaplasmal infections because it can theoretically provide extremely rapid turnaround time.

Serologic Diagnosis

The ubiquity of most genital mycoplasmas in adults makes interpretation of antibody titers difficult, and the mere existence of antibodies alone cannot be considered significant. However, infants with systemic infections of the central nervous system caused by *M. hominis* may mount a measurable serologic response. It has also been suggested that increases in titers of type-specific antibodies against certain ureaplasmal serovars may occur in women with pregnancy wastage and in infants with respiratory disease compared with titers in control patients *(65)*. More comparative data from well-characterized and carefully matched control populations are needed to fully assess the value of serologic diagnosis in these settings *(5)*. The relative hypogammaglobulinemic state of preterm neonates, those who are most likely to experience significant invasive disease caused by these organisms, adds to the complexity of interpreting serologic findings.

Serologic assays that have been described for *M. hominis, M. genitalium,* and *Ureaplasma* spp include indirect immunofluorescence assays, enzyme-linked immunoassays, microimmunofluorescence, and metabolic inhibition tests *(14)*. At the present time, no assays designed for genital mycoplasmas have been standardized and sold commercially in the United States, and serology cannot be recommended for routine diagnosis of neonatal or perinatal mycoplasmal or ureaplasmal infections.

CONCLUSIONS

As evidence mounts for a role for *M. hominis* and *Ureaplasma* spp in neonatal and perinatal diseases, the need for their accurate laboratory detection and identification becomes more important. The lack of diagnostic services has been a contributing factor to the general unfamiliarity with these organisms that is widespread among clinical microbiologists as well as physicians. Greater availability of commercially prepared media and reagents for use in mycoplasmal detection and identification has helped the situation somewhat, but it is important to remember that most of these products have not been compared rigorously to traditional nonproprietary methods for mycoplasma detection, and therefore their analytical sensitivities are largely unknown.

Several microbiology reference laboratories offer detection of mycoplasmas and ureaplasmas by culture. The Diagnostic Mycoplasma Laboratory at the University of Alabama at Birmingham offers specialized testing that includes culture and PCR. Cultures for mycoplasmas and ureaplasmas are also becoming more common in hospital microbiology laboratories located in major medical centers. Should a clinician feel it necessary to obtain diagnostic specimens for detection and identification of genital mycoplasmas, the most important factors to consider are how to collect and transport the specimen to ensure that any mycoplasmas that may be present can be preserved for cultural isolation.

Understanding the role of mycoplasmas and ureaplasmas in neonatal and perinatal disease will be facilitated if more physicians attempt to make microbiological diagnoses when their presence is suspected, and patients themselves may benefit when the etiology of such infections is established so that appropriate treatment can be rendered.

REFERENCES

1. Tully JG, Smith LG. Postpartum septicemia with *Mycoplasma hominis.* JAMA 1968;204:827–828.
2. Shurin PA, Alpert S, Bernard Rosner BA, Driscoll SG, Lee YH. Chorioamnionitis and colonization of the newborn infant with genital mycoplasmas. N Engl J Med 1975;293:5–8.
3. Klein JO, Buckland D, Finland M. Colonization of newborn infants by mycoplasmas. N Engl J Med 1969;280:1025–1030.
4. Elder HA, Santamarina BA, Smith S, Kass EH. The natural history of asymptomatic bacteriuria during pregnancy: the effect of tetracycline on the clinical course and the outcome of pregnancy. Am J Obstet Gynecol 1971;111:441–462.
5. Cassell GH, Waites KB, Crouse DT. Mycoplasmal infections. In: Remington JS, Klein JO, eds. Infectious Diseases of the Fetus and Newborn Infant, 5th ed. Philadelphia: Saunders, 2001:733–767.

6. Taylor-Robinson D, Ainsworth JG, McCormack WM. Genital mycoplasmas. In: Holmes KK, Mardh PA, Sparling PF, et al., eds. Sexually Transmitted Diseases, 3rd ed. New York: McGraw Hill, 1999:533–548.

7. Ursi D, Ursi JP, Ieven M, Docx M, Van Reempts P, Pattyn SR. Congenital pneumonia due to *Mycoplasma pneumoniae*. Arch Dis Child Fetal Neonatal Ed 1995;72:F118–F120.

8. Taylor-Robinson D. *Mycoplasma genitalium*—an up-date. Int J STD AIDS 2002;13:145–151.

9. Blanchard A, Hamrick W, Duffy L, Baldus K, Cassell GH. Use of the polymerase chain reaction for detection of *Mycoplasma fermentans* and *Mycoplasma genitalium* in the uro-genital tract and amniotic fluid. Clin Infect Dis 1993;17(Suppl 1):S272–S279.

10. Labbe AC, Frost E, Deslandes S, Mendonca AP, Alves AC, Pepin J. *Mycoplasma genitalium* is not associated with adverse outcomes of pregnancy in Guinea-Bissau. Sex Transm Infect 2002;78:289–291.

11. Lu GC, Schwebke JR, Duffy LB, et al. Midtrimester vaginal *Mycoplasma genitalium* in women with subsequent spontaneous preterm birth. Am J Obstet Gynecol 2001;185:163–165.

12. Kovachev E, Popova A, Protopopov F, Minkov R, Tsvetkova S. [Association between *Mycoplasma genitalium* and preterm labor]. Akush Ginekol (Sofia) 2002;41:26–29.

13. Luki N, Lebel P, Boucher M, Doray B, Turgeon J, Brousseau R. Comparison of polymerase chain reaction assay with culture for detection of genital mycoplasmas in perinatal infections. Eur J Clin Microbiol Infect Dis 1998;17:255–263.

14. Waites KB, Rikihisa Y, Taylor-Robinson D. *Mycoplasma* and *Ureaplasma*. In: Murray PR, Baron EJ, Jorgensen JH, Pfaller MA, Yolken RH, eds. Manual of Clinical Microbiology, 8th ed. Washington, DC: American Society for Microbiology, 2003:972–990.

15. Kim M, Kim G, Romero R, Shim SS, Kim EC, Yoon BH. Biovar diversity of *Ureaplasma urealyticum* in amniotic fluid: distribution, intrauterine inflammatory response and pregnancy outcomes. J Perinat Med 2003;31:146–152.

16. Zheng X, Watson HL, Waites KB, Cassell GH. Serotype diversity and antigen variation among invasive isolates of *Ureaplasma urealyticum* from neonates. Infect Immunol 1992;60:3472–3474.

17. Abele-Horn M, Wolff C, Dressel P, Pfaff F, Zimmermann A. Association of *Ureaplasma urealyticum* biovars with clinical outcome for neonates, obstetric patients, and gynecological patients with pelvic inflammatory disease. J Clin Microbiol 1997;35:1199–1202.

18. Naessens A, Foulon W, Breynaert J, Lauwers S. Serotypes of *Ureaplasma urealyticum* isolated from normal pregnant women and patients with pregnancy complications. J Clin Microbiol 1988;26:319–322.

19. Martinez MA, Ovalle A, Santa-Cruz A, Barrera B, Vidal R, Aguirre R. Occurrence and antimicrobial susceptibility of *Ureaplasma parvum* (*Ureaplasma urealyticum* biovar 1) and *Ureaplasma urealyticum* (*Ureaplasma urealyticum* biovar 2) from patients with adverse pregnancy outcomes and normal pregnant women. Scand J Infect Dis 2001;33:604–610.

20. Domingues D, Tavira LT, Duarte A, Sanca A, Prieto E, Exposto F. *Ureaplasma urealyticum* biovar determination in women attending a family planning clinic in Guine-Bissau, using polymerase chain reaction of the multiple-banded antigen gene. J Clin Lab Anal 2002;16:71–75.

21. Sanchez PJ. Perinatal transmission of *Ureaplasma urealyticum*: current concepts based on review of the literature. Clin Infect Dis 1993;17(Suppl 1):S107–S111.

22. Cassell GH, Davis RO, Waites KB, et al. Isolation of *Mycoplasma hominis* and *Ureaplasma urealyticum* from amniotic fluid at 16–20 weeks of gestation: potential effect on outcome of pregnancy. Sex Transm Dis 1983;10(4 Suppl):294–302.

23. Carey JC, Blackwelder WC, Nugent RP, et al. Antepartum cultures for *Ureaplasma urealyticum* are not useful in predicting pregnancy outcome. The Vaginal Infections and Prematurity Study Group. Am J Obstet Gynecol 1991;164:728–733.

24. Foulon W, Naessens A, Dewaele M, Lauwers S, Amy JJ. Chronic *Ureaplasma urealyticum* amnionitis associated with abruptio placentae. Obstet Gynecol 1986;68:280–282.

25. Gray DJ, Robinson HB, Malone J, Thomson RB Jr. Adverse outcome in pregnancy following amniotic fluid isolation of *Ureaplasma urealyticum*. Prenat Diagn 1992;12:111–117.
26. Andrews WW, Shah SR, Goldenberg RL, Cliver SP, Hauth JC, Cassell GH. Association of post-cesarean delivery endometritis with colonization of the chorioamnion by *Ureaplasma urealyticum*. Obstet Gynecol 1995;85:509–514.
27. Goncalves LF, Chaiworapongsa T, Romero R. Intrauterine infection and prematurity. Ment Retard Dev Disabil Res Rev 2002;8:3–13.
28. Martius J, Eschenbach DA. The role of bacterial vaginosis as a cause of amniotic fluid infection, chorioamnonitis, and prematurity—a review. Arch Obstet Gynecol 1990;247:1–13.
29. Taylor-Robinson D, Waites K, Cassell G. Genital mycoplasmas. In: Morse SA, Ballard RC, Holmes KK, Moreland AA, eds. Atlas of Sexually Transmitted Diseases and AIDS, 3rd ed. New York: Mosby, 2003:127–139.
30. Hillier SL, Nugent RP, Eschenbach DA, et al. Association between bacterial vaginosis and preterm delivery of a low-birth-weight infant. The Vaginal Infections and Prematurity Study Group. N Engl J Med 1995;333:1737–1742.
31. Donders GG, Van Bulck B, Caudron J, Londers L, Vereecken A, Spitz B. Relationship of bacterial vaginosis and mycoplasmas to the risk of spontaneous abortion. Am J Obstet Gynecol 2000;183:431–437.
32. Madan E, Meyer MP, Amortegui AJ. Isolation of genital mycoplasmas and *Chlamydia trachomatis* in stillborn and neonatal autopsy material. Arch Pathol Lab Med 1988;112:749–751.
33. Kundsin RB, Driscoll SG, Monson RR, Yeh C, Biano SA, Cochran WD. Association of *Ureaplasma urealyticum* in the placenta with perinatal morbidity and mortality. N Engl J Med 1984;310:941–945.
34. Quinn PA, Butany J, Chipman M, Taylor J, Hannah W. A prospective study of microbial infection in stillbirths and early neonatal death. Am J Obstet Gynecol 1985;151:238–249.
35. Cassell GH, Waites KB, Crouse DT, et al. Association of *Ureaplasma urealyticum* infection of the lower respiratory tract with chronic lung disease and death in very-low-birth-weight infants. Lancet 1988;2:240–245.
36. Wang EE, Frayha H, Watts J, et al. Role of *Ureaplasma urealyticum* and other pathogens in the development of chronic lung disease of prematurity. Pediatr Infect Dis J 1988;7:547–551.
37. Sanchez PJ, Regan JA. *Ureaplasma urealyticum* colonization and chronic lung disease in low birth weight infants. Pediatr Infect Dis J 1988;7:542–546.
38. Crouse DT, Odrezin GT, Cutter GR, et al. Radiographic changes associated with tracheal isolation of *Ureaplasma urealyticum* from neonates. Clin Infect Dis 1993;17(Suppl 1):S122–S130.
39. Payne NR, Steinberg SS, Ackerman P, et al. New prospective studies of the association of *Ureaplasma urealyticum* colonization and chronic lung disease. Clin Infect Dis 1993;17(Suppl 1):S117 S121.
40. Wang EE, Ohlsson A, Kellner JD. Association of *Ureaplasma urealyticum* colonization with chronic lung disease of prematurity: results of a metaanalysis. J Pediatr 1995;127:640–644.
41. Ollikainen J, Korppi M, Heiskanen-Kosma T, Heinonen K. Chronic lung disease of the newborn is not associated with *Ureaplasma urealyticum*. Pediatr Pulmonol 2001;32:303–307.
42. Heggie AD, Bar-Shain D, Boxerbaum B, Fanaroff AA, O'Riordan MA, Robertson JA. Identification and quantification of ureaplasmas colonizing the respiratory tract and assessment of their role in the development of chronic lung disease in preterm infants. Pediatr Infect Dis J 2001;20:854–859.
43. Smyth AR, Shaw NJ, Pratt BC, Weindling AM. *Ureaplasma urealyticum* and chronic lung disease. Eur J Pediatr 1993;152:931–932.

44. Saxen H, Hakkarainen K, Pohjavuori M, Miettinen A. Chronic lung disease of preterm infants in Finland is not associated with *Ureaplasma urealyticum* colonization. Acta Paediatr 1993;82:198–201.

45. Berger A, Witt A, Haiden N, Kretzer V, Heinze G, Kohlhauser C. Microbial invasion of the amniotic cavity at birth is associated with adverse short-term outcome of preterm infants. J Perinat Med 2003;31:115–121.

46. Galetto Lacour A, Zamora S, Bertrand R, et al. [Colonization by *Ureaplasma urealyticum* and chronic lung disease in premature newborn infants under 32 weeks of gestation]. Arch Pediatr 2001;8:39–46.

47. Waites KB, Katz B, Schelonka R. Mycoplasmas and ureaplasmas as neonatal pathogens. Clin Microbial Rev 2005. In press.

48. Ollikainen J. Perinatal *Ureaplasma urealyticum* infection increases the need for hospital treatment during the first year of life in preterm infants. Pediatr Pulmonol 2000;30:402–405.

49. Rudd PT, Cassell GH, Waites KB, Davis JK, Duffy LB. *Ureaplasma urealyticum* pneumonia: experimental production and demonstration of age-related susceptibility. Infect Immunol 1989;57:918–925.

50. Viscardi RM, Kaplan J, Lovchik JC, et al. Characterization of a murine model of *Ureaplasma urealyticum* pneumonia. Infect Immunol 2002;70:5721–5729.

51. Crouse DT, Cassell GH, Waites KB, Foster JM, Cassady G. Hyperoxia potentiates *Ureaplasma urealyticum* pneumonia in newborn mice. Infect Immunol 1990;58:3487–3493.

52. Waites KB, Sims PJ, Crouse DT, et al. Serum concentrations of erythromycin after intravenous infusion in preterm neonates treated for *Ureaplasma urealyticum* infection. Pediatr Infect Dis J 1994;13:287–293.

53. Waites KB, Duffy LB, Crouse DT, et al. Mycoplasmal infections of cerebrospinal fluid in newborn infants from a community hospital population. Pediatr Infect Dis J 1990;9:241–245.

54. Waites KB, Rudd PT, Crouse DT, et al. Chronic *Ureaplasma urealyticum* and *Mycoplasma hominis* infections of central nervous system in preterm infants. Lancet 1988;1:17–21.

55. Ollikainen J, Hiekkaniemi H, Korppi M, Katila ML, Heinonen K. *Ureaplasma urealyticum* cultured from brain tissue of preterm twins who died of intraventricular hemorrhage. Scand J Infect Dis 1993;25:529–531.

56. Rao RP, Ghanayem NS, Kaufman BA, Kehl KS, Gregg DC, Chusid MJ. *Mycoplasma hominis* and *Ureaplasma* species brain abscess in a neonate. Pediatr Infect Dis J 2002;21:1083–1085.

57. Miller TC, Sudhaker IB, Albers WH. Massive pericardial effusion due to *Mycoplasma hominis* in a newborn. Am J Dis Child 1982;136:271–272.

58. Glaser JB, Engelberg M, Hammerschlag M. Scalp abscess associated with *Mycoplasma hominis* infection complicating intrapartum monitoring. Pediatr Infect Dis 1983;2:468–470.

59. Hamrick HJ, Mangum ME, Katz VL. *Ureaplasma urealyticum* abscess at site of an internal fetal heart rate monitor. Pediatr Infect Dis J 1993;12:410–411.

60. Waites KB, Crouse DT, Philips JB, 3rd, Canupp KC, Cassell GH. Ureaplasmal pneumonia and sepsis associated with persistent pulmonary hypertension of the newborn. Pediatrics 1989;83:79–85.

61. Brus F, van Waarde WM, Schoots C, Oetomo SB. Fatal ureaplasmal pneumonia and sepsis in a newborn infant. Eur J Pediatr 1991;150:782–783.

62. Waites KB, Bebear CM, Robertson JA, Talkington DF, Kenny GE, eds. Cumitech 34, Laboratory Diagnosis of Mycoplasmal Infections. Washington, DC: American Society for Microbiology, 2001.

63. Waites KB, Canupp KC. Evaluation of BacT/ALERT system for detection of *Mycoplasma hominis* in simulated blood cultures. J Clin Microbiol 2001;39:4328–4331.

64. Waites KB, Talkington DF, Bebear CM. Mycoplasmas. In: Truant AL, ed. Manual of Commercial Methods in Clinical Microbiology. Washington, DC: American Society for Microbiology, 2002:201–224.

65. Quinn PA. Evidence of an immune response to *Ureaplasma urealyticum* in perinatal morbidity and mortality. Pediatr Infect Dis 1986;5(6 Suppl):S282–S287.

Patricia Whitley-Williams

THE ORGANISM

Candida spp are ubiquitous dimorphic yeasts that can exist as 2- to 5-μm round-oval cells called blastospores, which reproduce by budding. They have the ability to produce pseudohyphae, which are filamentous processes elongating from the cells. Fifty years ago, these round vegetative cells were considered nonpathogens. Some *Candida* spp, especially *Candida albicans*, exist as normal flora on skin and in the lower gastrointestinal (GI) tract and female genital tract. However, therapeutic and technological advances in medicine have enabled these yeasts to become true pathogens, especially in the immunocompromised hosts. In addition to causing insignificant and mild mucocutaneous infections in the normal host, these yeasts cause invasive and life-threatening disease affecting almost any organ.

Of the 200 *Candida* spp, *C. albicans* has been the most common, accounting for about 60–80% of neonatal infections. Other *Candida* spp that act as human pathogens include *Candida tropicalis, Candida pseudotropicalis, Candida lipolytica, Candida krusei, Candida guilliermondii, Candida parapsilosis, Candida lusitaniae, Candida globrata*, and *Candida stellatoidea*.

There are reports that infections in low birth weight infants caused by other *Candida* spp, such as *C. parapsilosis*, have increased. *C. parapsilosis* accounted for 29–60% of blood isolates in neonatal intensive care units, including one large multicenter study that demonstrated 60% prevalence between 1991 and 1995 *(1–3)*. *C. parapsilosis* and *C. albicans* account for 90% of *Candida* blood isolates in low birth weight infants. *C. parapsilosis* appears to be less virulent than *C. albicans* because of its inability to produce phagocytosis-resistant pseudohyphae and its poor adherence and penetration of human endothelium. The mortality rate in one study from *C. albicans* was 26% compared to 4% from *C. parapsilosis (1,2)*.

TRANSMISSION

The majority of neonatal *Candida* infections are acquired either through vertical transmission or by nosocomial spread. Electrophoretic karyotyping and pulsed field gel electrophoresis have been used to demonstrate the mode of transmission of some *Candida* spp. There is some evidence to suggest that most *C. albicans* infections in

From: *Infectious Disease: Congenital and Perinatal Infections: A Concise Guide to Diagnosis*
Edited by: C. Hutto © Humana Press Inc., Totowa, NJ

preterm infants are transmitted vertically *(1,3–5)*. The timing of vertical transmission may occur prenatally or at the time of delivery.

Intrauterine infection or true congenital infection occurs as a result of an ascending maternal infection and may lead to placentitis or chorioamnionitis. Fewer than 100 cases of congenital candidiasis have been reported in the literature *(6)*. Histopathological evidence of fungi within umbilical or chorionic vessels supports the diagnosis of fetal candidemia in congenital candidiasis. Hematogenous spread of the infection to the fetus via the umbilical vein is extremely rare and has been reported in only three cases of congenital candidiasis *(6)*. The rare occurrence of fetal candidemia supports the fact that the placenta is a highly effective barrier against these fungi. Congenital infection results more often in cutaneous than in disseminated candidiasis; however, the latter occurs more often in premature infants.

Perinatal or neonatal candidiasis, which is acquired as a result of passage through an infected birth canal, can result in infection in the newborn period. The most common presentation is mucocutaneous candidiasis in the form of oral thrush or perineal dermatitis. Disease occurs for the most part in infants who were colonized at the time of birth or within the first several weeks after birth. Disseminated disease, which is far less common than mucocutaneous candidiasis, occurs in the first 30–90 days of life and is more likely to occur in preterm colonized infants. Rarely does neonatal candidiasis produce an invasive fungal dermatitis, as is seen in congenital cutaneous candidiasis. Severe pulmonary disease as a result of aspiration of infected vaginal secretions is rare *(6)*.

Intimate contact such as breast-feeding with an infected mother as well as nosocomial spread may lead to postnatal candidiasis. In an earlier study, environmental contamination with *Candida* on chest tubes, ventilators, water reservoirs, breast milk, umbilical or central line catheters, or isolette walls could not be documented, although it does occur *(5)*. Hospital personnel carry *C. parapsilosis* as the most common *Candida* species on their hands. Inadequate hand washing has allowed horizontal transmission of this organism, especially among the very low birth weight infants, and has been the cause of several nursery outbreaks *(4,7)*.

COLONIZATION

The fungal colonization rate for low birth weight infants (<1500 g) ranges from 19 to 47% in the first 24 hours of life *(3,5,8)*. In one study, the most common site of early colonization (i.e., at birth or first 24 hours of life) was the GI tract, as demonstrated by positive rectal fungal cultures. At birth, 86% had rectal colonization, followed by 60% with tracheal colonization and 57% with oropharyngeal colonization *(5)*. The endotracheal acquisition at birth represents aspiration of the yeast during labor and delivery. Oropharyngeal acquisition at birth was not as frequent as rectal acquisition. At 1–2 weeks of age, the detection of yeast in the rectum and oropharynx was less likely. Late colonization was more often detected in the groin cultures. By 2 weeks of age, 64–85% of low birth weight neonates were colonized with *Candida* in the groin sites.

Colonization rates were higher for *C. parapsilosis* (56%) than *C. albicans* (44%) in one study in which surface cultures were obtained between the first and second weeks, third and fourth weeks, and fifth and sixth weeks of age *(9)*. In several studies, *C. parapsilosis* colonization occurred after the first or second week of life and could not be accounted for by a maternal reservoir *(3,4,9)*. However, this was not true in one study in which *C. parapsilosis* colonization occurred early in the first day or week of life

(5). C. tropicalis, however, tends to appear as a colonizer later, after the first 2 weeks of life, and therefore tends to appear as a pathogen in late-onset disease (>7 days of age).

PREDISPOSING FACTORS IN MATERNAL INFECTION

Candida vulvovaginitis occurs in about 25% of pregnant women; however, this is usually not associated with obstetrical complications *(10,11)*. Although infrequent, ascending infections from the vagina and cervix can occur, leading to infection of the placenta. Because of the presence of chorioamnionitis or funisitis, candidemia and sepsis may occur in the pregnant woman, but this is rare. Invasive disease would be unlikely unless the mother was immunosuppressed. Such conditions would include human immunodeficiency virus, immunosuppressive therapy, prolonged corticosteroid or broad-spectrum antibiotic use, burns, trauma, and indwelling vascular and urinary catheters.

PREDISPOSING FACTORS IN FETAL AND NEONATAL INFECTION

Despite its presence in 25% of all pregnant women, isolation of *Candida* from the placenta is rare *(12,13)*. Baley reported an incidence of less than 1% *(14)*. In the presence of chorioamnionitis, fetal infection can occur and presents as congenital cutaneous candidiasis (CCC). Risk factors for congenital infection include early preterm birth, the presence of a foreign body such as an intrauterine device or cervical sutures, and possibly diagnostic amniocentesis *(6,12)*. Factors that do not appear to play a role in congenital candidiasis are maternal age, prolonged rupture of membranes, diabetes, urinary tract infection, parity, and antibiotic, tocolytic, or corticosteroid therapy *(15)*. The role of congenital candidiasis in precipitating preterm labor or premature rupture of membranes remains unknown and warrants further investigation *(16,17)*.

There are many factors that may make the neonate more susceptible to fungal infections. These include an immature immune system, low birth weight, prematurity, congenital immunodeficiency, indwelling vascular and urinary catheters, prolonged broad-spectrum antibiotic use, intralipid and parenteral nutrition, and early fungal colonization of the GI tract. At the end of the 20th century, the incidence of candidemia and its relationship to colonization has been studied.

The overall incidence of neonatal candidemia is 7.7% in low birth weight colonized infants *(5)*. The incidence of candidemia in the low birth weight infants has increased over the last 20 years. In one study, the rate of candidemia in 1407 infants weighing less than 1000 g increased from 10.4 cases per 1000 admissions in 1981–1985 to 98.9 per 1000 in 1991–1995 *(1)*. The mean age of onset of candidemia ranged from 15 to 173 days of age, with mean ages of 43–47 days in some studies *(1,2)*. The incidence of candidemia was 0.2% (7/3033) in infants with birth weights above 2500 g admitted to the neonatal intensive care nursery *(18)*. This risk is much lower than that for low birth weight infants. The most frequent underlying condition in these term infants was a major congenital malformation, which occurred in half of the infants with fungal sepsis.

Colonization has been shown to be a significant risk factor for mucocutaneous and invasive candidiasis. In one study, one third of the colonized infants developed mucocutaneous candidiasis, and 7.7% developed systemic fungal disease *(5)*. In another study of 383 low birth weight infants, the overall incidence of invasive disease was 4.5%, and for mucocutaneous candidiasis, it was 7.8%. Invasive disease developed in 32% of the infants with mucocutaneous candidiasis compared to 2% without *(19)*.

The largest prospective multicenter cohort study was conducted in six level-III neonatal intensive care nurseries in diverse geographical areas from 1993 to 1995 to determine the incidence and associated risk factors for candidemia in 2847 infants *(20)*. The overall risk for candidemia was lower than previous reports (1.2%). The significant risk factors identified included preterm, low 5-minute Apgar score, disseminated intravascular coagulation, prior use of intralipid, parenteral nutrition, central venous catheters, H_2 blockers, intubation, or length of stay for more than 7 days. Although GI tract colonization was not identified as an independent risk factor, almost half of the patients who developed candidemia had preceding colonization. In fact, enteral feeds may be protective and prevent or decrease GI colonization.

Some studies have looked at other factors, such as the nursery environment *(5)*. There was no evidence of environmental contamination found in chest tubes, ventilators, water reservoirs, breast milk, umbilical or central line catheters, or isolette walls documented, but it probably does occur. Vaginal delivery (compared to cesarean section) did not seem to be a risk factor. The only statistically significant factor was a grade 3 or 4 intraventricular hemorrhage (for infants delivered vaginally) *(5)*. These infants tended to be sicker.

A univariate analysis of factors associated with colonization in a study of 116 low birth weight infants showed no significant difference between colonized and noncolonized infants. These factors included birth weight, gestational age, duration of nursery stay, vaginal delivery, steroid administration, or duration of intubation. Infants with colonization had a significantly longer duration of antimicrobial therapy, parenteral nutrition, and intralipid infusions. The duration of use of intravascular catheters approached significance *(3)*.

Because of the increasing occurrence of *C. parapsilosis*, the risk of invasive disease associated with colonization of the GI tract in newborns was investigated *(9)*. Of 82 colonized, low birth weight infants, 6% developed *C. parapsilosis* septicemia. There was an association with umbilical artery catheters and absence of enteral feeds. In that particular nursery, enteral feeds were not given if an umbilical artery catheter was in place.

Colonization of the urinary tract and respiratory tract may be risk factors for invasive candidiasis in the newborn. In one study, almost 15% of the infants with urinary tract colonization developed invasive disease *(5)*. There is evidence to suggest that endotracheal colonization, especially in the first week of life, is a marker for invasive disease in low birth weight infants. These infants were 10 times more likely to develop invasive disease. It is unclear whether the trachea is a portal of entry or is a marker of high fungal burden *(8)*.

PRENATAL EVALUATION

Any pregnant woman with a vaginal discharge or inflamed vulvovaginal area should be evaluated for *Candida*. *Candida* vulvovaginitis is the second most common cause of vaginitis after bacterial vaginosis. Many women are asymptomatic, but the classic signs are a profuse, pruritic, thick, white, curdlike discharge associated with dysuria, dyspareunia, and pruritus ani. The diagnosis of *Candida* vulvovaginitis is a clinical diagnosis that is confirmed by culture and microscopic detection of the yeast. A drop of the cervicovaginal fluid should be immersed in a 10% potassium hydroxide (KOH) preparation on a glass slide with a coverslip for microscopic examination. Sometimes, this slide is heated before examining it under the microscope. The presence of ovoid budding yeast cells 3–7 μm in diameter, seen sometimes with pseudohyphae, can make a presumptive diagnosis. The diagnosis is confirmed by isolating *Candida* from the cervicovaginal secretions cultured on Sabouraud's dextrose agar, which is commercially available. If bacterial contamination of the specimen is expected, then chloramphenicol should be used in the culture medium. Cycloheximide, which prevents fungal overgrowth, should not be used because it may inhibit some strains of *Candida*.

Candida is an unlikely pathogen in the immunocompetent pregnant woman. If the mother is immunosuppressed or has other risk factors for systemic candidiasis and is symptomatic, a workup should be initiated. If a pregnant woman who is immunocompetent has signs of systemic infection, such as fever, shock, or respiratory distress, or focal signs, a full sepsis work should be done. This would include multiple blood cultures, midstream clean catch or catheterized urine sample for urinalysis and culture, complete blood cell count and differential, liver function tests, and chest x-ray. Attempts to isolate *Candida* from blood and any other affected areas, such as cerebrospinal fluid, joint fluid abscess formation, bone marrow, bronchial alveolar lavage washings, skin lesions, tissue biopsy specimens, urine, and placenta should be made.

The isolation of *Candida* from urine, sputum, or bronchial washings does not always confirm the diagnosis. *Candida* isolated from respiratory and urinary cultures, especially in the presence of bacteria, may reflect contamination from oral or vaginal flora. Quantitative urine cultures are not helpful.

The lysis-centrifugation blood culture method (Isolator system), which is the most sensitive method for detection of bacteria in blood cultures, can detect almost all clinically significant yeast isolates. Therefore, *Candida* can be easily detected and isolated from routine blood cultures. Blood isolation may take from 24 to 72 hours. On the agar plate, *Candida* colonies are white or cream-colored colonies, with filamentous extensions coming from the edges of the colonies indicating the formation of pseudohyphae. *C. albicans* may undergo a transformation when placed in human serum for several hours. These new forms, chlamydospores, have cylindrical extensions called germ tubes. Because this is unique to *C. albicans*, a positive germ tube test confirms the diagnosis of *C. albicans* infection. Determining which *Candida* species has been isolated is important in invasive disease because of possible resistance. For example, *C. krusei* is known to be resistant to fluconazole. Routine susceptibility testing is not recommended. These tests are not always done in hospital laboratories, may not be reliable, and may be difficult to interpret.

Because the yield from cultures may be low in patients who are immunocompromised, tissue diagnosis may be required to confirm the diagnosis. The presence of yeast cells or pseudohyphae on histologic sections helps to confirm the diagnosis. The presence of pseudohyphae suggests tissue invasion rather than colonization; however, blastospores or yeast cells can be virulent as well. Diagnosis should be made in conjunction with the clinical picture and other diagnostic tests, such as urinalysis, radiographic imaging of the lungs or kidneys, or endoscopy, to rule out esophagitis or tissue biopsy. The isolation of *Candida* from cultures and histological detection of *Candida* in tissue specimens confirms the diagnosis. The pregnant woman should be treated for vaginal or invasive candidiasis. Preliminary studies do not justify the use of antifungal chemoprophylaxis to prevent invasive candidiasis in the newborn. Whether chemoprophylaxis is beneficial needs further study.

FETAL EVALUATION

Although sampling of amniotic fluid obtained by transabdominal amniocentesis for prenatal detection of *Candida* may allow earlier diagnosis and intervention for invasive neonatal candidiasis as well as obstetrical intervention, this is not routinely recommended. Further investigation regarding obstetrical and perinatal management of mother and fetus is needed for the detection of *Candida* in amniotic fluid. The use of antifungal agents for chemoprophylaxis in the mother for preventing CCC or neonatal candidiasis and the use of oxytocin vs the continuation of tocolytic administration need further study.

PERINATAL EVALUATION

Although intrauterine infection is rare, chorioamnionitis may lead to preterm labor, congenital and neonatal infections, *Candida* sepsis, and endometritis. In intrauterine infection, gross examination of the placenta and umbilical cord will reveal a yellow exudate on the placental surface and areas of necrosis and discrete, yellow macular lesions along the cord near the funicular vessels. Histological examination of the cord and placenta may reveal spores and pseudohyphae on periodic acid-Schiff stain, Gomori methenamine silver stains, toluidine blue, or Gram stain. There is an inflammatory infiltrate of neutrophils, lymphocytes, and histiocytes as well as microabscess formation.

NEONATAL EVALUATION

Maternal *Candida* vulvovaginitis may result in colonization of the newborn or mucocutaneous, invasive candidiasis or congenital candidiasis. Congenital candidiasis can present in infants as CCC or invasive disease *(6,12,17,21)*. CCC is a severe cutaneous candidiasis that is far less common.

Mucocutaneous candidiasis consists of oral thrush or diaper dermatitis or both. Oral thrush typically presents on the days 7–10 of life as whitish patches (resembling milk curds) anywhere on the oral mucosa. The lesions can extend to the posterior pharynx but most often are located on the buccal mucosa, tongue, and palate. Scraping of these lesions results in a denuded erythematous base. Microscopic examination of these scrapings placed in 10% KOH suspension on a glass slide reveals blastospores or ovalround yeast cells and pseudohyphae. The diagnosis of oral thrush is based on clinical findings. Even though this is a presumptive diagnosis, routine culturing or microscopic examination of the scrapings is not necessary unless the thrush is persistent or atypical.

Candida dermatitis appears as 1- to 3-mm vesicular or pustular lesions on an erythematous base in the perineum, axillae, and neck folds. These discrete lesions can coalesce to form large patches of inflamed, denuded skin, especially in the perineal area. Again, the diagnosis is a clinical one unless the lesions are atypical or persistent or there is evidence of systemic disease.

Invasive candidiasis in the newborn infant presents as acute respiratory distress usually after the first 2 weeks of life. This may be accompanied by apnea, bradycardia, temperature instability, metabolic acidosis, coagulopathy, and other focal signs. It may lead to meningitis, endocarditis, brain abscesses, pneumonia, endophthalmitis, renal and hepatic abscesses, and other organ involvement. Infants with *C. albicans* fungemia (compared to *C. parapsilosis*) are more likely to present early with hypoxemia, respiratory distress requiring intubation, shock, and bradycardia and thrombocytopenia. They were also more likely (46 vs 2%) to have positive cultures from sites other than the bloodstream, including abscess fluid, cerebrospinal fluid, ascitic fluid, and sputum *(2)*. Therefore, in any low birth weight infant with respiratory distress and history of prolonged antibiotic therapy, parenteral nutrition, intralipid infusions, or with indwelling intravascular catheters, fungal sepsis should be suspected.

Infants with CCC typically present on the first day of life with a generalized rash consisting of erythematous macules, papules, or pustules on a 5- to 10-mm erythematous base. Generalized erythema can be seen initially, which then can evolve into a severe skin eruption with discrete papules or vesicles and sometimes bullae. The eruption occurs predominantly on the back, extensor surfaces, skin folds, palms, and soles, but the perineum area is spared. The rash in very low birth weight infants can rapidly progress to bullae, erosion, and desquamation resembling burns or scalded skin. This is associated with an extreme leukemoid reaction. The nails may also be involved and appear opaque, raised, and rough. With the loss of the skin barrier, the preterm infant is at risk for dehydration and secondary bacterial infections. The differential includes staphylococcal pustulosis, bullous impetigo, syphilis, neonatal pustular melanosis, toxic epidermolysis bullosa, incontinentia pigmenti, neonatal listeriosis, herpes simplex, or varicella-zoster. CCC may also involve multiple organ systems, leading to hemorrhage and necrosis of the heart, lungs, kidneys, spleen, and other organs.

A definitive diagnosis of *Candida* infection in the newborn is made by isolation of the organism from culture of a sterile site or demonstration of the organism in tissue specimens. A sepsis workup should be performed in any infant suspected of having congenital candidiasis or *Candida* sepsis. This includes a blood culture, urinalysis, urine culture, complete blood count, lumbar puncture, and chest x-ray. A buffy coat culture can also be done to isolate *Candida*. Urine samples should be obtained for culture by suprapubic aspiration if possible. Straight bladder catheterization is an alternative method for obtaining the urine but may be contaminated with normal or colonizing flora. The cerebrospinal fluid evaluation should include cell count, Gram stain, culture, protein, glucose, and KOH preparation. Demonstration of spores and pseudohyphae in tissue, urine, and skin scrapings should be attempted.

It is recommended that daily blood cultures be done until sterilization of the blood has been achieved, which may take several days. In one study, as many as 60% of infants with neonatal candidemia had persistently positive cultures (>72 hours after initiation of antifungal therapy) *(22)*. These infants were more likely to have focal complications. Therefore, if *Candida* cannot be eliminated from the blood stream after 48–72 hours or if clinically indicated, an evaluation for focal sites of infection is recommended. An electrocardiogram and echocardiogram should be done to rule out fungal endocarditis. Magnetic resonance imaging or computeed axial tomography scan of the brain should be obtained to rule out brain abscesses. An abdominal or renal ultrasound should be performed to look for abscesses in the kidney, spleen, and liver. A computed tomographic scan of the abdomen and pelvis may provide further delineation of intra-abdominal or renal involvement or may be indicated for the purpose of localization for biopsy or drainage of an abscess. An ophthalmological examination should be performed to rule out retinitis or endophthalmitis. Diagnostic procedures such as bronchoscopy; biopsies of liver, lung, or bone; aspiration or incision and drainage of abscesses; and bone marrow aspiration should be performed if clinically indicated to obtain specimens for culture, Gram stain, KOH prep, and histological examination with special stains (periodic acid-Schiff, Gomori methenamine silver, toluidine blue). Indwelling vascular devices should be removed.

DIRECT DIAGNOSTIC ASSAYS FOR EVALUATING THE MOTHER AND INFANT

A number of immunological and serologic diagnostic tests have been investigated because of the difficulty with interpreting the isolation of *Candida* from the urinary and respiratory tracts as well as confirming the diagnosis of invasive candidiasis, especially in immunocompromised hosts. Some of these tests look promising; however, most are not commercially available for routine use. Several rapid antigen detection assays are available, including latex particle agglutination (LPA), enzyme immunoassay, and radioimunoassay. Most assays detect mannan as the main *Candida* antigen. Some of these tests have a high rate of false negatives. The LPA is the easiest to perform and has been shown to be useful in quantitation of *Candida*. Using a titer of 1:4 or above as a positive result, it has an excellent specificity of more than 90% but at best a sensitivity of only 70%. The LPA is more useful for monitoring response to therapy than diagnosis because there is some correlation with decreasing titers and successful antifungal treatment. The enzyme immunoassay is a rapid and quantitative test for *Candida* antigen that has excellent specificity but has poor sensitivity and cannot provide species information and therefore is not very useful.

Antibody tests are not routinely recommended because there is a high rate of false negatives, especially in the immunocompromised patients. Complement fixation and indirect immunofluorescent antibody tests are not very helpful in the diagnosis of disseminated disease. Deoxyribonucleic acid probes are used as a rapid diagnostic test for vulvovaginal candidiasis with excellent specificity (99%) and good sensitivity (75%). *Candida* skin tests are not useful and should not be used because they cannot distinguish between colonization and invasive disease. Assays to measure levels of D-arabinitol, a metabolite of pathogenic *Candida* species in the urine and serum, have been developed but are expensive and difficult to perform. The measurement of the D/L-arabinitol ratio appears to be of diagnostic value in invasive disease. This test looks promising but is still under investigation.

Candida species can be rapidly detected in urine, blood, and sputum by polymerase chain reaction (PCR); however, detection may not mean invasive disease in a colonized patient. Detection of *Candida* by PCR using clinical isolates followed by restriction fragment length patterns looks promising for rapid diagnosis of disseminated candidiasis. These tests are not routinely available and are under further investigation. In an outbreak, analysis of the isolates can be accomplished by two genotyping methods: electric field gel electrophoresis and PCR-based direct sequencing.

REFERENCES

1. Kossoff EH, Buescher ES, Karlowicz MG. Candidemia in a neonatal intensive care unit: trends during 15 years and clinical features of 111 cases. Pediatr Infect Dis J 1998;17P:504–508.
2. Huang YC, Lin TY, Lien RI, et al. Candidemia in special care nurseries: comparison of *Albicans* and *Parapsilosis* infection. J Infect 2000;40:171–175.

3. Huang YC, Li CC, Lin TY, et al. Association of fungal colonization and invasive disease in very low birth weight infants. Pediatr Infect Dis J 1998;17:819–822.

4. Waggoner-Fountain LA, Whit Walker M, Hollis RJ, et al. Vertical and horizontal transmission of unique *Candida* species to premature newborns. Clin Infect Dis 1996;22:803–808.

5. Baley JE, Kliegman RM, Boxerbaum B, Fanaroff AA. Fungal colonization in very low birth weight infants. Pediatrics 1986;78:225–232.

6. Schwartz DA, Reef S. *Candida albicans* placentitis and funisitis: early diagnosis of congenital candidemia by histopathologic examination of umbilical cord vessels. Pediatr Infect Dis J 1990;9:661–665.

7. Saxen H, Virtanen M, Carlson P, et al. Neonatal *Candida parapsilosis* outbreak with a high case fatality rate. Pediatr Infect Dis J 1995;14:776–781.

8. Rowen JL, Tate JM, Neonatal Candidiasis Study Group. Management of neonatal candidiasis. Pediatr Infect Dis J 1998;17:1007–1011.

9. El-Mohandes AE, Johnson-Robbins L, Keiser JF, Simmens SJ, Aure MV. Incidence of *Candida parapsilosis* colonization in an intensive care nursery population and its association with invasive fungal disease. Pediatr Infect Dis J 1994;13:520–524.

10. Maudsley RF, Brix GA, Hinton NA, Robertson EM, Bryans AM, Haust MD. Placental inflammation and infection. A prospective bacteriologic and histologic study. Am J Obstet Gynecol 1966;95:648–659.

11. Kam L, Giacoia G. Congenital cutaneous candidiasis. Am J Dis Child 1975;129:1215–1218.

12. Darmstadt GL, Dinulos JG, Miller Z. Congenital cutaneous candidiasis: clinical presentation, pathogenesis, and management guidelines. Pediatrics 2000;105:438–444.

13. Maudsley RF, Brix GA, Hinton NA, Robertson EM, Bryans AM, Haust MD. Placental inflammation and infection. A prospective bacteriologic and histologic study. Am J Obstet Gynecol 1966;95:648–659.

14. Baley JE: Neonatal candidiasis: The current challenge. Clin Perinatol 1991;18:263–268.

15. Whyte R, Hussain Z, DeSa D. Antenatal infections with *Candida* species. Arch Dis Child 1982; 57:528–535.

16. Meis PJ, Goldenberg RI, Mercer B, et al. The preterm prediction study: significance of vaginal infections. Am J Obstet Gynecol 1995;173:1731–1736.

17. Van Winter JT, Ney JA, Ogburn PL, Johnson RV. Preterm labor and congenital candidiasis: a case report. J Reproduct Med 1994;39:987–990.

18. Rabalais GP, Samiec TD, Bryant KK, Lewis JJ. Invasive candidiasis in infants weighing more than 2500 grams at birth admitted to a neonatal intensive care unit. Pediatr Infect Dis J 1996; 15:348–352.

19. Faix RG, Kovarik SM, Shaw TR, Johnson RV, Mucocutaneous and invasive candidiasis among very low birth weight (<1500 grams) infants in intensive care nurseries: a prospective study. Pediatrics 1989;83:101–107.

20. Saiman L, Ludington E, Pfaller M, et al. Risk factors for candidemia in neonatal intensive care unit patients. Pediatr Infect Dis J 2000;194:319–324.

21. Rowen JL, Reuch MA, Kozinetz CA, Adams JM, Baker CJ. Endotracheal colonization with *Candida* enhances risk of systemic candidasis in very low birth weight neonates. J Pediatr 1994;124:789–794.

22. Chapman RL, Faix RG. Persistently positive cultures and outcome in invasive neonatal candidiasis. Pediatr Infect Dis J 2000;19:822–827.

Masako Shimamura

EPIDEMIOLOGY

Malaria is a global parasitic disease caused by four species of *Plasmodium*: *Plasmodium falciparum, Plasmodium vivax, Plasmodium ovale, and Plasmodium malariae*. Approximately 40% of the world's population live in malaria-endemic areas, and an estimated 300–500 million cases occur annually. The majority of deaths occur in infants and children (WHO Special Programme for Research and Training in Tropical Diseases Web site: http://www.who.int/tdr/diseases/malaria/direction.htm). Progress in the diagnosis and treatment of malaria has been hampered by its prevalence mainly in impoverished areas of the world, limiting patient access to health care and funds for research. Malaria was eradicated in the United States during the 1950s via a combination of mosquito control programs and aggressive antimalarial treatment of infected individuals *(1)*. However, cases in the United States continue to be reported annually. Most cases are described in recent immigrants, but rarely cases occur through blood transfusions, congenital transmission, or cryptic transmission in patients without identifiable exposure to malaria *(2)*.

PLASMODIUM LIFE CYCLE

Plasmodium is a unicellular protozoan in the order Kinetoplastida, which also includes the pathogenic parasites *Toxoplasma* and *Trypanosoma. Plasmodium* requires an insect host, the Anopheles mosquito, and a mammalian host during the sexual and asexual life cycle stages, respectively. *Plasmodium* species exhibit restricted host specificity, such that species causing human malaria are unable to survive in nonhuman hosts. Conversely, *Plasmodium* species infecting other mammals are not capable of causing human disease. This host range limitation facilitated the eradication of malaria in previously endemic areas of the United States as no animal reservoirs persisted after *Plasmodium* was eliminated from the human population.

On entry into the human circulatory system via the bite of an infected mosquito, *Plasmodium* sporozoites rapidly attach to and enter hepatocytes. During this hepatic or exo-erythrocytic stage, sporozoites undergo asexual reproduction within hepatocytes over 5–15 days, ultimately lysing the host cell to release merozoites into the bloodstream. A proportion of *P. vivax* and *P. ovale* sporozoites do not replicate but remain inert as hypnozoites within hepatocytes, retaining the ability to reactivate and cause

From: *Infectious Disease: Congenital and Perinatal Infections: A Concise Guide to Diagnosis*
Edited by: C. Hutto © Humana Press Inc., Totowa, NJ

relapses months or even years after initial infection. Such forms are responsible for clinical disease long after an individual has left an endemic area and may cause congenital malaria in offspring of women experiencing unsuspected reactivations during pregnancy. In contrast, *P. falciparum* and *P. malariae* do not maintain liver latency and do not cause disease recrudescence after acute infection. However, *P. malariae* has been reported to persist at low levels in the bloodstream for years and thus may cause congenital malaria in children born to asymptomatic mothers *(1,3)*.

Once liberated from hepatocytes into the bloodstream, merozoites rapidly invade circulating erythrocytes. *P. vivax* utilizes the Duffy blood group antigen as a receptor *(4)*, whereas the receptors utilized by the other *Plasmodium* species remain undetermined. *P. vivax* and *P. ovale* infect only reticulocytes; *P. malariae* infects only old red blood cells (RBCs), thus limiting the degree of parasitemia and severity of clinical disease associated with these infections. In contrast, *P. falciparum* is capable of infecting erythrocytes of any age, reaching high parasitemias, and often causing life-threatening disease. After entering the erythrocyte, intraerythrocytic parasites undergo further asexual replication, filling and eventually rupturing the host RBC. The intraerythrocytic life cycle is characteristically 48–72 hours, depending on the *Plasmodium* species. These cycles of synchronized erythrocyte lysis are responsible for the classically described quotidian and tertian fevers experienced in clinical malaria. Clinical disease resolves with antimalarial treatment or the development of strain-specific antibodies. However, these antibodies do not protect against reinfection, thus allowing patients in endemic areas to experience multiple episodes of clinical malaria throughout their lives *(1,3)*.

Finally, some intraerythrocytic parasites develop into sexual gametocytes. When ingested by a mosquito feeding on the human host, the gametocytes undergo sexual reproduction in the mosquito gut to form diploid zygotes that mature and undergo meiosis into haploid sporozoites, which are again capable of infecting humans. Each species of *Plasmodium* forms a morphologically distinctive gametocyte. In patients from geographic areas harboring multiple *Plasmodium* species, definitive diagnosis of the species infecting a given human patient requires identification of the gametocyte on a blood smear. Research laboratories are capable of performing species-specific polymerase chain reaction (PCR) from whole blood, but this technique is not commercially available *(5,6)*.

CLINICAL MANIFESTATIONS: ADULTS AND CHILDREN

Acute malaria manifests during the erythrocytic phase of infection. Symptoms in immunologically naïve hosts are initially nonspecific and include fevers, rigors, headache, myalgias, lethargy, abdominal pain, and vomiting. In children, symptoms may present acutely and in a rapidly progressive fashion with seizures, hypoglycemia, severe anemia, and hypotension. The physical examination may reveal hepatosplenomegaly, but despite hemolysis, jaundice is not frequently observed. Cerebral malaria, characterized by unarousable coma caused by sludging of parasitized erythrocytes in cerebral capillaries, is a severe complication of falciparum malaria and is fatal if untreated.

In contrast, partially immune hosts (i.e., patients living in malaria-endemic areas) may have asymptomatic circulating parasitemia. Others may have intermittent fevers without localizing signs or severe disease. In these cases, interpretation of positive smears must be made with caution as parasitemia may not indicate clinical disease *(1,3)*. Tests are not available to identify reinfection of partially immune patients with new strains to which the host is not immune.

CONGENITAL MALARIA

Risk and Pathogenesis

Congenital malaria is thought to be a rare occurrence, with a historically reported incidence of 0.3% in immune mothers and up to 7.4% of nonimmune mothers *(7)*. More recent studies have shown incidence rates of 7–17% when testing infant blood after delivery *(8,9)*. Studies utilizing cord blood as a marker for neonatal malaria transmission are of limited significance as it has been shown that cord blood parasitemia does not correlate with development of congenital malaria *(10,11)*. It is thought that transmission of malaria from mother to infant occurs at the time of delivery via breakdown of maternofetal placental blood barriers during parturition *(12,13)*.

Because the exact timing of neonatal infection is clinically difficult to determine, *congenital malaria* in this review refers to all malaria that is felt to be acquired vertically either *in utero* or peripartum from the mother and not from the bite of an infected mosquito. In general, the fetus *in utero* appears to be relatively resistant to *Plasmodium* infection. Factors preventing infection are thought to include the high percentage of fetal hemoglobin and low oxygen tension in fetal circulation and the function of the placenta as a barrier and filter for the parasites *(12,14)*. However, little research has been performed to investigate the clinical and molecular aspects of congenital malaria.

Pregnant women are more susceptible to malaria than nonpregnant individuals. It is thought that the immune suppression associated with pregnancy contributes to malarial disease severity *(15)*. Primigravidas demonstrate fever and heavy parasitemias, particularly during the first trimester, even when previously immune *(15,16)*. A prospective study of 60 primigravid women in Nigeria showed that malaria parasitemia incidence and density of infection was higher in pregnant women compared to the same women before pregnancy and to a control group of similar age *(17)*. Malaria during pregnancy contributes to maternal anemia and low birth weight in neonates *(12,18,19)*. Stillbirth, spontaneous abortion, and severe maternal disease may also occur with maternal infection in areas of low endemicity *(15,16)*.

Clearly, the placenta plays a major role in preventing congenital malaria. It is well documented that the placenta may harbor a high parasite load even in the absence of maternal peripheral parasitemia *(7,20,21)*. It is thought that the placenta may preferentially sequester parasitized erythrocytes via preferential cytoadherence mediated by *Plasmodium*-encoded surface antigens *(22)*. However, despite this high local parasite load, numerous studies of placentas and infants demonstrated a low rate of transmission to the infant from infected placentas *(10,23–25)*. The mechanism of this protection is not well understood *(12)*.

Clinical Presentation: Mothers and Infants

Most studies of congenital malaria in endemic areas are limited by the lack of medical resources in those areas of the world. However, reports from the US Centers for Disease Control and Prevention in the 1990s documented the clinical presentation and course of 24 infants born in the United States who clearly contracted congenital malaria from maternal transmission *(2,26–34)*. In these cases, infants generally presented with fever 3–8 weeks after delivery, although some who developed symptoms in the first week of life were not diagnosed until later. Two infants were born prematurely. It is not clear whether maternal malaria precipitated the preterm delivery, although both mothers had positive blood smears at delivery. Most infants also presented with symptoms of poor feeding, irritability, or lethargy. Anemia and thrombocytopenia were reported in several cases, although other infants reportedly had normal laboratory parameters. The diagnosis was made in all infants by thick and thin blood smears. *P. vivax* malaria was reported for 18 infants (75%), *P. falciparum* malaria was found in 4 infants (17%), and *P. malariae* was detected in 2 infants (8%). Most infants were treated with chloroquine. Other treatment regimens included chloroquine with primaquine (4 cases), quinine or intravenous quinidine (2 cases), and mefloquine (1 case). All infants recovered and no deaths were reported. No infant was treated immediately after delivery, even when the mother was found to be parasitemic during delivery. Interestingly, 1 infant diagnosed with congenital malaria had an asymptomatic, unaffected twin who never required antimalarial treatment.

Mothers of these infants with congenital malaria all originally lived in malaria-endemic areas. Most had immigrated to the United States either shortly before or during pregnancy. However, 3 mothers had left the malarious region 2–8 years prior to the pregnancy and had no subsequent malaria exposure. Some mothers reported receiving treatment abroad for malaria during pregnancy, but the type and duration of treatment were not documented. Some mothers took chloroquine for prophylaxis or treatment of malaria during pregnancy. At the time of delivery, most mothers were asymptomatic. Two mothers had symptoms (fever, anemia, thrombocytopenia) at the time of delivery but only received treatment for malaria peri- and postpartum. Neither of those infants received malaria treatment after delivery. At the time of their infants' diagnosis, mothers' smears were reported as negative in 9 cases, positive in 8 cases, and unreported in 7 cases. Additional testing of some mothers revealed positive serologies against the *Plasmodium* species infecting the infant as well as positive serologies against other species not found in the infant. One mother whose smears were negative underwent blood PCR testing, which was also negative.

Findings from this small case series generally reflect findings noted in other case series reviews and individual case reports of congenital malaria occurring in nonendemic countries *(13,35–40)*. In nonendemic countries, the diagnosis of congenital malaria is rarely made at the time of delivery but is suspected when clinical symptoms arise several weeks after delivery. It is likely that in malaria-endemic countries, infants presenting with congenital malaria in the first few weeks of life cannot be distinguished from those with postnatally acquired malaria. Therefore, it is quite difficult to determine a true incidence of congenital malaria transmission in endemic areas, and as a consequence it most likely is underreported.

DIAGNOSIS

The mainstay of malaria diagnosis remains the thick and thin blood smears. In this technique, one drop of blood is obtained from the patient, preferably from a capillary-rich site such as the finger or earlobe rather than from venipuncture because of the preferential sequestration of parasitized erythrocytes in capillary beds. The drop is placed on a slide and smeared using a second slide, with the thickness of the smear determined by the size of the smear and the angle of the second slide. The thick smear is stained unfixed, and the thin smear is fixed in methanol before staining with Field's, Wright's or Giemsa stain *(2,41,42)*.

The thick smear is used for screening large numbers of erythrocytes for the presence of malarial inclusions to make the diagnosis. The sensitivity of the thick film can be as little as 5–50 parasites/µL of blood or 0.0001–0.001% of RBCs infected, although in field studies lower sensitivities are obtained *(42,43)*. The early trophozoite or "ring" is the form typically seen in circulation. Visualization of the gametocyte or sexual form identifies the *Plasmodium* species and is more easily detected in the thin smear. The thin smear is also used to estimate percentage parasitemia, which is the number of infected erythrocytes compared to total RBCs per high-power field.

For *P. vivax*, *P. ovale,* and *P. malariae* species, only erythrocytes of a certain age are infected, and maximum parasitemias reach approx 2%. In *P. falciparum* malaria, all erythrocyte stages are infected and parasitemias may become quite high. Parasitemias above 2–5% are considered potentially life-threatening, and those above 10% may require exchange transfusion *(43)*. In endemic areas, children demonstrate higher parasitemias than adults, presumably because of partial immunity in adults. Nonnative, nonimmune travelers may also develop high parasitemias and serious illness *(1)*. For accurate diagnosis, the thick-and-thin smear require an experienced technician but minimal equipment and reagents, so smears are commonly used in malaria-endemic countries. Conversely, technicians in nonendemic countries may lack expertise in identifying malarial forms in RBCs and may have difficulty determining the diagnosis if parasitemia is low.

The diagnosis of congenital malaria is usually made by examination of the infant's thick-and-thin smear. As discussed, often the mother does not demonstrate symptoms or peripheral parasitemia. Thick and thin smears of maternal blood should be examined for parasitemia, but these are often negative in the setting of congenital malaria. The placenta is frequently infected histologically, and cord blood may also be smear positive, but by the time congenital malaria is suspected, these may not be available for evaluation. Furthermore, as noted, a positive placenta or cord blood supports but does not define the diagnosis of congenital malaria. *Plasmodium*-specific antibodies may also be tested in the mother. A negative maternal antibody test rules out congenital malaria in the infant, but a positive test only provides evidence of past maternal infection and does not necessarily indicate active maternal infection or congenital transmission. Maternal antibodies to each *Plasmodium* species may be distinguished and may identify the species infecting the infant.

Diagnosis: Recent Assays

New rapid tests have been developed to diagnose malaria and are discussed next. It should be emphasized that none of these tests have been approved for the diagnosis of congenital malaria. Therefore, results obtained from such tests in the newborn should be interpreted with caution and should be performed in consultation with experts in pediatric infectious diseases.

To simplify the microscopic analysis of blood smears, fluorescent dyes such as acridine orange have been used to identify parasite nucleic acids within erythrocytes because uninfected RBCs lack nuclei (reviewed in refs. *42* and *43*). Staining may be performed directly on thick films or on capillary blood tubes *(44,45)*. In the latter technique, blood is centrifuged to separate leukocytes and platelets from erythrocytes (centrifugal quantitative buffy coat or QBC II, Becton Dickinson, Franklin Lakes, NJ). Parasitized erythrocytes concentrate below the leukocytes and are stained with the fluorochrome. Disadvantages of these techniques include the need for fluorescence microscopy, an appropriate centrifuge for the quantitative buffy coat method, and the need for training in the identification of parasitized erythrocytes and distinction from fluorescent artifacts and Howell-Jolley bodies. The sensitivity and specificity of these assays are highly variable, depending on the conditions (research vs field trials), *Plasmodium* species encountered, and the fluorochrome used *(46–49)*. Another limitation of this technique compared to traditional thick and thin smears is the inability to distinguish the *Plasmodium* species, an important consideration in areas where several species are prevalent.

Other tests utilize commercial antibodies to detect *Plasmodium* antigens in blood (reviewed in refs. *42* and *43*). In these immunochromatographic or dipstick tests, antibodies specific for the *Plasmodium* protein of interest capture the target antigen in blood, then migrate along a nitrocellulose membrane, where a second *Plasmodium*-specific antibody bound to the membrane captures the labeled antigen-antibody complex. As a positive control, an antibody directed against the first capture antibody is placed at the distal end of the dipstick and becomes positive when the liquid phase antibody in buffer has migrated along the entire membrane. Three commercial tests, the ParaSight-F (Becton Dickinson), ICT Pf/Pv (Amrad ICT, Sydney, Australia), and PATH Falciparum Malaria IC test (PATH, Seattle, WA), screen for the presence of the histidine-rich protein 2, a surface and secreted protein produced by *P. falciparum*. The OptiMAL dipstick test (Flow Inc., Portland, OR) detects *Plasmodium* lactate dehydrogenase (pLDH), a glycolytic enzyme found in all four *Plasmodium* species. This assay incorporates antibodies that recognize pLDH from all *Plasmodium* species as well as antibodies specific for *P. falciparum* pLDH, thus permitting distinction of *P. falciparum* malaria cases from those caused by the other species.

All of these immunochromatographic assays have undergone testing in both endemic and nonendemic areas. Field trials in Indonesia and Thailand comparing the ParaSight-F test to conventional microscopy showed sensitivities of 93–95% and specificities of 95–98% *(50,51)*. False positives were noted in patients recently treated for malaria. In children with uncomplicated malaria in the Gambia, West Africa, the Parasight-F test had a sensitivity and specificity of 96 and 90%, respectively, compared to microscopy *(52)*. Field testing of the ICT Pf/Pv assay yielded similar results *(53)*. In Honduras, the OptiMAL test compared to microscopy had sensitivities of 88–94% and specificities of 99–100% depending on the infecting *Plasmodium* species *(54)*.

These tests have also been studied in febrile travelers returning from malaria endemic areas, a situation perhaps resembling that of congenital malaria in nonendemic countries. In these studies, comparisons were made between the ICT Malaria Pf/Pv, PATH *Falciparum* Malaria IC, OptiMAL, and conventional microscopic techniques in Kuwait, Germany, Canada, London, Italy, and Australia *(55–60)*. In these conditions, the rapid diagnostic tests generally performed well in comparison to traditional microscopy but had false-negatives at low parasitemias and occasionally also at very high parasitemias, as well as inconsistent results in mixed infections. Therefore, the use of dipstick tests was recommended in addition to, not in place of, the thick-and-thin smear in this situation.

Finally, PCR has been utilized to identify malaria infections in blood. Primers recognizing species-specific sequences in the small-subunit 18S ribosomal ribonucleic acid and circumsporozoite genes have been developed to distinguish the infecting *Plasmodium* species *(5,6,61,62)*. Nested and reverse transcription PCR permit identification of infections at very low (five parasites or less per microliter of blood) parasitemias with high sensitivity and specificity *(42)*. PCR also performed better in species identification than conventional microscopy in patients with mixed infections *(5,63)*. However, these assays are not commercially available, and all studies have been performed using primers and conditions developed and utilized solely by individual researchers. Furthermore, equipment and personnel requirements for PCR, as well as difficulties in controlling for contamination, make this an impractical test for widespread applications in remote and resource-poor areas of the world.

PCR is the only rapid diagnostic technique that has undergone any study to diagnose congenital malaria. Adachi et al. performed PCR and conventional microscopy on samples from 298 asymptomatic neonates in Tanzania and identified 1 infant positive by PCR and negative by smear, 1 infant negative by PCR and positive by smear, and 1 infant positive by both methods *(64)*. It is concluded that PCR may be a useful screening technique for asymptomatic newborns at risk for congenital malaria in highly endemic areas, but that PCR does not replace conventional microscopy for diagnosis in symptomatic neonates. Rubio et al. described three infants born in a nonendemic country who were diagnosed with congenital malaria shortly after delivery *(65,66)*. All infants had both positive smears and PCR results. However, PCR detected a mixed infection in two infants, which was not suspected by smear. Based on these limited studies, it is possible that PCR may in the future become clinically utilized in conjunction with thick-and-thin smears in making the diagnosis of congenital malaria.

CONCLUSIONS

Congenital malaria is a rare occurrence in malaria-nonendemic countries and requires a high degree of clinical suspicion to attain the diagnosis. Even a remote maternal history of residence in a malaria endemic area is the key risk factor. Conversely, maternal symptoms do not necessarily correlate with congenital transmission. Prompt diagnosis and treatment of affected infants result in good outcomes without long-term morbidity. In developing nations, the incidence of congenital malaria is not well documented and may be higher than historically reported *(7)*. As the treatment is similar for congenital and acquired malaria in the neonate, this distinction may not have substantial clinical relevance in malaria-endemic areas. Recently developed methods for the diagnosis of malaria in adults may soon be utilized in young infants to detect congenital malaria, but this area will require further study.

REFERENCES

1. Mandell G, Bennett J, Dolin R. Principles and Practice of Infectious Diseases, 5th ed., Vol. 2. New York: Churchill Livingstone, 2000:2817–2830.
2. Causer L, Newman RD, Barber AM, et al. Malaria surveillance—United States, 2000. MMWR Surveill Summ 2002;51:9–21.

3. Cook G. Manson's Tropical Diseases, 20th ed. London: Saunders, 1996:1087–1164.
4. Miller L, Mason SJ, Clyde DF, McGinniss MH. The resistance factor to *Plasmodium vivax* in blacks. The Duffy-blood-group genotype, FyFy. N Engl J Med 1976;295:302–304.
5. Snounou G, Viriyakosol S,Jarra W, Thaithong S, Brown KN. Identification of the four human malaria parasite species in field samples by the polymerase chain reaction and detection of a high prevalence of mixed infections. Mol Biochem Parasitol 1993;58:283–292.
6. Rubio J, Post RJ, van Leeuwen WM, Henry MC, Lindergard G, Hommel M. Alternative polymerase chain reaction method to identify *Plasmodium* species in human blood samples: the semi-nested multiplex malaria PCR (SnM-PCR). Trans R Soc Trop Med Hyg 2002;96(Suppl 1):S199–S204.
7. Covell G. Congenital malaria. Trop Dis Bull 1950;47:1147–1167.
8. Nyirjesy P, Kavasya T, Axelrod P, Fischer PR. Malaria during pregnancy: neonatal morbidity and mortality and the efficacy of chloroquine chemoprophylaxis. Clin Infect Dis 1993;16:127–132.
9. Ndyomugyenyi R, Magnussen P. Chloroquine prophylaxis, iron/folic-acid supplementation or case management of malaria attacks in primigravidae in western Uganda: effects on congenital malaria and infant haemoglobin concentrations. Ann Trop Med Parasitol 2000;94:759–770.
10. Marshall D. The transplacental passage of malaria parasites in the Solomon Islands. Trans R Soc Trop Med Hyg 1983;77:470–473.
11. Nguyen-Dinh P, Steketee RW, Greenberg AE, Wirima JJ, Mulenda O, Williams SB. Rapid spontaneous postpartum clearance of *Plasmodium falciparum* parasitaemia in African women. Lancet 1988;2:751–752.
12. Loke Y. Transmission of parasites across the placenta. Adv Parasitol 1982;21:155–228.
13. Hulbert T. Congenital malaria in the United States: report of a case and review. Clin Infect Dis 1992;14:922–926.
14. Wilson R, Pasvol G, Weatherall D. Invasion and growth of *Plasmodium falciparum* in different types of human erythrocyte. Bull WHO 1977;55:179–186.
15. Walter P, Garin Y, Blot P. Placental pathologic changes in malaria. A histologic and ultrastructural study. Am J Pathol 1982;109:330–342.
16. Watkinson M, Rushton D. Plasmodial pigmentation of placenta and outcome of pregnancy in West African mothers. Br Med J Clin Res 1983;287:251–254.
17. Beeson J, Reeder JC, Rogerson SJ, Brown GV. Parasite adhesion and immune evasion in placental malaria. Trends Parasitol 2001;17:331–337.
18. Bruce-Chwatt L. Malaria in African infants and children in Southern Nigeria. Ann Trop Med Parasitol 1952;46:173–200.
19. Jelliffe E. Low birth-weight and malarial infection of the placenta. Bull WHO 1968;38:69–78.
20. Logie D, McGregor IA, Rowe DS, Billewicz WZ. Plasma immunoglobulin concentrations in mothers and newborn children with special reference to placental malaria: studies in the Gambia, Nigeria, and Switzerland. Bull WHO. 1973;49: 547–554.
21. McGregor I. Epidemiology, malaria and pregnancy. Am J Trop Med Hyg 1984;33:517–525.
22. Brabin B. An analysis of malaria in pregnancy in Africa. Bull WHO 1983;61:1005–1016.
23. Gilles H, Lawson JB, Sibelas M, Voller A, Allan N. Malaria, anaemia and pregnancy. Ann Trop Med Parasitol 1969;63:245–263.
24. McGregor I, Wilson M, Billewicz W. Malaria infection of the placenta in the Gambia, West Africa; its incidence and relationship to stillbirth, birthweight and placental weight. Trans R Soc Trop Med Hyg 1983;77:232–244.
25. Fleming A. Tropical obstetrics and gynaecology. 1. Anaemia in pregnancy in tropical Africa. Trans R Soc Trop Med Hyg 1989;83:441–448.
26. Zucker J, Barber AM, Paxton LA, et al. Malaria surveillance—United States, 1992. MMWR Surveill Summ 1995;44:1–17.

27. Barat L, Zucker JR, Barber AM, et al. Malaria surveillance—United States, 1993. MMWR Surveill Summ 1997;46:27–47.
28. Kachur S, Reller ME, Barber AM, et al. Malaria surveillance—United States, 1994. MMWR Surveill Summ 1997;46:1–18.
29. Williams H, Roberts J, Kachur SP, et al. Malaria surveillance—United States, 1995. MMWR Surveill Summ 1999;48:1–23.
30. Holtz T, Kachur SP, MacArthur JR, et al. Malaria surveillance—United States, 1998. MMWR Surveill Summ 2001;50:1–20.
31. Mungai M, Roberts J, Barber AM, et al. Malaria surveillance—United States, 1996. MMWR Surveill Summ 2001;50:1–24.
32. MacArthur J, Levin AR, Mungai M, et al. Malaria surveillance—United States, 1997. MMWR Surveill Summ 2001;50:25–43.
33. Newman R, Barber AM, Roberts J, Holtz T, Steketee RW, Parise ME. Malaria surveillance—United States, 1999. MMWR Surveill Summ 2002;51:15–28.
34. Filler S, Causer LM, Newman RD, et al. Malaria surveillance—United States, 2001. MMWR Surveill Summ 2003;52:1–14.
35. Lee W, Singh M, Tan C. A recent case of congenital malaria in Singapore. Singapore Med J 1996;37:541–543.
36. Edwards B. Congenital malaria [comment]. N Engl J Med 1997;336:71–72.
37. Lane R. Congenital malaria [comment]. N Engl J Med 1997;336:71–72.
38. Ahmed A, Cerilli L, Sanchez P. Congenital malaria in a preterm neonate: case report and review of the literature. Am J Perinatol 1998;15:19–22.
39. Comellini L, Tozzola A, Baldi F, et al. *Plasmodium vivax* congenital malaria in a newborn of a Zairian immigrant. Ann Trop Paediatr 1998;18:41–43.
40. Kuyucu N, Yarali N, Sonmezisik G, Yilmaz S, Tezic T. Congenital malaria: a case report. Turk J Pediatr 1999;41:103–106.
41. Warrell D, Gilles H. Essential Malariology. New York: Oxford University Press, 2002:78.
42. Moody A. Rapid diagnostic tests for malaria parasites. Clin Microbiol Rev 2002;15:66–78.
43. Hanscheid T. Diagnosis of malaria: a review of alternatives to conventional microscopy. Clin Lab Haematol 1999;21:235–245.
44. Levine R, Wardlaw S, Patton C. Detection of haematoparasites using quantitative buffy coat analysis tubes. Parasitol Today 1989;5:132–134.
45. Kawamoto F. Rapid diagnosis of malaria by fluorescence microscopy with light microscope and interference filter. Lancet 1991;337:200–202.
46. Wongsrichanalai C, Pornsilapatip J, Namsiripongpun V, et al. Acridine orange fluorescent microscopy and the detection of malaria in populations with low-density parasitemia. Am J Trop Med Hyg 1991;44:17–20.
47. Baird J, Purnomo, Jones T. Diagnosis of malaria in the field by fluorescence microscopy of QBC capillary tubes. Trans R Soc Trop Med Hyg 1992;86:3–5.
48. Hemvani N, Chitnis DS, Dixit DS, Asolkar MV. Acridine orange stained blood wet mounts for fluorescent detection of malaria. Indian J Pathol Microbiol 1999;42:125–128.
49. Htut Y, Aye KH, Han KT, Kyaw MP, Shimono K, Okada S. Feasibility and limitations of acridine orange fluorescence technique using a malaria diagnosis microscope in Myanmar. Acta Med Okayama 2002;56:219–222.
50. Banchongaksorn T, Yomokgul P, Panyim S, Rooney W, Vickers P. A field trial of the ParaSight-F test for the diagnosis of *Plasmodium falciparum* infection. Trans R Soc Trop Med Hyg 1996;90:244–245.
51. Taylor W, Widjaja H, Basri H, et al. Assessing the Parasight-F test in northeastern Papua, Indonesia, an area of mixed *Plasmodium falciparum* and *Plasmodium vivax* transmission. Am J Trop Med Hyg 2002;66:649–652.
52. Bojang K. The diagnosis of *Plasmodium falciparum* infection in Gambian children, by field staff using the rapid, manual, ParaSight-F test. Ann Trop Med Parasitol 1999;93:685–687.

53. Wongsrichanalai C, Arevalo I, Laoboonchai A, et al. Rapid diagnostic devices for malaria: field evaluation of a new prototype immunochromatographic assay for the detection of *Plasmodium falciparum* and non-*falciparum Plasmodium*. Am J Trop Med Hyg 2003;69:26–30.

54. Palmer C, Lindo JF, Klaskala WI, et al. Evaluation of the OptiMAL test for rapid diagnosis of *Plasmodium vivax* and *Plasmodium falciparum* malaria. J Clin Microbiol 1998;36:203–206.

55. Iqbal J, Sher A, Hira PR, Al-Owaish R. Comparison of the OptiMAL test with PCR for diagnosis of malaria in immigrants. J Clin Microbiol 1999;37:3644–3646.

56. Jelinek T, Grobusch MP, Schwenke S, et al. Sensitivity and specificity of dipstick tests for rapid diagnosis of malaria in nonimmune travelers. J Clin Microbiol 1999;37:721–723.

57. Mills C, Burgess DC, Taylor HJ, Kain KC. Evaluation of a rapid and inexpensive dipstick assay for the diagnosis of *Plasmodium falciparum* malaria. Bull WHO 1999;77:553–559.

58. Moody A, Hunt-Cooke A, Gabbett E, Chiodini P. Performance of the OptiMAL malaria antigen capture dipstick for malaria diagnosis and treatment monitoring at the Hospital for Tropical Diseases, London. Br J Haematol 2000;109:891–894.

59. Gatti S, Berruzzi AM, Bisoffi Z, et al. Multicentre study, in patients with imported malaria, on the sensitivity and specificity of a dipstick test (ICT Malaria Pf/Pv) compared with expert microscopy. Ann Trop Med Parasitol 2002;96:15–18.

60. Playford E, Walker J. Evaluation of the ICT malaria Pf/Pv and the OptiMal rapid diagnostic tests for malaria in febrile returned travellers. J Clin Microbiol 2002;40:4166–4171.

61. Sethabutr O, Brown AE, Panyim S, Kain KC, Webster HK, Echeverria P. Detection of *Plasmodium falciparum* by polymerase chain reaction in a field study. J Infect Dis 1992;166:145–148.

62. Kawamoto F, Miyake H, Kaneko O, et al. Sequence variation in the 18S rRNA gene, a target for PCR-based malaria diagnosis, in *Plasmodium ovale* from southern Vietnam. J Clin Microbiol 1996;34:2287–2289.

63. Brown A, Kain KC, Pipithkul J, Webster HK. Demonstration by the polymerase chain reaction of mixed *Plasmodium falciparum* and *P. vivax* infections undetected by conventional microscopy. Trans R Soc Trop Med Hyg 1992;86:609–612.

64. Adachi M, Manji K, Ichimi R, et al. Detection of congenital malaria by polymerase-chain-reaction methodology in Dar es Salaam, Tanzania. Parasitol Res 2000;86:615–618.

65. Rubio J, Benito A, Berzosa PJ, et al. Usefulness of seminested multiplex PCR in surveillance of imported malaria in Spain. J Clin Microbiol 1999;37:3260–3264.

66. Rubio J, Roche J, Berzosa PJ, Moyano E, Benito A. The potential utility of the Semi-Nested Multiplex PCR technique for the diagnosis and investigation of congenital malaria. Diagn Microbiol Infect Dis 2000;38:233–236.

Index